Gastric Cardiac Cancer

Qin Huang
Editor

Gastric Cardiac Cancer

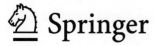 Springer

Editor
Qin Huang
Harvard Medical School/Brigham and Women's Hospital
Veterans Affairs Boston Healthcare System
West Roxbury
Massachusetts
USA

ISBN 978-3-319-79113-5   ISBN 978-3-319-79114-2   (eBook)
https://doi.org/10.1007/978-3-319-79114-2

Library of Congress Control Number: 2018943619

Printed on acid-free paper

This Springer imprint is published by the registered company Springer International Publishing AG part of Springer Nature.
The registered company address is: Gewerbestrasse 11, 6330 Cham, Switzerland

Preface

This book is intended to be used by physicians, patients, and translational research scientists as an easy-to-use practical guide when dealing with gastric cardiac cancer.

Gastric cardiac cancer arises in cardiac mucosa located primarily in the proximal stomach and occasionally invading into the distal esophagus. In recent years, this poorly understood cancer has been the focus of intense investigation on mechanisms of pathogenesis, genomic profile, classification, diagnosis, prognosis, staging, and clinical management. As such, a growing body of high-quality evidence has been accumulated for better clinical management. It is time for a specialized, concise reference on this cancer for clinicians and patients alike.

Because of uncertainty in tumorigenesis mechanisms, there are no universally accepted clinical practice guidelines on gastric cardiac cancer. The best clinical management strategy, we believe, is a multidisciplinary approach, including a team of healthcare subspecialists in gastroenterology, pathology, radiology, abdominal surgery, thoracic surgery, medical oncology, radiation oncology, and palliative care. The pertinent essential information on gastric cardiac cancer in these medical fields is included in this book. The manner of presentation of the information in this book will, we hope, help the reader to quickly master the essential characteristics of this cancer as described and illustrated with numerous endoscopic, gross, and microscopic photographs, and drawings. We hope this book will facilitate efficient communication and the decision-making process by the multidisciplinary team for appropriate patient triage and treatment.

A plain, simple language, without medical jargon, is utilized throughout the book so that patients and their family members and friends may find the materials presented understandable and useful when they face the challenge of this potentially fatal cancer.

We believe that with joint efforts from clinical healthcare professionals, patients and their family members, and translational research scientists, gastric cardiac cancer could be cured in the future. We would appreciate feedback from our readers regarding the usefulness of this book in their clinical practice and research on this cancer.

The views expressed in the book do not necessarily represent the views of the Veterans Affairs or the United States Government.

West Roxbury, MA, USA   Qin Huang

Acknowledgment

Special thanks are given to Raj K. Goyal, M.D., M.B.B.S, of Harvard Medical School and Veterans Affairs Boston Healthcare System; Robert D. Odze, M.D., F.R.C.P.C., of Harvard Medical School and Brigham and Women's Hospital; and Gregory Y. Lauwers, M.D., previously at Harvard Medical School and Massachusetts General Hospital in Boston, USA, for their strong support and guidance over the past 13 years to our clinicopathologic investigation on gastric cardiac cancer.

This book could not have been written without generous support and assistance of physicians working at the Veterans Affairs Boston Healthcare System and Harvard Medical School in Boston, USA; the Nanjing Drum Tower Hospital in Nanjing; and the Changzhou Second Hospital in Changzhou, P. R. China.

Contents

Contributors

Valia Boosalis Department of Hematology, VA Boston Healthcare System, Jamaica Plain, MA, USA

Xiangshan Fan Department of Pathology, The Affiliated Drum Tower Hospital, Nanjing University Medical School, Nanjing, Jiangsu, People's Republic of China

Qian Geng Department of Oncology, the Affiliated Changzhou No.2 People's Hospital of Nanjing Medical University, Changzhou, Jiangsu, People's Republic of China

Jason S. Gold Brigham and Women's Hospital/Harvard Medical School, Boston, MA, USA

VA Boston Healthcare System, Boston, MA, USA

Yu Gong Department of Gastrointestinal Surgery, Affiliated Changzhou No 2 Peoples Hospital Nanjing Medical University, Changzhou, Jiangsu, People's Republic of China

Kun (Kim) Huang Department of Radiation Oncology, Harvard Medical School, Boston University School of Medicine, VA Boston Healthcare System, Jamaica Plain, MA, USA

Lily Huang Beth Israel Deaconess Medical Center, Boston, MA, USA

Qin Huang Pathology and Laboratory Medicine, Veterans Affairs Boston Healthcare System, West Roxbury, MA, USA

Harvard Medical School and Brigham and Women's Hospital, Boston, MA, USA

Hua Jiang Department of Oncology, Affiliated Changzhou Second Hospital of Nanjing Medical University, Changzhou, People's Republic of China

Edward Lew Harvard Medical School, VA Boston Healthcare System and Brigham and Women's Hospital, Boston, MA, USA

Rui Li Soochow University First Hospital, Soochow University, Soochow, People's Republic of China

Tingshan Lin Nanjing Drum Tower Hospital, Nanjing, People's Republic of China

A. Travis Manasco Department of Anesthesiology, Washington University in St. Louis School of Medicine, Barnes Jewish Hospital, St. Louis, MO, USA

Hiroshi Mashimo VA Boston Healthcare System and Brigham and Women's Hospital, Harvard Medical School, Boston, MA, USA

Xingchu Ni Department of Radiotherapy, Affiliated Changzhou No 2 People's Hospital, Nanjing Medical University, Changzhou, Jiangsu, People's Republic of China

Xiaolin Pu Department of Oncology, the Affiliated Changzhou No.2 People's Hospital of Nanjing Medical University, Changzhou, Jiangsu, People's Republic of China

Jun Qian Department of General Surgery, Center of Gastrointestinal Surgery, Changzhou No 2 People's Hospital, Affiliated Hospital of Nanjing Medical University, Changzhou, Jiangsu, People's Republic of China

Dongtao Shi Department of Gastroenterology, Soochow University First Hospital, Soochow University, Soochow, People's Republic of China

Qi Sun Department of Pathology, Nanjing Drum Tower Hospital, Nanjing, Jiangsu, People's Republic of China

Liming Tang Department of Gastroenterology, Changzhou Second Hospital, Nanjing Medical University, Changzhou, People's Republic of China

Guifang Xu Nanjing Medical University, Nanjing Drum Tower Hospital, Nanjing, People's Republic of China

Kequn Xu Department of Oncology, Affiliated Changzhou Second People's Hospital of Nanjing Medical University, Changzhou, People's Republic of China

Kun Yan VA North California Healthcare System, Mather, CA, USA

Yang Yang Nanjing Drum Tower Hospital, Nanjing University, Nanjing, People's Republic of China

Chenggong Yu Department of Gastroenterology, Nanjing Drum Tower Hospital, The Affiliated Hospital of Nanjing University Medical School, Nanjing, Jiangsu, People's Republic of China

Hongbo Yu Department of Pathology and Laboratory Medicine, VA Boston Healthcare System, West Roxbury, MA, USA

Harvard Medical School, Brigham and Women's Hospital, Boston, MA, USA

Ellen Hui Zhan Harvard Medical School, VA Boston Healthcare System, Boston, MA, USA

Chapter 1
The Esophagogastric Junction

Qin Huang

Introduction

By convention, the esophagogastric junction (EGJ) line is the line between the strat-ified squamous epithelium-lined distal esophagus and the columnar mucosa-lined proximal gastric cardia, where the tubular esophagus ends and the saccular stomach begins. In general, the definition of the EGJ can be anatomical, physiological, endo-scopic, and histological. By anatomy, the structure above the EGJ belongs to the distal esophagus, and the tissue below the EGJ constitutes the gastric cardia within a narrow region of 1–4 cm in the longitudinal length. The muscular structure in the EGJ region consists of smooth muscle layers and functions as the lower esophageal sphincter (LES), which can be better evaluated by physiologic manometric methods for pressure changes across the EGJ. In some patients with diseases involving the EGJ region, the LES is degenerated and becomes loose and relaxed, which causes dilatation of the distal esophagus and EGJ, forming hiatal hernia that has become rampant primarily in the elderly Caucasian male population. The mucosal EGJ in a normal human without severe gastroesophageal reflux disease overlaps the squamo-columnar junction (SCJ) (Fig. 1.1); but in patients with hiatal hernia and circumfer-ential columnar-lined esophagus, the SCJ is frequently displaced proximally, separated from the mucosal EGJ proximally to various extends (Fig. 1.2). In addi-tion to hiatal hernia, a number of other diseases arise in the EGJ region and make a confident designation of the mucosal EGJ difficult and challenging. In a retrospec-tive comparison study in Japan [1], the patients with superficial EGJ cancers arising in the distal esophagus above the EGJ had significantly worse reflux esophagitis and

Q. Huang
Pathology and Laboratory Medicine, Veterans Affairs Boston Healthcare System,
West Roxbury, MA, USA

Harvard Medical School and Brigham and Women's Hospital,
Boston, MA, USA

© Springer International Publishing AG, part of Springer Nature 2018
Q. Huang (ed.), *Gastric Cardiac Cancer*, https://doi.org/10.1007/978-3-319-79114-2_1

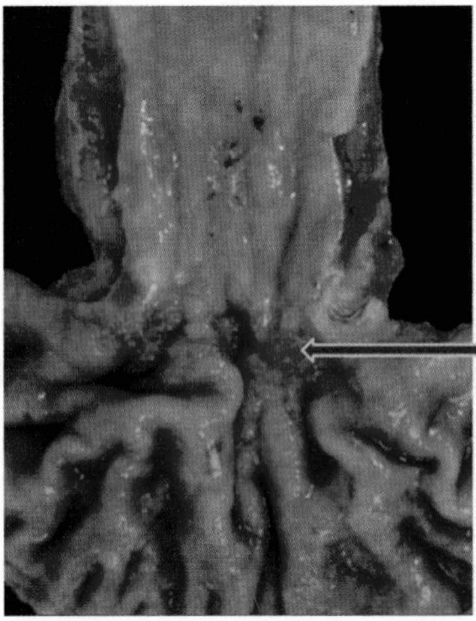

Fig. 1.1 The mucosal junction between the distal end of the pearly white esophageal squamous mucosa and the proximal end of gastric longitudinal brownish mucosal folds defines the mucosal esophagogastric junction (EGJ) that overlaps the squamocolumnar junction (SCJ) and the angle of His in a normal person. Adopted from [4]

Fig. 1.2 In an elderly American Caucasian male patient with hiatal hernia and severe reflux esophagitis, the SCJ is displaced proximally and separated away from the mucosal esophagogastric junction (EGJ). The mucosa between the SCJ and EGJ in this situation is termed columnar-lined esophagus grossly [4]

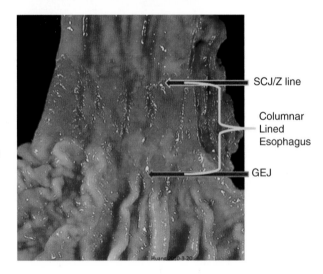

hiatus hernia but less atrophic gastritis than those with the cancer below the EGJ. In another study comparing clinicopathologic features of EGJ cancers between Chinese and American patients, investigators found significantly more severe chronic active gastric carditis and dysplasia below the EGJ, but no intestinal metaplasia and dysplasia above the EGJ in the distal esophagus in Chinese than in American Caucasian patients whose tumor epicenters were above the EGJ [2]. These results illustrate significant differences between cancers arising above or below the EGJ in different ethnic populations. Therefore, it is of paramount importance for accurate designation of the EGJ as a prerequisite for any meaningful studies and effective management of diseases and classification of cancers occurring in the EGJ region. At present, there are no universally accepted gold standards for accurate designation of the EGJ. However, several landmarks have been generally used worldwide to define the macroscopic, endoscopic, and microscopic EGJ [3, 4].

Angle of His

In a surgical resection specimen from the EGJ region, the peritoneal reflection of the stomach onto the diaphragm, i.e., the incisura, is known as the angle of His [5]. This landmark for designation of the EGJ is usable clinically only when the disease damage in the EGJ region is minimal and the patient does not have hiatal hernia [6]. Therefore, the clinical utility of the angle of His to define the EGJ is marginal. In patients with severe hiatal hernia, the entire LES is damaged to various extends, and this landmark is also affected. When a malignant tumor arises in the EGJ region, this landmark is most likely destroyed and becomes useless for clinical classification of the tumor origin in the esophagus versus in the stomach [6, 7]. In a recent autopsy study by Austrian surgeons in 50 consecutive cases, the EGJ was found normally located intra-abdominally in all cases with a mean distance to the angle of His of 3.6 cm (range, 2.7–4.6 cm) [8]. This finding may help surgical management of patients with diseases involving the EGJ region.

Proximal End of Gastric Longitudinal Mucosal Folds

The American Gastroenterology Association guidelines define the proximal end of gastric longitudinal mucosal folds as the endoscopic landmark of the mucosal EGJ (Figs. 1.1 and 1.2), [9] which has been widely followed worldwide except for Japan, despite the fact that this landmark has not been validated by histology. The initial autopsy study showed that the most proximal margin of gastric longitudinal mucosal folds was closely associated with the muscular EGJ [10]. For this reason, McClave et al. [11] were the first to find that the endoscopic SCJ was located within 2 cm of the proximal end of these gastric folds in a normal person; in the patient with hiatal hernia, the proximal end of these gastric folds provided "a fixed, reproducible, anatomic landmark at endoscopy" and could be used as the mucosal EGJ that was, they believed, equivalent to the muscular EGJ. Therefore, the diagnosis of columnar-lined esophagus (Fig. 1.2) can be made when a biopsy is obtained at the site greater than 2 cm above the proximal end of gastric longitudinal mucosal folds within a hiatal hernia sac [11]. Since then, the conclusion of this endoscopic study has become the standard of practice. Because of the widespread presence of hiatal hernia in the West, the accuracy of this endoscopic landmark for the true mucosal EGJ has been questioned [12, 13]. For instance, the gastric mucosal folds can be artificially flattened at endoscopy with over-inflation of the stomach and also changed during respiration and gagging. As such, almost all endoscopic studies that employ this endoscopic criterion of the EGJ are potentially flawed [14], and the biopsy at the so-called EGJ almost always shows columnar-lined esophagus [13]. In a correlation study for the hypothesis that the proximal end of gastric longitudinal mucosal folds was at the same level as the endoscopic SCJ and the angle of His, Wallner [15] labeled the SCJ endoscopically with India ink and then measured the distance between this ink mark and the angle of His in seven resection specimens.

The author reported a disparity of <5 mm and, therefore, concluded that the proximal end of gastric longitudinal mucosal folds is indeed very close to the true EGJ at endoscopy. The major limitation to this conclusion is the lack of histology validation since all seven cases had cancers in the distal esophagus or in the proximal stomach. In fact, the image shown in his paper exhibited typical columnar-lined esophagus [15].

At present, the best endoscopic mucosal landmark of the EGJ has not been universally accepted, although the proximal end of the gastric longitudinal mucosal fold is considered very close to the true EGJ, which remains to be validated histologically.

Distal End of Esophageal Longitudinal Palisading Vessels

In Japan, the distal end of esophageal palisading vessels is considered more accurate as the endoscopic landmark of the mucosal EGJ than the proximal end of gastric longitudinal mucosal folds. In the distal esophagus, there are many parallel longitudinal veins running in the lamina propria and ending at the mucosal junction with the gastric cardia (Fig. 1.3). These veins are visible endoscopically as palisading vessels in a conscious person [16] and also identifiable in columnar-lined esophagus. Because these palisading veins (Fig. 1.4) are absent in the stomach, the Japanese Society of Esophageal Diseases authorized the definition of the distal end of the esophageal longitudinal vessels as the mucosal EGJ in 2000 [16]. As such, the diagnosis of columnar-lined esophagus and Barrett's esophagus can be made endoscopically in Japan. These esophageal mucosal veins can be best visualized during deep inspiration of a conscious person but sometime invisible, especially in patients

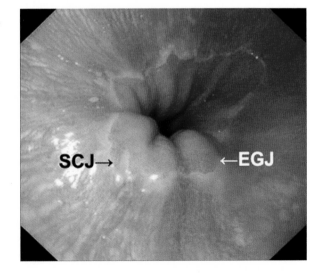

Fig. 1.3 At endoscopy in a normal adult Chinese man, the distal end of the pearly whitish esophageal squamous mucosa forms the squamocolumnar junction (SCJ) and meets the proximal end of reddish gastric longitudinal mucosal folds as the true mucosal esophagogastric junction (EGJ). The esophageal longitudinal vessels (veins) are clearly visible in the distal esophagus running parallel longitudinally toward the SCJ/EGJ

Fig. 1.4 Esophageal veins
(arrows) run underneath
the squamous epithelium
as palisading veins

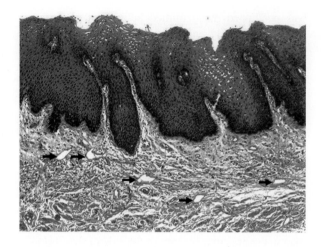

with active esophagitis or in resected or autopsy esophageal specimens [17]. This is the major reason why endoscopists in North America and Europe do not use this criterion for the mucosal EGJ in their practice. In the aforementioned clinical situations in Japan, the patients are treated with proton pump inhibitors before endoscopy to minimize active esophagitis-induced mucosal edema that makes the longitudinal vessels murky at endoscopy [17]. In the patient with columnar-lined esophagus, these veins must be scrutinized for clear identification of the distal ends of the veins, i.e., the mucosal EGJ, during deep inspiration in order to making an accurate diagnosis of columnar-lined esophagus endoscopically [17].

According to the Japanese guideline, any columnar mucosa proximal to the distal ends of esophageal longitudinal palisading vessels is classified as Barrett's esophagus, and the patient is subjected to endoscopic surveillance. This guideline has been challenged by the results of a histology study in 42 resection specimens in Japanese patients on investigation of the relationship between the mucosal EGJ and the distal end of these palisading veins [18]. The authors analyzed the still images of the mucosal EGJ and found that the endoscopically defined distal ends of esophageal longitudinal vessels were <5 mm distal to the SCJ in over 95% of cases and the mucosa in between was columnar in a narrow zone. The authors doubted that the columnar mucosa in this narrow zone had any increased risk of esophageal cancer development but overdiagnosed as columnar-lined esophagus/Barrett's esophagus in Japan [18].

In a comparison study on the relationship among the distal end of esophageal longitudinal vessels, the proximal end of gastric mucosal folds, and the most distal end of deep esophageal glands and ducts, Sato et al. [19] systematically investigated the entire EGJ in 87 consecutive resection specimens from Japanese patients with esophageal squamous cell carcinoma. They used the CD31 immunostain to identify the distal end of esophageal longitudinal veins in the lamina propria and evaluated the correlation between the distal end of esophageal veins and conventional EGJ landmarks. They reported that the most distal end of esophageal longitudinal veins was positioned distal immediately to other landmarks of EGJ, not at the true EGJ. Interestingly enough, both SCJ and EGJ are not a straight line but U- or V-shaped with the distance at the lesser curvature of the stomach significantly longer than that at the greater curvature. This unique shape of the EGJ has not been described in the literature. According to the authors, the unusual U- or V-shaped EGJ line results from unique interaction between the esophageal longitudinal and circular muscles with the gastric innermost oblique muscle layer along with longitudinal-middle circular muscle layers. At the EGJ, the gastric innermost oblique muscle layer becomes sling fibers with roots in the greater curvature side of the EGJ. These sling fibers function as hooks around the notch between the distal esophagus and gastric fundus, forming parallel fibers to the lesser curvature and disappearing gradually around the angle of His. This forms the basis of the U- or V-shaped mucosal EGJ line [19]. In Barrett's esophagus, Sato et al. also discovered that columnar-lined esophagus was significantly more severe in the lesser curvature than in the greater curvature of the side of the EGJ [19].

The results of the histology studies carried out solely in Japan suggest that the distal end of esophageal longitudinal veins may not be as accurate as the proximal end of gastric longitudinal mucosal folds to define the true mucosal EGJ line, because of overestimation of columnar-lined esophagus. Further investigation and validation studies are needed for the gold standard of the true mucosal EGJ.

Squamocolumnar Junction

In a normal adult person without reflux esophagitis, the macroscopic mucosal EGJ is at the same level as the microscopic SCJ (Figs. 1.1 and 1.3). This mucosal EGJ/SCJ line is not straight between the esophagus and stomach; rather, it is serrated, zigzag, also known as the Z line (but it should not be termed as the "dentate line," referring to the junction between the anus and the rectum). This Z line is unstable with three types of histology patterns: (a) an abrupt transition between esophageal squamous epithelium and gastric columnar mucosa; (b) an overlapping of gastric cardiac glands that continuously extend from the cardia into the distal esophagus underneath the squamous epithelium, forming superficial esophageal glands [20, 21], i.e., the so-called "buried" glands; this pattern can be seen in 80–95% of Japanese patients [22, 23]; and (c) moving upwards proximally, separating from the EGJ. The distance between the SCJ and the EGJ defines the length of columnar-lined esophagus (Fig. 1.2). In an autopsy study in 50 consecutive elderly Japanese patients (mean age, 80 years old), the SCJ was found at the same level as the angle of His in 28% of cases, and the distance between the SCJ and the angle of His ranged from 0 to 10 mm. None of the cases showed an upshift of the SCJ toward the proximal esophagus [22]. This finding has been confirmed in Chinese patients. In an endoscopic study of 145 Chinese patients, Law et al. [24] performed biopsies at or immediately below the SCJ that showed a normal appearance in 94% of cases and none upshifted proximally. Thus, the mucosal EGJ is indeed at the same level as SCJ in almost all Chinese adult subjects. This conclusion has been validated by a histology study of the EGJ in 44 resection specimens in adult Chinese patients [25]. In that study, the investigators microscopically examined the entire EGJ region in 31 resection cases, using the most distal end of squamous mucosa, multilayered epithelium, and deep esophageal glands and ducts as the histology landmarks of the mucosal EGJ line. They confirmed that the SCJ was truly at the same level as the EGJ in all cases they studied.

The SCJ may be displaced proximally and move upwards from the mucosal EGJ in Caucasian patients because of the presence of Barrett's esophagus. In those patients, the SCJ cannot be used as a gold standard for the true mucosal EGJ line to guide the endoscopic study in a general practice setting. However, in Japanese and Chinese populations, the SCJ overlaps the mucosal EGJ in most subjects at endoscopy (Fig. 1.3). It remains unknown the relationship among the SCJ, the distal end of esophageal palisading veins, and the proximal end of gastric longitudinal mucosal folds in these populations.

Histologic Landmarks of Mucosal Esophagogastric Junction

At present, distinction between the proximal stomach and the distal esophagus in a small biopsy specimen from the EGJ region is heavily dependent upon the endoscopist's impression as to the precise location of the biopsy site. Unfortunately, in addition to the problematic endoscopic landmark definition of the mucosal EGJ discussed above, many additional confounding factors such as hiatal hernia, respiratory movement of the subject, active or ulcerative esophagitis, etc., make an accurate endoscopic determination of precise biopsy sites almost impossible. Recent studies in histopathology have characterized the morphologic features of the mucosal EGJ and defined the following histological criteria on the mucosal EGJ line as the distal end of (1) squamous epithelium or islands (Fig. 1.5), (2) deep esophageal glands/ducts (Figs. 1.6 and 1.7), (3) multilayered epithelium (Fig. 1.8) and hybrid glands, and (4) double-layered mucosa [3, 16, 26–28]. In addition, conspicuous atrophy and fibrosis are commonly seen in the distal esophagus (Fig. 1.9), but not in the gastric cardia. In the distal esophagus, the squamous mucosa and deep esophageal glands and ducts are unique because they are absent in the stomach [3, 21, 29, 30]. Therefore, these histology landmarks are currently used as the best markers of the esophagus to help define the true histologic EGJ line. In patients with extensive columnar-lined esophagus, the squamous epithelium may frequently become fragmented in small patches and islands (Fig. 1.5). These small squamous epithelial islands surrounded with columnar mucosa in a small endoscopic biopsy specimen are indicative of the esophageal origin (Figs. 1.5 and 1.10) [3, 27]. Other landmarks

Fig. 1.5 A squamous epithelial island (yellow arrow) is surrounded by columnar-lined esophagus (blue arrow) from an American Caucasian male patient with reflux disease and moderate chronic inflammation in the background

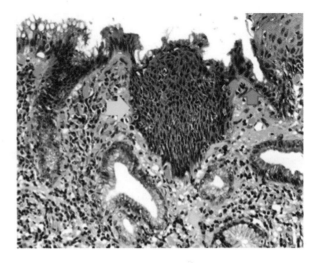

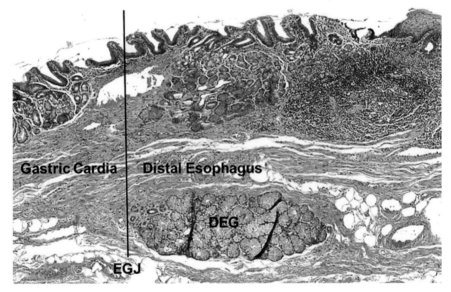

Fig. 1.6 The distal end of a deep esophageal gland (DEG) defines the esophagogastric junction (EGJ). The gastric cardia is on the left. The distalmost esophageal squamous epithelium is replaced by columnar-lined esophagus, consisting of mucoxyntic glands. Note a prominent lymphoid follicle on the left in the distal esophagus in this 62-year-old Chinese man

for the esophagus include (1) the double-layered muscularis mucosa (Fig. 1.11), which can be identified in the distalmost esophagus [26] but found nonspecific for the esophagus because it is also seen in hiatal hernia and post-radiation/sclerotherapy [22], and (2) the multilayered epithelium, which was found to be the precursor

Fig. 1.7 A biopsy specimen at the esophagogastric junction from a 57-year-old American Caucasian man shows focal intestinal metaplasia and a deep esophageal gland duct (blue arrow), indicating the origin of the biopsy in the distal esophagus

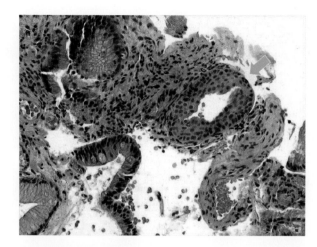

Fig. 1.8 Multilayered epithelium (MLE) is characterized by columnar epithelial cells on the surface, immunoreactive to MUC5AC (right upper), and squamoid cells at the bottom, immunoreactive to p63 (left lower) [4]

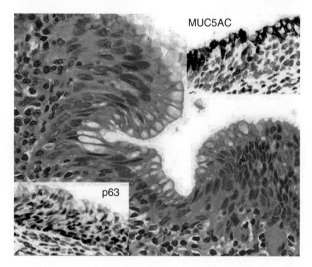

of columnar-lined esophagus and Barrett's esophagus and is present only in the distal esophagus, presumably as a result of reflux-induced esophageal injury [14, 30]. However, inter-observer variability among expert gastrointestinal pathologists is also high for this morphologic marker [3]. In addition, the presence of mucosal crypt architectural disarray, mucosal atrophy, and hybrid glands has been common in columnar-lined esophagus, but these markers also suffer a high inter-observer variability among pathologists [3], disqualifying them as the definitive histology markers of the histology EGJ. At present, the best histology markers of the mucosal EGJ line are the distal end of (a) squamous epithelium, (b) deep esophageal glands/ducts, and (c) multilayered epithelium [4].

Fig. 1.9 Markedly atrophic columnar-lined mucosa in the distalmost esophagus of the esophagogastric region in an elderly male patient with a long history of gastroesophageal reflux disease. Note the sparsely distributed mucous glands embedded in a hyperplastic fibromuscular stroma with moderate chronic inflammation

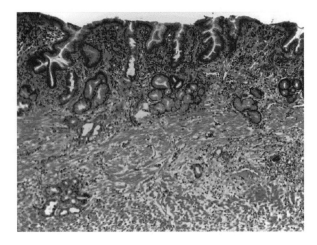

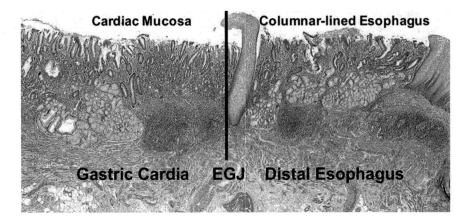

Fig. 1.10 The distal end of a squamous island defines the esophagogastric junction (EGJ) in this 65-year-old Chinese man. In the gastric cardia on the left of the EGJ line, mucous glands grow in both tubular and compound acinar patterns. The same type of mucous glands is present in the same growth patterns, in the distal esophagus, also known as superficial esophageal mucous glands or "buried" glands. Because of the replacement of esophageal squamous epithelium with mucous glands, the distal esophageal mucosa now becomes so-called columnar-lined esophagus. It is entirely possible that the disappearance, due to toxin insult, of the overlying normal esophageal squamous epithelium exposes the underlying naïve superficial esophageal mucous glands. The entire process may not be the results of a "metaplastic" process because of the identical growth pattern of the same mucous glands in the gastric cardia and the adjacent distal esophagus. Note the marked chronic inflammation with multiple lymphoid follicles in the EGJ region. No intestinal metaplasia is detected in both organs

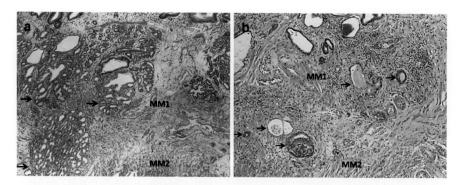

Fig. 1.11 Double-layered muscularis mucosae (MM1 and MM2) in the gastric cardia. Between the two layers of muscularis mucosae is the loose fibrovascular connective tissue with myxoid edematous changes (**a**). Note that cardiac mucous glands grow in a lobular fashion and are deeply seated in the muscularis mucosae (arrows) (**a**). Oftentimes, individual mucous glands (arrows) may present also in the hyperplastic, thickened muscularis mucosae, mimicking invasive well-differentiated tubular adenocarcinoma (**b**). Note the absence of desmoplastic stromal reaction and other malignant features for invasive adenocarcinoma

Histopathologic Interpretation of Mucosal Biopsy at Z Line

Histopathologic determination of the diseases present at the Z line is critically important for patient clinical management because of the different pathology and cancer risk between Barrett's esophagus in the distal esophagus above the EGJ and chronic gastric carditis below the EGJ. The Z line may be at the same position as the true mucosal EGJ, as seen in most Japanese and Chinese subjects (Fig. 1.12), or represents the SCJ that is upshifted proximally because of the short- or long-segment of Barrett's esophagus, as frequently observed in American Caucasian patients. As shown in Table 1.1, Barrett's esophagus at present is the only proven risk factor for distal esophageal adenocarcinoma, while chronic gastric carditis is an inflammatory disease with much lower risk for carcinoma development. As such, an accurate pathologic diagnosis of a mucosal biopsy at the Z line dictates appropriate patient management strategy.

By histology, both Barrett's esophagus and chronic gastric carditis share some common features such as chronic inflammation and pancreatic metaplasia, but mucosal erosion (Fig. 1.13) and atrophy are more commonly associated with the former, while lymphoid follicle is frequently seen in the latter, especially in Chinese patients. Intestinal metaplasia consists of complete, i.e., the small intestinal type, and incomplete, i.e., the colonic type, categories. The complete type is more commonly seen in chronic gastric carditis, but both complete and incomplete types are frequently detected in Barrett's esophagus. Regardless, the key histology features

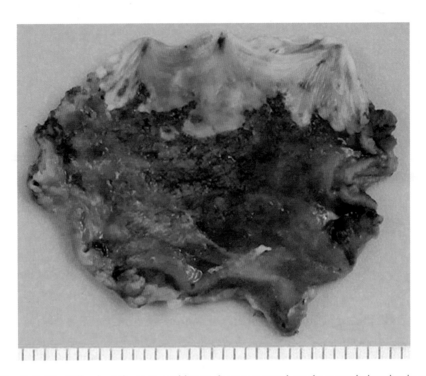

Fig. 1.12 The Z line is at the same position as the true mucosal esophagogastric junction in an endoscopic resection specimen after formalin fixation. Note the zigzag irregular border between the whitish-gray esophageal squamous epithelium and gray-brown gastric cardiac mucosa, reflecting the dynamic, versatile changes in this area, not necessarily indicating Barrett's esophagus (Courtesy of Qi Sun, M.D., M.S. of the Nanjing Drum Tower Hospital in China)

Table 1.1 Comparison between Barrett's esophagus and chronic gastric carditis

Feature	Barrett's esophagus	Gastric carditis
Gender and age	Male > female, >60 years	Equal gender, <60 years
Primary cause	Gastroesophageal reflux disease	*H. pylori* infection, others
Endoscopic columnar-lined esophagus	Common, >1 cm in length, more circumferential	Uncommon, <1 cm in length, more tongue or islands
Histopathology	Chronic inflammation, erosion, atrophy	Chronic inflammation, lymphoid follicle
Intestinal metaplasia (goblet cells)	Both complete and incomplete types	Mainly complete type
Esophageal markers: squamous island, deep esophageal gland duct, multilayer epithelium	Present	Absent
Cancer risk	High	Low
Clinical management strategy	Proton pump inhibitor	Anti-*H. pylori* therapy and others
Endoscopic surveillance	Required	Not required

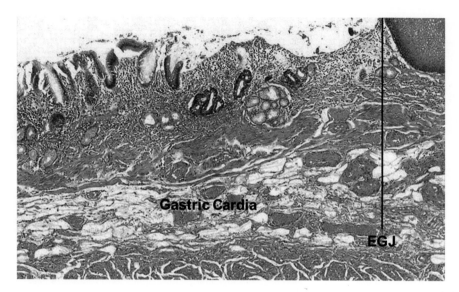

Fig. 1.13 Conspicuous gastric cardiac mucosal erosion is present immediately adjacent to the distal end (the esophagogastric junction, EGJ) of esophageal squamous mucosa in this 65-year-old man without a history of Barrett's esophagus. Moderate chronic inflammation is evident in the gastric cardia, but intestinal metaplasia is absent in mucous glands

for a diagnosis of Barrett's esophagus should include the findings of esophageal landmarks such as squamous islands (Fig. 1.5), deep esophageal glands/ducts (Figs. 1.6 and 1.7), and multilayered epithelium (Fig. 1.8). Because of the high cancer risk in Barrett's esophagus for development of distal esophageal adenocarcinoma, it is prudent for the pathologist to review the upper endoscopy findings of the patient for the evidence of columnar-lined esophagus, especially, its length (over 1 cm) and gross morphology, before making a final diagnosis of Barrett's esophagus. In a patient without the evidence of conspicuous columnar-lined esophagus at endoscopy, the finding of intestinal metaplasia in a few glands underneath squamous epithelium or associated with squamous islands is insufficient for the diagnosis of Barrett's esophagus. This is because both reflux disease and *H. pylori* infection can cause chronic inflammation and intestinal metaplasia. In cases without the evidence of histology markers of the esophagus, a simple description is appropriate along with the statement on the presence or absence of intestinal metaplasia and dysplasia in a pathology report. In most patients, ultrashort columnar-lined esophagus in the length shorter than 1 cm in the island or tongue pattern (Fig. 1.14) is very common in daily clinical practice because of the versatile nature of cells in the EGJ region. In a Chinese population, columnar-lined esophagus can be detected in most cases of surgical resection specimens for gastric cardiac carcinoma; however, in about 97% of such cases, the length of columnar-lined esophagus is shorter than 1 cm [25]. In fact, the British Society of Gastroenterology guidelines on the diagnosis of Barrett's esophagus states: "An oesophagus in which any portion of the nor-

Fig. 1.14 Focal island-like columnar-lined esophagus (arrow) in the distalmost esophagus detected in a 61-year-old man without a history of gastroesophageal reflux disease is not diagnostic of Barrett's esophagus

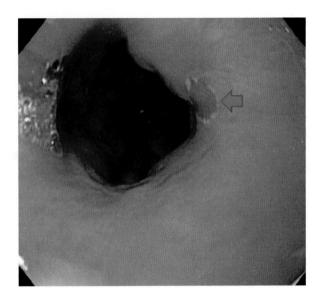

mal distal squamous epithelial lining has been replaced by metaplastic columnar epithelium, which is clearly visible endoscopically (≥1 cm) above the GOJ [31]." Thus, it is prudent for the pathologist to be cautious for making the diagnosis of Barrett's esophagus identified in the distal esophagus within 1 cm above the EGJ.

Recent molecular studies reveal the existence of a discrete population of residual embryonic cells in the EGJ region, which have the capacity of multi-directional differentiations under various stromal microenvironments [32]. In response to toxic insult to the naïve squamous epithelium, these embryonic cells at the EGJ are capable of reprograming their genetic transcription pathways, migrating toward the damaged squamous epithelium to repair, frequently in the form of new columnar epithelium with the molecular and morphologic characteristics of Barrett's esophagus. Therefore, the final differentiation of these cells depends upon "competitive interactions between cell lineages driven by opportunity" [32]. As such, a pathologic diagnosis of Barrett's esophagus may be rendered for a columnar-lined esophageal lesion over 1 cm above the EGJ in the distal esophagus.

Fibromuscular Hypertrophy

In the EGJ region, the muscularis mucosae consists of smooth muscle that runs longitudinally, rather than in the circular and longitudinal fashions as in the corpus stomach. In the adult population, smooth muscle of the muscularis mucosae in the EGJ is markedly thickened as a result of fibromuscular hypertrophy, in which

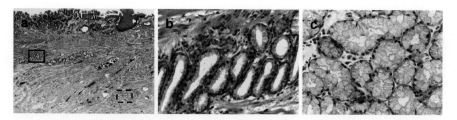

Fig. 1.15 Marked fibromuscular hypertrophy in the esophagogastric junction in (**a**) is associated with scattered cardiac mucous glands squared with solid lines, which are enlarged in (**b**) and exhibit pale eosinophilic mucous glands. The squared area with broken lines in (**a**), located in the right lower corner, is enlarged in (**c**) as deep esophageal glands with bluish hue

scattered cardiac glands are frequently present, and should not be confused with deep esophageal glands that are located below the muscularis mucosae as primarily serous glands with an alkaline blue hue, not cardiac mucous glands above and within the muscularis mucosae with a pale pink (neutral pH) appearance in nature on a routine hematoxylin-eosin stain (Fig. 1.15). These displaced cardiac mucous glands should not be misinterpreted as well-differentiated tubular adenocarcinoma invading into the muscularis mucosae or submucosa. Sometimes, hypertrophic muscularis mucosae become double-layered with the fibrovascular, edematous tissue in between (Fig. 1.11b), which may cause incorrect pathology staging as the muscularis propria invasion (pT2), rather than invasion into the muscularis mucosae (M3, pT1a).

Embryonic Development

The embryonic development of the most important structures involved in the diseases of the EGJ region, such as the most distal squamous epithelium, multilayered epithelium, esophageal glands and ducts, and proximal (distal superficial esophageal) and distal (gastric cardiac) mucous mucosa, remains poorly understood. Our preliminary studies on fetal autopsy materials show the following histologic characteristics:

1. The most distal esophageal squamous epithelium consists of both ciliated glandular and primitive squamous elements that are present as early as gestational age week 26 and best illustrated at week 30 (Fig. 1.16).
2. The primitive deep esophageal glands are discernable at gestational week 33 and present at week 35 (Fig. 1.17).
3. The presence of primitive proximal superficial esophageal mucous glands is identifiable at gestational week 35 (Fig. 1.18).

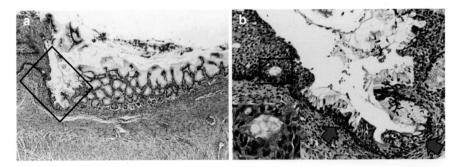

Fig. 1.16 Histologic characteristics of the fetal esophagogastric junction at gestational week 30. As shown in (**a**), the distalmost esophageal epithelium becomes multilayered, which is highlighted with a square and enlarged in (**b**), showing the columnar epithelium on the top and squamoid epithelial cells (arrows) in the bottom. The squared gland-like structure in (**b**) is enlarged in the insert in the left lower corner, illustrating the ciliated surface

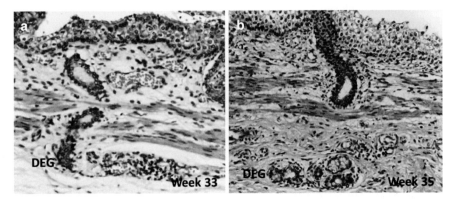

Fig. 1.17 The presence of primitive fetal deep esophageal glands (DEG) underneath the muscularis mucosae starts at gestational week 33 (**a**) and becomes lobular at week 35. Note the ciliated epithelium on the surface of the distal esophagus in (**a**)

Fig. 1.18 The earliest presence of primitive fetal proximal superficial esophageal mucous glands (arrows) in the esophagogastric junction is visible at gestational week 35

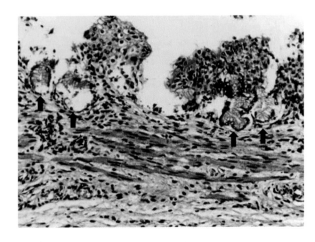

These findings suggest that the embryonic development of the EGJ region is dynamic with both glandular and squamoid differentiations, as well as occasional ciliated gland-like structures, and almost universal presence of the multilayered epithelium. Those preliminary observations require validation by thorough investigations with large samples.

Summary

The EGJ is a dynamic region with a diverse population of cells that are capable of continuous differentiation in different directions in response to the changes in local microenvironments. As a result, various diseases in this region may manifest in genetically different vulnerable populations. Therefore, accurate identification of the EGJ line dictates disease classification and appropriate patient management but is difficult at upper endoscopy and also in histopathology. At present, the proximal gastric longitudinal mucosal folds remain the most appropriate EGJ mucosal marker at endoscopy and the distal ends of squamous epithelium, multilayered epithelium, and deep esophageal glands/ducts as the widely accepted histology landmarks of the EGJ line.

References

 1. Jin L, Yoshida M, Kitagawa Y, et al. Subclassification of superficial cardia cancer in relation to the endoscopic esophagogastric junction. J Gastroenterol Hepatol. 2008;23(Suppl 2):S273–7.
 2. Huang Q, Fan XS, Agoston AT, et al. Comparison of gastroesophageal junction carcinomas in Chinese versus American patients. Histopathology. 2011;59(2):188–97.
 3. Srivastava A, Odze RD, Lauwers GY, Redston M, Antonioli DA, Glickman JN. Morphologic features are useful in distinguishing Barrett esophagus from carditis with intestinal metaplasia. Am J Surg Pathol. 2007;31(11):1733–41.
 4. Huang Q. Definition of the esophagogastric injunction: a critical mini review. Arch Pathol Lab Med. 2011;135:384–9.
 5. Goyal RK. Columnar cell-lined (Barrett's) esophagus: a historical perspective. In: Spechler SJ, Goyal RK, editors. Barrett's esophagus, pathophysiology, diagnosis and management. New York: Elsevier; 1985. p. 1–18.
 6. Misumi A, Murakami A, Harada K, Baba K, Akagi M. Definition of carcinoma of the gastric cardia. Langenbecks Arch Chir. 1989;374(4):221–6.
 7. Huang Q, Zhang LH. The histopathologic spectrum of carcinomas involving the gastroesophageal junction in the Chinese. Int J Surg Pathol. 2007;15:38–52.
 8. Shamiyeh A, Szabo K, Granderath FA, Syré G, Wayand W, Zehetner J. The esophageal hiatus: what is the normal size? Surg Endosc. 2010;24(5):988–91.
 9. Sharma P, McQuaid K, Dent J, et al. AGA Chicago Workshop. A critical review of the diagnosis and management of Barrett's esophagus: the AGA Chicago Workshop. Gastroenterology. 2004;127(1):310–30.
10. Bombeck CT, Dillard DH, Nyhus LM. Muscular anatomy of the junction and the role of phrenoesophageal ligament. Autopsy study of sphincter mechanism. Ann Surg. 1966;164:643–54.
11. McClave SA, Boyce HW Jr, Gottfried MR. Early diagnosis of columnar-lined esophagus: a new endoscopic diagnostic criterion. Gastrointest Endosc. 1987;33:413–6.
12. Chandrasoma PT, Lokuhetty DM, Demeester PT, et al. Definition of histopathologic changes in gastroesophageal reflux disease. Am J Surg Pathol. 2000;24:344–51.

13. Ringhofer C, Lenglinger J, Izay B, et al. Histopathology of the endoscopic esophago-gastric junction in patients with gastroesophageal reflux disease. Wien Klin Wochenschr. 2008;120(11–12):350–9.
14. Wieczorek TJ, Wang HH, Antonioli DA, Glickman JN, Odze RD. Pathologic features of reflux and Helicobacter pylori-associated carditis: a comparative study. Am J Surg Pathol. 2003;27(7):960–8.
15. Wallner B. Endoscopically defined gastroesophageal junction coincides with the anatomical gastroesophageal junction. Surg Endosc. 2009;23(9):2155–8.
16. Takubo K, Aida J, Sawabe M, et al. The normal anatomy around the oesophagogastric junction: a histopathologic view and its correlation with endoscopy. Best Pract Res Clin Gastroenterol. 2008;22(4):569–83.
17. Takubo K, Vieth M, Aida J, et al. Differences in the definitions used for esophageal and gastric diseases in different countries. Digestion. 2009;80:248–57.
18. Ogiya K, Kawano T, Ito E, et al. Lower esophageal palisade vessels and the definition of Barrett's esophagus. Dis Esophagus. 2008;21(7):645–9.
19. Sato T, Kato Y, Matsuura M, Gagner M. Significance of palisading longitudinal esophagus vessels: identification of the true esophagogastric junction has histopathological and oncological considerations. Dig Dis Sci. 2010;55(11):3095–101.
20. DeNardi FG, Riddle RH. In: Sternberg SS, editor. Histology for pathologists. 2nd ed. New York: Raven Press; 1997. p. 461–80.
21. Huang Q, Zhang LH. Histopathological features of diseases in esophageal glands in the region of the gastroesophageal junction in Chinese patients with gastric cardiac cancer involving the esophagus. Pathol Lab Med Int. 2010;2:33–40.
22. Takubo K, Arai T, Sawabe M, et al. Structures of the normal esophagus and Barrett's esophagus. Esophagus. 2003;1:37–47.
23. Nakanishi Y, Saka M, Eguchi T, Sekine S, Taniguchi H, Shimoda T. Distribution and significance of the oesophageal and gastric cardiac mucosae: a study of 131 operation specimens. Histopathology. 2007;51(4):515–9.
24. Law S, Lam KY, Chu KM, Wong J. Specialized intestinal metaplasia and carditis at the gastroesophageal junction in Chinese patients undergoing endoscopy Specialized Intestinal Metaplasia. Am J Gastroenterol. 2002;97:1924–9.
25. Fan XS, Feng AN, Lauwers GY, Huang Q. Esophageal columnar metaplasia is common in the distal esophagus of Chinese patients. Gastroenterology. 2010;138(5 Suppl 1):S-758.
26. Takubo K, Sasajima K, Yamashita K, Tanaka Y, Fujita K. Double muscularis mucosae in Barrett's esophagus. Hum Pathol. 1991;22(11):1158–61.
27. Takubo K, Vieth M, Aryal G, et al. Islands of squamous epithelium and their surrounding mucosa in columnar-lined esophagus: a pathognomonic feature of Barrett's esophagus? Hum Pathol. 2005;36(3):269–74.
28. Owen DA. Stomach (chapter 20). In: Sternberg SS, editor. Histology for pathologists. 2nd ed. New York: Raven Press; 1997. p. 481–93.
29. Chandrasoma P, Makarewicz K, Wickramasinghe K, Ma Y, Demeester T. A proposal for a new validated histological definition of the gastroesophageal junction. Hum Pathol. 2006;37(1):40–7.
30. Glickman JN, Chen YY, Wang HH, Antonioli DA, Odze RD. Phenotypic characteristics of a distinctive multilayered epithelium suggests that it is a precursor in the development of Barrett's esophagus. Am J Surg Pathol. 2001;25(5):569–78.
31. Fitzgerald RC, di Pietro M, Ragunath K, et al. British Society of Gastroenterology. British Society of Gastroenterology guidelines on the diagnosis and management of Barrett's oesophagus. Gut. 2014;63:7–42.
32. Wang X, Ouyang H, Yamamoto Y, et al. Residual embryonic cells as precursors of a Barrett's-like metaplasia. Cell. 2011;145(7):1023–35.

Chapter 2
Cardiac Mucosa

Qin Huang

Introduction

Gastric cardiac carcinoma (GCC) arises in cardiac mucosa located predominantly in the proximal stomach, where the mucosa is composed of primarily mucous glands, also known as cardiac glands. In a healthy human, cardiac glands are composed of predominantly mucous cells, scattered parietal cells, a few undifferentiated cells in the neck, and rare endocrine cells in the base, but no chief cells [1–3]. When the number of parietal cells increases, often in the basal half of gastric mucosa, oxyntic glands admix with mucous glands to form mucoxyntic glands (Fig. 2.1).

In general, cardiac glands show two major growth patterns: (a) tubular, similar to gastric pyloric glands, and (b) compound acinar or racemose glands, mimicking the duodenal Brunner's glands. Like pyloric and Brunner's glands, cardiac glands secrete mucus that forms a protective blanket on the gastric mucosal surface. At the subcellular level, these mucous cells are equipped with short microvilli at the apical surface and secretory granules in the apical cytoplasm, which can be highlighted with periodic acid Schiff reaction for carbohydrates but negative on the Alcian blue stain at pH 2.5 or lower (Fig. 2.2), which is similar to the staining pattern of mucous cells elsewhere in the stomach [1, 2]. Anatomically, cardiac and mucoxyntic glands are mainly concentrated around the esophagogastric junction (EGJ) in a narrow zone and also clustered in small numbers at the upper or rarely in other parts of the esophagus [2–4]. In the distal esophagus, cardiac glands may be present underneath the squamous mucosa above the muscularis mucosae, also known as superficial esophageal glands or "buried" glands (Fig. 2.3) [4–8].

Q. Huang
Pathology and Laboratory Medicine, Veterans Affairs Boston Healthcare System, West Roxbury, MA, USA

Harvard Medical School and Brigham and Women's Hospital, Boston, MA, USA

© Springer International Publishing AG, part of Springer Nature 2018
Q. Huang (ed.), *Gastric Cardiac Cancer*, https://doi.org/10.1007/978-3-319-79114-2_2

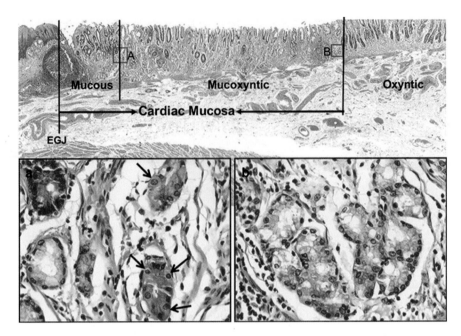

Fig. 2.1 The gastric cardia is located distal to the esophagogastric junction (EGJ) that is defined as the distal end of squamous epithelium in this case. Note a prominent lymphoid follicle across the EGJ line in this Chinese patient. A few cardiac mucous glands on the left of the EGJ line are present underneath the squamous epithelium, also known as superficial esophageal glands or "buried" glands. The gastric cardia shows two types of glands: pure mucous glands, i.e., cardiac mucous glands, and mucoxyntic glands. The squared area labeled A is enlarged in the left lower panel, showing the presence of parietal cells (arrows) and starting the mucoxyntic mucosa. The squared area labeled B is enlarged in the right lower panel, showing pure mucous glands. The glands between A and B constitute mucoxyntic glands. On the most right is the oxyntic mucosa, composed of pure oxyntic glands of the gastric corpus and fundus

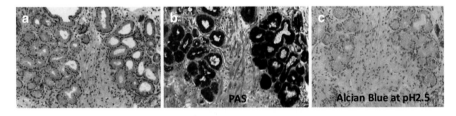

Fig. 2.2 Cardiac mucous cells grow in lobules (**a**). Those mucous cells are intensely reactive to a periodic acid Schiff (PAS) stain in (**b**) but negative to an Alcian blue stain at pH 2.5 in (**c**)

Traditional teaching holds that cardiac and mucoxyntic glands are congenital in nature and constitute the cardiac mucosa in the most proximal part of the stomach as a transition zone of 10–40 mm in length, which abuts proximally with the esophageal squamous mucosa and distally with gastric fundic-type oxyntic glands [2–4]. Recent research results mainly from the Chandrasoma group in the United States

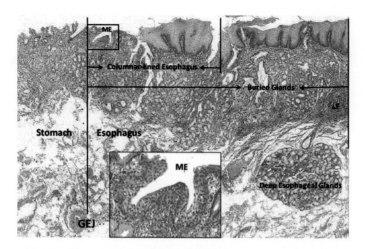

Fig. 2.3 Cardiac mucosa extends from the gastric cardia to the superficial distal esophagus in the same, uninterrupted growth pattern. The distal end of multilayered epithelium defines esophago-gastric junction (EGJ). Mild chronic inflammation is present in both organs. One lymphoid follicle (LF) is present on the far right. Note the identical mucous glands in both gastric cardiac and distal esophageal regions. Adapted from [8]

challenge this doctrine [9–11]. They reported that in the EGJ region of unselected adult autopsies, cardiac glands were present in only 29% of cases and mucoxyntic glands in 44%; even in selected autopsies with the entire EGJ examined microscopi-cally, cardiac glands were detected in only 44% of cases. Recent autopsy studies further found that the length of the cardiac mucosa was, in fact, not 10–40 mm, but varied between 1 and 4 mm in pediatric patients [9, 12], and about 5 mm in most adults in the Caucasian population [9, 13]. Therefore, cardiac glands, regardless of whether or not present in the proximal stomach or in the distal esophagus, are believed to be an acquired metaplastic lesion [11]. As such, cardiac mucosa was no longer considered by some authorities to be part of the proximal stomach but the distal esophagus [9–11, 14]. In supporting of this notion, some study results from Europe and North America also show similar clinical, molecular, and pathologic features of adenocarcinomas arising in the EGJ region [15–17]. In the seventh can-cer staging manual issued by the American Joint Committee on Cancer and International Union against Cancer in 2010, the entire section of gastric cardiac cancer was removed from the chapter of the stomach into that of the esophagus [18]. The manual requires using the esophageal cancer staging criteria for pathologic staging of cancers arising in the proximal gastric cardia [18]. This dramatic para-digm shift caused considerable confusions among clinicians on patient management and also invited extensive worldwide scientific investigations on the true property of cardiac mucosa. As a result, an overwhelming body of scientific evidence derived from worldwide well-designed investigations supports the congenital nature of proximal gastric cardiac mucosa that shows, however, various lengths among differ-ent ethnic populations at different ages [19].

Embryos and Fetuses

In 1961, Salenius published a histological study on gastric mucosal development at different gestational ages [20]. The formation of gastric pits was found at gestational Week 8 in all portions of the stomach except for the pylorus and cardia. Parietal cells were the first differentiated glandular cells, while pyloric and cardiac glands started to develop at Week 13 [20]. These findings were confirmed by the data from a similar study in 2003 [21]. Using the periodic acid Schiff-Alcian blue stain, the investigators showed the presence of cardiac glands in all embryonic specimens [21]. In their report, cardiac glands formed a single layer of the epithelium lined with tall columnar cells with mucus-filled apical cytoplasm containing both neutral and sialylated mucins, which differed from parietal cells conspicuously on hematoxylin-eosin stained sections. Only neutral mucin was present in most superficial foveolar cardiac glands. From the gestational age of Week 15 onwards, these mucous cells started to form cardiac glands that open into pits. At Week 23, the squamous mucosa with ciliated epithelium is replaced by columnar mucous epithelium, constituting primitive cardiac mucosa (Fig. 2.4). At Week 27, the length of primitive cardiac mucosa increases (Fig. 2.5). Therefore, the primitive esophageal mucosa was positioned proximally to cardiac glands. In the last trimester, cardiac glands were further differentiated. At Week 41, all cardiac glands secreted neutral mucin. The authors emphasized that cardiac glands, thus cardiac mucosa, were present on all sections of all cases (Table 2.1) [21].

This conclusion is similar to, but differs to some extent, from that of an earlier fetal study in 2001 [22]. In that report with routine histology sampling, cardiac and mucoxyntic glands in the transition zone between the esophageal squamous mucosa and gastric fundic-type oxyntic mucosa were found in 6% and 52% of cases, respectively. Both studies found that the number of cardiac glands increased with increasing gestational age [21, 22]. In 2003, Park et al. studied the same transition zone with either hematoxylin-eosin or periodic acid Schiff stain (Table 2.1) [23]. In their hands, this transition zone measured <0.4 mm in length, always contained oxyntic cells, but lacked cardiac glands in 20% of Korean cases. This observation is slightly

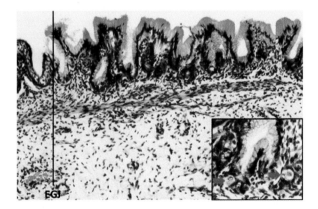

Fig. 2.4 Cardiac mucosa is present at the embryonic age of Week 20 in this fetus. The distal end of the squamous epithelium defines the esophagogastric junction (EGJ). On the right, the gastric cardia is lined with mucous glands; rare parietal cells are discernable at the enlarged insert (arrows)

Fig. 2.5 Primitive cardiac mucosa with pure mucous glands can be identified in the fetal gastric cardia, on the left of the esophagogastric junction (EGJ) at the gestational age of Week 27. The squared area is enlarged in the image below to illustrate the presence of oxyntic glands on the left with the presence of parietal cells (arrows). Note the adjacent mucous glands on the right show no evidence of the parietal cells

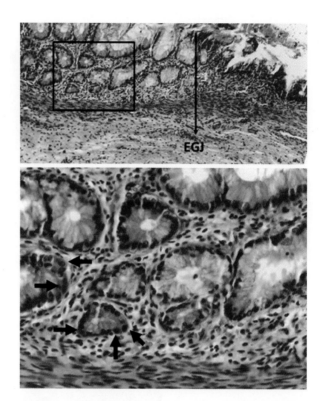

Table 2.1 Ontogeny of cardiac mucosa in humans [19]

Ethnic population	N	Gestational age (weeks)	Absence (%)	Cardiac mucosa presence (%)	Length (mm)	Relation to age	Ref.
American	134	13–41	0	100	NA	NA	20
American	31	15–39	0	45–66	NA	Increased	22
Korean	15	18–34	22	78	NA	Not related	23
European	12	15–41	0	100	0.3–0.6	Decreased	21

Note: *N* number, *NA* not available, *Ref* reference

different from that reported by De Hertogh et al., who described that the "cardiac mucosa was distal to, or straddled, the angle of His in all cases" [21].

At present, the results of all, but one, studies confirmed the presence of cardiac glands and thus cardiac mucosa in the transition zone of the proximal stomach between esophageal squamous epithelium and gastric oxyntic glands in all embryos and fetuses (Table 2.1). The data confirm the congenital nature of cardiac glands and cardiac mucosa in the most proximal stomach at this stage of human development. It must be emphasized that the entire EGJ region is unstable. As shown in Figs. 2.6 and 2.7, cardiac mucous glands are frequently interspersed early at gestational age of Week 23 in the distal embryonic squamous esophageal epithelium that is ciliated (Fig. 2.7). This dynamic region is plastic and varies in length with age and the changes in the local microenvironment.

Fig. 2.6 In the esophagogastric junction region of a fetus at the gestational age of Week 23, multiple mucous glands are inserted in the primitive distal squamous epithelium (arrows) or above the squamoid epithelial cells (*), mimicking "multilayered epithelium"

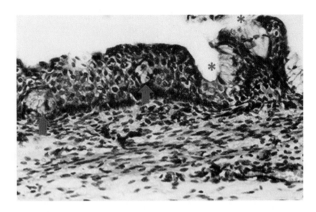

Fig. 2.7 In the fetus, the surface of the primitive esophagus is lined with cilia. The ciliated surface epithelium sometimes forms gland-like structures with ciliated luminal surface (arrows) in this fetus at the gestational age of Week 23

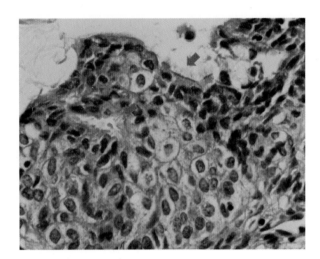

Pediatric Population

Several groups of investigators carried out the investigations mainly in pediatric autopsy cases (Table 2.2). In 2000, Chandrasoma et al. [9] in a prospective study with the entire EGJ examined microscopically reported the absence of cardiac mucosa in about half cases; even in the other half cases, the length of cardiac mucosa was very short (mean length, 0.3 mm). This study was criticized for poor specimen preparation and obvious autolysis demonstrated in the images the authors published [9, 24]. In a well-designed and well-executed study [12], Kilgore et al. systematically investigated the histology of the entire EGJ on period acid Schiff-stained sections in consecutive autopsy cases without reflux esophagitis, Barrett esophagus, antiacid medications, or *H. pylori* infection. They reported the findings of a normal squamocolumnar junction (SCJ), as the landmark of the EGJ, and the presence of cardiac glands in all cases, exclusively on the gastric side of the SCJ/EGJ. In their

Table 2.2 The existence of cardiac mucosa in pediatric population (≤20 year female)[a]

Ethnic population	Tissue type	EGJ	N	Age (years)	Absence (%)	Presence (%)	Cardiac mucosa length (range) (mm)	Relation to age	Ref.
American	Autopsy	Entire	7	3–18	43	57	0.3 (0.07–0.7)	?	9
American	Autopsy	Entire	30	Neonate–18	0	100	1.8 (1–4)	?	12
American	Autopsy	Entire	45	Neonate–17	2	98	NA	Increased	22
American	Biopsy	Selected	74	1–19	0	100	NA	?	25
American	Autopsy	Selected	100	Neonate–18	0	100	1 (0.1–3)	?	26
Korean	Autopsy	Entire	8	Neonate–15	22	78	0.17 (0.1–0.27)	Not related	23

Note: *N* number, *Ref* references, *EGJ* esophagogastric junction, *?* unknown
[a]Reproduced with permission from [19] © John Wiley and Sons Inc.

study, the length of cardiac mucosa was 1.8 mm on average (Table 2.2). The short-coming of their study was the lack of controls and clinicopathologic information [19, 24]. In similar autopsy studies in newborns, infants, and young children-adolescents, investigators reported the presence of cardiac mucosa distal to the SCJ in almost all cases and concluded that cardiac mucosa was congenital in nature [22, 25]. In a retrospective study of endoscopic mucosal biopsies at the place 1 mm below the SCJ, Glickman et al. reported the presence of cardiac mucosa in all pediatric cases, including cardiac glands in 81% and mixed mucoxyntic glands in 19% [26]. In no case did the authors identify pure oxyntic glands immediately below the SCJ. They concluded that cardiac mucosa was congenital in the pediatric population. However, because of the overwhelming presence of inflammation in 88% of the cases and the absence of proper controls without inflammation, the authors could not determine with certainty the nature of cardiac glands with regard to as physiologic gastric components or as pathologic metaplastic changes in response to gastric acid insults or *H. pylori* infection [26].

At present, all, but two [9, 23], studies in pediatric subjects show the histological evidence of the presence of cardiac glands and cardiac mucosa on the gastric side of the EGJ as a congenital, not acquired, gastric structure; but the length of cardiac mucosa is short, less than 2 mm on average (Table 2.2). All studies used the distal end of squamous mucosa, i.e., the SCJ, as the mucosal EGJ, which may be potentially problematic [27]. In both fetal and pediatric populations, the length of cardiac mucosa increases with age [28].

Adults in North America and Europe

In adults, the status of cardiac glands and cardiac mucosa in the proximal stomach remains a hot topic of research (Table 2.3). A series of studies by the Chandrasoma group showed the morphologic evidence of the absence of gastric cardiac glands in a substantial number of adult American patients. For example, in an endoscopic histological study of the mucosal tissues biopsied above and below the EGJ in adults with 24-h pH monitoring and measurement of lower esophageal sphincter pressure, they reported the absence of cardiac glands in 26% of cases and a statistically significant association of the presence of cardiac glands with reflux esophagitis, as evidenced with an esophageal luminal acidic pH < 4, low lower esophageal sphincter pressure, the presence of hiatal hernia, and active esophagitis [29]. In a subsequent endoscopic biopsy study within 40 mm of the EGJ, they further showed a strong correlation between the length of cardiac mucosa and the amount of acid exposure in the esophagus [10]. The results of this study were disputed with regard to the biopsy site, because it was not clear whether or not their biopsies included the SCJ and the possibility of sampling errors in the proximal gastric fundic region was obvious [24, 26]. In addition, the absence of controls without inflammation makes their arguments weak. In a retrospective autopsy study with one selected EGJ section examined microscopically in each case, the same investigators reported a

Table 2.3 The existence of cardiac mucosa in adult populations (≥20 years) [19]

Ethnic population	Tissue type	EGJ	N	Absence (%)	Cardiac mucosa presence (%)	Length (mm)	Ref.
American	Biopsy	Selected	334	26	74	NA	29
American	Biopsy	Selected	71	0	100	<20	10
American	Autopsy	Selected	66	18	82	<5	9
American	Autopsy	Entire	11	0	100	5	9
American	Biopsy	Selected	903	39	61	1–40.0	11
American	Biopsy	Selected	226	15	85	NA	33
European	Resection	Entire	36	3	97	5 (1–15)	13
European	Biopsy	Selected	63	0	100	NA	24
Japanese	Biopsy	Selected	182	0	100	NA	34
Japanese	Resection	Entire	56	0	100	NA	34
Japanese	Resection	Entire	131	0	100	13 (2–64)	30
Chinese	Biopsy	Selected	100	27[a]	73	NA	36
Chinese	Resection	Entire	44[b]	0	100	7 (3–19)	5

Note: *N* number, *Ref* references, *EGJ* esophagogastric junction, *NA* not available
[a] Pure cardiac glands with no information on mucoxyntic glands
[b] 13 cases were selected and 31 with the entire EGJ examined microscopically

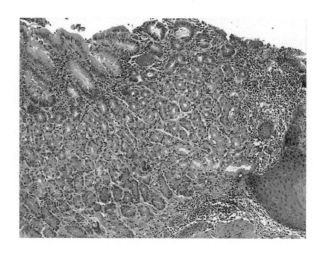

Fig. 2.8 The gastric cardia in this 75-year-old male patient shows pure oxyntic mucosa immediately abutting the distal esophageal squamous mucosa with no evidence of mucous glands in the cardia. Note chronic inflammation in the background, severe at the place adjacent to the squamous epithelium with focal erosion and apparent dropouts of gastric glands

complete absence of cardiac glands in 67% of cases (Fig. 2.8) and similar results (64%) from 11 prospective autopsies with the entire EGJ examined microscopically [9]. The authors concluded that cardiac glands were acquired as an early metaplastic response to inflammation and gastric acid insult. This study was also criticized for poor preparation of autopsy EGJ specimens and obvious autolysis present in the images that authors published [24, 30]. In 2003, the Chandrasoma group published their histology study results on consecutive endoscopic biopsies at the EGJ [11]. In that study, they defined cardiac and mucoxyntic glands as "abnormal" columnar mucosa that had a length of 1–40 mm, while the columnar mucosa with pure oxyntic glands was considered as "normal" gastric glands. They reported the cases with pure oxyntic, cardiac, and mucoxyntic glands in 39%, 43%, and 18%, respectively, and the prevalence of intestinal metaplasia increased with the increasing length of cardiac mucosa. They concluded that, "cardiac mucosa is absent in over 50% of the general population. When present, its extent is in the 1–9 mm range in over 95% of the general population and approximately 85% of a population undergoing endoscopy" [11, 31]. These investigators advocate defining the proximal end of gastric fundic-type oxyntic mucosa as the true mucosal EGJ and the entire gastric cardia as the damaged, degenerated, and dilated distal esophagus [14].

Several groups of investigators from Europe and North America conducted a series of studies, trying to confirm or refute the findings by the Chandrasoma group. In 2002, German pathologists, Sarbia et al. systemically investigated histology of the entire EGJ in surgical resection specimens for squamous cell carcinoma in patients with no gross evidence of the columnar-lined esophagus [13]. They defined the EGJ as the macroscopic junction between brown-red gastric mucosa and pear-gray esophageal mucosa. The authors reported the detection of cardiac and mucoxyntic glands in 97% of cases with a mean length of 5 mm (range 1–15 mm). They did not identify any case that showed a direct transition of gastric fundic-type oxyntic glands to the esophageal squamous mucosa. In addition, they also reported the findings of intra-esophageal presence of cardiac and mucoxyntic glands above the deep esophageal glands in 25% of cases. However, in as high as 61% of cases in their report were squamous islands present adjacent to cardiac or mucoxyntic glands, which indicates that their analysis, at least in part, was actually carried out in the tissues taken from the distal esophagus, not in the proximal stomach, since squamous islands are indicative of the esophagus [27, 32].

To contribute to the debate on the existence of gastric cardiac glands and cardiac mucosa, Marsman et al. conducted an endoscopic biopsy study in 63 of 198 unselected subjects with biopsies at or immediately below the endoscopically normal appearing SCJ that was defined as the EGJ [24]. They reported a uniform presence of cardiac mucosa in the proximal stomach, including cardiac glands in 62% of cases and mucoxyntic glands in 38%. Therefore, they concluded that cardiac glands and cardiac mucosa were congenital, not metaplastic [24]. Their conclusion was confirmed in a similar study of volunteer healthcare workers in the United States [33].

Thus far, all studies show the consistent presence of cardiac glands and cardiac mucosa on the gastric side of the EGJ in most, but not all, patients, which is slightly different from that shown in fetal and pediatric populations. The length of cardiac mucosa in this transitional zone is short, about 5 mm in length on average. The absence of cardiac mucosa in over 39% of adult Americans, as reported by the Chandrasoma group, has not been confirmed by most investigators. It should be noted that most studies used the SCJ as the landmark of the EGJ, which may be a potential source of errors [27].

Adults in Japan and China

Interestingly enough, the data from published investigations on cardiac mucosa in the EGJ region from Japan and China are different from those of the studies conducted in North America and Europe. In Japan, Misumi et al. studied the relationship between the mucosal EGJ [34], which was defined as the distal end of esophageal longitudinal vessels, and cardiac glands in endoscopic biopsies from patients without reflux esophagitis, ulcer, hiatal hernia, or tumors in the esophagus and stomach. They also systemically mapped cardiac glands in the entire EGJ region in additional resection specimens for esophageal or gastric carcinoma. They reported the presence of cardiac glands in an area between 7.5 mm proximal and 13 mm distal to the EGJ. In histology, cardiac mucosa straddled the EGJ about 10 mm proximally and 20 mm distally [34]. In a histology study also in Japan, Nakanishi et al. investigated the entire EGJ macro- and microscopically in 131 surgical resection specimens for upper and middle esophageal squamous cell carcinomas [30]. They reported the presence of cardiac glands in the proximal stomach in all cases and superficial esophageal cardiac glands in 95% of cases with the mean lengths of 13 mm and 4 mm and ranges of 2–64 mm and 1–26 mm, respectively. The results clearly indicate the presence of both proximal gastric and superficial esophageal cardiac glands and cardiac mucosa in all Japanese subjects. The superficial esophageal cardiac glands are believed to protect the squamous mucosa from acidic injury [7]. Indeed, the Japanese Research Society of Gastric Cancer defines the gastric cardia as the region where cardiac glands and cardiac mucosa are located [35].

Recent endoscopic and histological study results in the Chinese population are similar to those reported in the Japanese population. For example, Law et al. performed endoscopic biopsies at or immediately below the SCJ that showed a normal appearance in 94% of cases and none with the SCJ shifted proximally toward the esophagus [36]. The authors reported the presence of pure cardiac glands in 73% of cases in the proximal stomach below the SCJ/EGJ line but did not describe the status of mucoxyntic glands [36]. In another histology study of the EGJ in 44 resection specimens for gastric cardiac cancer in Chinese patients with 31 cases having the entire EGJ examined microscopically, Fan et al. used the most distal end of squamous mucosa along with deep esophageal glands and ducts as the landmarks of the EGJ to investigate the distribution of cardiac glands [5, 27]. They found that cardiac glands distributed not only distally in the proximal stomach with a mean length of 7 mm (range 3–20 mm) but also proximally underneath the squamous epithelium into the distal superficial esophagus with a mean length of 7 mm (range 3–18 mm). In their report, chronic inflammation was present in 95% of cases and 64% with *H. pylori* infection [5]. The major limitations of their study included small sample size and the potential confounding factor of cancer involvement in the tissues their studied.

Apparently, the results from recent studies in Japanese and Chinese populations show a universal presence of cardiac glands in the proximal stomach and also in the distal superficial esophagus with approximate lengths of about 13 mm distally and 7 mm proximally from the EGJ, which differs substantially from the data reported in the Caucasian population in Europe and North America. The major limitations of these studies include (1) the lack of universally accepted histological landmarks to define the EGJ in the early studies [37], (2) the absence of controls without chronic inflammation or cancer involvement in the EGJ region, and (3) the use of biopsy tissues in many studies.

Cardiac Glands in Distal Esophagus

In the distal esophagus above the EGJ, cardiac glands may present underneath the squamous epithelium as "buried glands" (Fig. 2.9) after successful repair of toxin-damaged squamous mucosa in Caucasian patients [38]. In contrast, the concept of "buried glands" is barely reported in East Asians because of the rarity of Barrett's esophagus [39]. However, these glands are frequently found in the distal esophagus in Chinese patients, but not associated with premalignant diseases such as Barrett's esophagus, unlike seen in American Caucasian patients [8, 39–42]. In a histopathology study of these glands in the distal esophagus, investigators identified

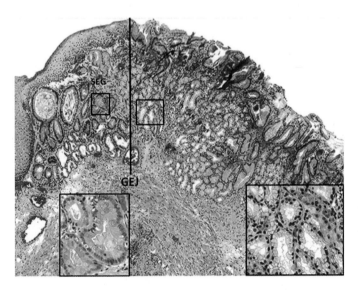

Fig. 2.9 The distal end of esophageal squamous epithelium is the esophagogastric junction (EGJ) line. On the right is gastric cardia, composed of pure mucous glands. On the left are the same mucous glands, also known as "buried" glands or superficial esophageal glands, in the same growth pattern as those in gastric cardia but show intestinal metaplasia evidenced by the presence of goblet cells. The background stroma shows minimal chronic inflammation in this 65-year Caucasian man

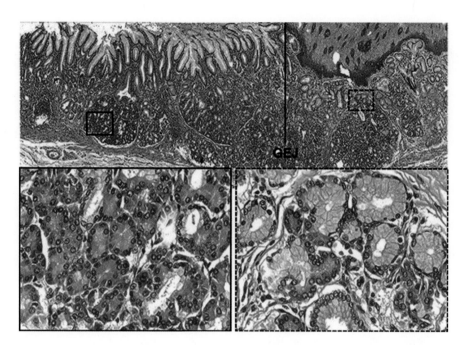

Fig. 2.10 The same cardiac mucous glands are present in gastric cardia and in superficial distal esophagus in a predominantly compound lobular growth pattern with extensive pancreatic metaplasia

181 consecutive gastric cardiac carcinoma resection cases with the tissue from the distal esophagus and studied the distribution and pathology of those cardiac glands [8]. Among those cases, 149 were unselected with one EGJ section for evaluation and 32 selected with the entire EGJ examined microscopically [8]. In 114 eligible cases, the presence of cardiac glands in the distal esophagus was found in 110 (96.5%) cases. These mucous glands were associated with chronic inflammation (95%), lymphoid follicle (85%), *H. pylori* infection (42%), intestinal metaplasia (25%), pancreatic metaplasia (36%) (Fig. 2.10), and dysplasia (10%). Columnar-lined esophagus was identified in 65% of cases with an average length of 4 mm (range, 1–13 mm). Interestingly enough, about 97% of cases with columnar-lined esophagus were within 10 mm in the longitudinal length above the EGJ [8]. The data clearly demonstrate a predominance of *H. pylori* infection-associated chronic inflammation-related diseases in the superficial esophageal cardiac mucosa within 10 mm above the EGJ in this Chinese patient population.

Heterogeneity of Cardiac Glands

In the gastric cardia, cardiac glands are lobulated in different sizes and compositions. In general, those glands are composed of primarily mucous cells and occasional parietal cells. Overall, those glands demonstrate mucous proteins that are histochemically positive for PAS and immunoreactive to MUC6, but not MUC5, MUC2, and CDX2 (Fig. 2.11).

Among lobules of cardiac glands are the glands with duct-like structures showing basal lining cells underneath columnar mucous cells. The mucus of columnar cells in those duct-like glands exhibits blue alkaline reaction to a histochemical Alcian blue stain at pH 2.5. By immunohistochemistry, the basal cells of the lobules are immunoreactive to p63 (Fig. 2.12), suggestive of the features of stem cells [43].

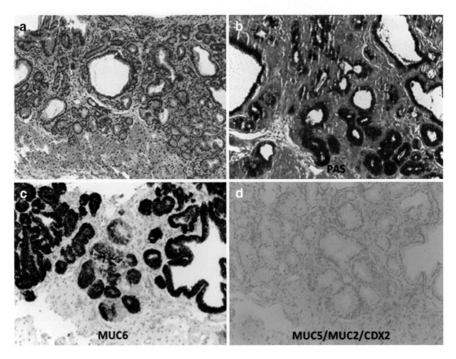

Fig. 2.11 Cardiac mucosa (**a**) is composed of a heterogeneous group of lobulated mucous glands, some of which are dilated and vary in size and composition. However, almost all mucous cells in the cardia exhibit strong histochemical reactivity to a PAS stain (**b**) and show strong immunoreactivity to MUC6 (**c**), but not MUC5, MUC2, or CDX2 (**d**)

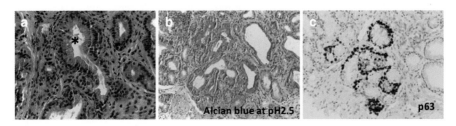

Fig. 2.12 Some cardiac glands show a duct-like, multilayered structure (*) with luminal mucous cells and underneath immature squamoid cells (**a**). By a histochemical Alcian blue stain at pH 2.5, these luminal mucous cells exhibit blue alkaline reaction in contrast to the negative reaction of the adjacent cardiac mucous glands (**b**). Immunohistochemically, the underneath immature squamoid cells are immunoreactive to p63 (**c**)

The presence of those heterogeneous cardiac glands in the cardia may have significant implication in pathology of this region.

Stem Cells

Recent scientific studies from several laboratories have gradually uncovered the mystery of stem cells in the stomach. It is now recognized that Lgr5+ stem cells are mainly located at the bottom of a gastric unit and distribute primarily in the gastric cardia along with villin+ stem cells (Fig. 2.13). Mutation of those stem cells may be responsible for tumorigenesis of chromosomal instable adenocarcinomas of the stomach and distal esophagus [44]. In addition, there exist residual embryonic stem cells in the cardiac/EGJ region [45]. These opportunistic stem cells have the potential to differentiate into different types of cells in response to the changes in local microenvironment toward squamous or columnar or even mesenchymal cells to repair damage and restore normal function [45]. Conceivably, malignant mutations in those residual embryonic cells in the cardiac/EGJ region may be responsible for a wide histopathologic spectrum of malignancy [46]. At present, those stem cells remain elusive as to biomarkers, morphologic features, function, and pathologic characteristics, once mutated as cancer stem cells (Fig. 2.14).

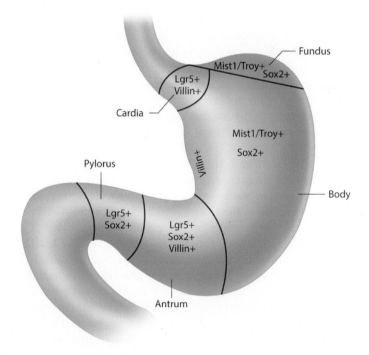

Fig. 2.13 Gastric stem cells are distributed in two distinct groups: (1) primarily with Lgr5+, villin+ stem cells in the gastric cardia, lesser curvature, antrum, and pylorus and (2) mainly with Troy+ and mist1+ stem cells in the gastric corpus and fundus. Modified from [44]

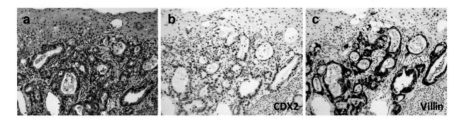

Fig. 2.14 Well-moderately differentiated tubular adenocarcinoma of the gastric cardia invading into the distal esophagus (**a**) is immunoreactive to CDX2 (**b**) and villin (**c**) in a 63-year-old Chinese man without a history of gastroesophageal reflux disease and the morphologic evidence of Barrett's esophagus both at upper endoscopy and in the resection specimen (Courtesy of Yuqing Cheng, M.D. of the Chang Zhou Second Hospital, China)

Summary

The results of the most recent studies in fetal, pediatric, and adult populations confirm the presence of cardiac mucosa in the proximal stomach as a congenital structure in a much shorter length than previously believed and various distribution patterns among different ethnic populations. In general, the length of cardiac mucosa increases with age. The data from the studies carried out in the European and American Caucasian populations suggests that the length of cardiac mucosa in the distal esophagus is influenced mainly by age, chronic inflammation, and reflux disease. In contrast, in the Japanese and Chinese populations, in whom reflux disease is not as common and as severe as in the Caucasians, cardiac glands and cardiac mucosa are almost always present not only in the gastric cardia but also in the distal superficial esophagus underneath the squamous epithelium. These differences between Caucasians and East Asians may be related to different clinicopathologic characteristics of carcinomas occurring in this region between these two different ethnic patient populations [37]. It appears that cardiac mucosa straddles the EGJ and encases the distal end of the esophageal squamous epithelium, conceivably providing the esophageal squamous mucosa with protective mucus against insults of various reflux toxic chemicals. The differences in the length and distribution patterns of cardiac mucosa may explain at least partially the reasons why the incidence of distal esophageal diseases such as Barrett's esophagus and adenocarcinoma remains rare in East Asia, but epidemic in Europe and North America [39–42]. In fact, many Caucasian patients without a history of severe gastroesophageal reflux disease do present for the first time with the diagnosis of Barrett dysphagia or distal esophageal adenocarcinoma at upper endoscopy with a biopsy [42]. On the other hand, gastric cardiac carcinoma is very common in the Chinese population in whom the length of cardiac mucosa is also much longer than that in the Caucasian population, but the distal esophageal adenocarcinoma remains rare. Therefore, cardiac mucosa appears to be the origin of cancer for both Barrett's adenocarcinoma above the EGJ in Caucasian patients and gastric cardiac carcinoma below the EGJ in Chinese patients [37, 40, 42]. It is also important to know that the EGJ region is plastic and dynamic with the morphologic features of both squamous and columnar (among others) epithelial differentiation potentials from the fetal developmental stage to the mature adult in whom residual embryonic stem cells may be responsible for directing the repair and adaptive responses. This provides the ontogenetic basis for understanding a wide histopathologic spectrum of gastric cardiac carcinoma [37].

References

1. Krause WJ, Ivey KJ, Baskin WN, MacKercher PA. Morphological observations on the normal human cardiac glands. Anat Rec. 1978;192(1):59–71.
2. Fawcett D. Chapter 25: The esophagus and stomach. In: Bloom W, Fawcett DW, editors. A textbook of histology. 12th ed. New York: Chapman and Hall; 1994. p. 593–616.
3. Takubo K, Arai T, Sawabe M, et al. Structures of the normal esophagus and Barrett's esophagus. Esophagus. 2003;1:37–47.
4. Owen DA. Stomach. In: Sternberg SS, editor. Histology for pathologists. 2nd ed. New York: Raven Press; 1997. p. 481–93.
5. Fan XS, Feng AN, Zhang LH, Lauwers G, Huang Q. Esophageal columnar metaplasia is common in the distal esophagus of Chinese patients. Gastroenterology. 2010;138(5 Suppl 1):S758.
6. Huang Q, Zhang LH. Histopathologic features of esophageal glands in the region of the gastroesophageal junction in Chinese patients with gastric cardiac cancer involving the esophagus. Pathol Lab Med Int. 2010;2:33–40.
7. Yagi K, Nakamura A, Sekine A, Umezu H. The prevalence of esophageal cardiac glands: relationship with erosive esophagitis and nonerosive reflux disease (NERD) in Japanese patients. Endoscopy. 2006;38(6):652–3.
8. Sun Q, Huang Q, Feng AN, et al. Columnar-lined esophagus in Chinese patients with proximal gastric carcinomas. J Dig Dis. 2013;14(1):22–8.
9. Chandrasoma PT, Der R, Ma Y, Dalton P, Taira M. Histology of the gastroesophageal junction: an autopsy study. Am J Surg Pathol. 2000;24(3):402–9.
10. Chandrasoma PT, Lokuhetty DM, Demeester PT, et al. Definition of histopathologic changes in gastroesophageal reflux disease. Am J Surg Pathol. 2000;24:344–51.
11. Chandrasoma PT, Der R, Ma Y, Peters J, Demeester T. Histologic classification of patients based on mapping biopsies of the gastroesophageal junction. Am J Surg Pathol. 2003;27(7):929–36.
12. Kilgore SP, Ormsby AH, Gramlich TL, et al. The gastric cardia: fact or fiction. Am J Gastroenterol. 2000;95:921–4.
13. Sarbia M, Donner A, Gabbert HE. Histopathology of the gastroesophageal junction: a study on 36 operation specimens. Am J Surg Pathol. 2002;26(9):1207–12.
14. Chandrasoma P, Makarewicz K, Wickramasinghe K, Ma Y, Demeester T. A proposal for a new validated histological definition of the gastroesophageal junction. Hum Pathol. 2006;37(1):40–7.
15. Wijnhoven BP, Siersema PD, Hop WC, et al. Adenocarcinomas of the distal oesophagus and gastric cardia are one clinical entity. Rotterdam Oesophageal Tumour Study Group. Br J Surg. 1999;86:529–35.
16. Dolan K, Morris AI, Gosney JR, Field JK, Sutton R. Three different subsite classification systems for carcinomas in the proximity of the GEJ, but is it all one disease? J Gastroenterol Hepatol. 2004;19(1):24–30.
17. Chandrasoma P, Wickramasinghe K, Ma Y, et al. Adenocarcinomas of the distal esophagus and "gastric cardia" are predominantly esophageal carcinomas. Am J Surg Pathol. 2007;31:569–75.
18. American Joint Committee on Cancer. Chapter 10: Esophagus and esophagogastric junction. In: AJCC cancer staging manual. 7th ed. New York: Springer; 2009. p. 103–15.

19. Huang Q. Controversies of cardiac glands in the proximal stomach: a critical review. J Gastroenterol Hepatol. 2011;26:450–5.
20. Salenius P. On the ontogenesis of the human gastric epithelial cells. A histologic and histochemical study. Acta Anat (Basal). 1962;50(Suppl 46):S1–S76.
21. De Hertogh G, Van Eyken P, Ectors N, Tack J, Geboes K. On the existence and location of cardiac mucosa: an autopsy study in embryos, fetuses, and infants. Gut. 2003;52(6):791–6.
22. Zhou H, Greco MA, Daum F, Kahn E. Origin of cardiac mucosa: ontogenic consideration. Pediatr Dev Pathol. 2001;4(4):358–63.
23. Park YS, Park HJ, Kang GH, Kim CJ, Chi JG. Histology of gastroesophageal junction in fetal and pediatric autopsy. Arch Pathol Lab Med. 2003;127(4):451–5.
24. Marsman WA, van Sandick JW, Tytgat GN, ten Kate FJ, van Lanschot JJ. The presence and mucin histochemistry of cardiac type mucosa at the esophagogastric junction. Am J Gastroenterol. 2004;99(2):212–7.
25. Derdoy JJ, Bergwerk A, Cohen H, Kline M, Monforte HL, Thomas DW. The gastric cardia: to be or not to be? Am J Surg Pathol. 2003;27(4):499–504.
26. Glickman JN, Fox V, Antonioli DA, Wang HH, Odze RD. Morphology of the cardia and significance of carditis in pediatric patients. Am J Surg Pathol. 2002;26(8):1032–9.
27. Huang Q. Definition of the esophagogastric junction. Arch Pathol Lab Med. 2011;135(3):384–9.
28. Peitz U, Vieth M, Malfertheiner P. Carditis at the interface between GERD and Helicobacter pylori infection. Dig Dis. 2004;22(2):120–5.
29. Oberg S, Peters JH, DeMeester TR, et al. Inflammation and specialized intestinal metaplasia of cardiac mucosa is a manifestation of gastroesophageal reflux disease. Ann Surg. 1997;226(4):522–30.
30. Nakanishi Y, Saka M, Eguchi T, Sekine S, Taniguchi H, Shimoda T. Distribution and significance of the oesophageal and gastric cardiac mucosae: a study of 131 operation specimens. Histopathology. 2007;51(4):515–9.
31. Chandrasoma P. Controversies of the cardiac mucosa and Barrett's esophagus. Histopathology. 2005;46:361–73.
32. Takubo K, Vieth M, Aryal G, Honma N, et al. Islands of squamous epithelium and their surrounding mucosa in columnar-lined esophagus: a pathognomonic feature of Barrett's esophagus? Hum Pathol. 2005;36(3):269–74.
33. El-Serag HB, Graham DY, Rabeneck L, Avid A, Richardson P, Genta RM. Prevalence and determinants of histological abnormalities of the gastric cardia in volunteers. Scand J Gastroenterol. 2007;42(10):1158–66.
34. Misumi A, Murakami A, Harada K, Baba K, Akagi M. Definition of carcinoma of the gastric cardia. Langenbecks Arch Chir. 1989;374(4):221–6.
35. Japanese Research Society for Gastric Cancer. The general rules for gastric cancer. Jpn J Surg. 1973;3:61–71.
36. Law S, Lam KY, Chu KM, Wong J. Specialized intestinal metaplasia and carditis at the gastroesophageal junction in Chinese patients undergoing endoscopy. Am J Gastroenterol. 2002;97(8):1924–9.
37. Huang Q, Fan XS, Agoston AT, et al. Comparison of gastroesophageal junction carcinomas in Chinese versus American patients. Histopathology. 2011;59(2):188–97.
38. Mörk H, Barth T, Kreipe HH, et al. Reconstitution of squamous epithelium in Barrett's oesophagus with endoscopic argon plasma coagulation: a prospective study. Scand J Gastroenterol. 1998;33(11):1130–4.
39. Huang Q, Fang DC, Yu CG, Zhang J, Chen MH. Barrett's esophagus-related diseases remain uncommon in China. J Dig Dis. 2011;12(6):420–7.
40. Huang Q, Shi J, Sun Q, et al. Distal esophageal carcinomas in Chinese patients vary widely in histopathology, but adenocarcinomas remain rare. Hum Pathol. 2012;43(12):2138–48.
41. Hongo M, Nagasaki Y, Shoji T. Epidemiology of esophageal cancer: Orient to Occident. Effects of chronology, geography and ethnicity. J Gastroenterol Hepatol. 2009;24(5):729–35.

42. Spechler SJ. Cardiac mucosa, Barrett's oesophagus and cancer of the gastro-oesophageal junction: what's in a name? Gut. 2017;66(8):1355–7. https://doi.org/10.1136/gutjnl-2016-311948. pii: gutjnl-2016-311948.
43. Reis-Filho JS, Schmitt FC. Taking advantage of basic research: p63 is a reliable myoepithelial and stem cell marker. Adv Anat Pathol. 2002;9(5):280–9.
44. Huang Q, Zou XP. Clinicopathology of early gastric carcinoma: an update for pathologists and gastroenterologists. Gastrointest Tumors. 2017;3(3–4):115–24.
45. Wang X, Ouyang H, Yamamoto Y, et al. Residual embryonic cells as precursors of a Barrett's-like metaplasia. Cell. 2011;145:1023–35.
46. Huang Q, Zhang LH. The histopathologic spectrum of carcinomas involving the gastroesophageal junction in the Chinese. Int J Surg Pathol. 2007;15(1):38–52.

Chapter 3
Epidemiology and Risk Factors

Qin Huang and Edward Lew

Introduction

Gastric cancer can be classified, according to anatomic sites, as cardia and non-cardia subtypes. Recent population-based worldwide epidemiology studies demonstrate considerable geographic variations in the incidence of gastric cancer, especially gastric cardiac carcinoma (Fig. 3.1) [1, 2]. High-quality data derived from cancer registries in Europe, North America, Japan, China, and many other Asian countries have shown a steady rising incidence of gastric cardiac carcinoma in East Asian populations, while the rate has plateaued or decreased in Caucasian populations. Risk factors for gastric cardiac carcinoma and the reasons for the increase in this fatal cancer in certain populations remain poorly understood, unlike that of distal gastric non-cardiac cancer, which is primarily associated with *H. pylori* infection with a worldwide decreasing trend. Moreover, there are also geographic and ethnic differences in the incidence of distal esophageal adenocarcinoma, which continues to increase in Caucasian populations but remains relatively uncommon in East Asian populations [1–11].

Q. Huang (✉)
Pathology and Laboratory Medicine, Veterans Affairs Boston Healthcare System,
West Roxbury, MA, USA

Harvard Medical School and Brigham and Women's Hospital,
Boston, MA, USA

E. Lew
Harvard Medical School, VA Boston Healthcare System and Brigham and Women's Hospital,
Boston, MA, USA
e-mail: Edward.Lew@va.gov

© Springer International Publishing AG, part of Springer Nature 2018
Q. Huang (ed.), *Gastric Cardiac Cancer*, https://doi.org/10.1007/978-3-319-79114-2_3

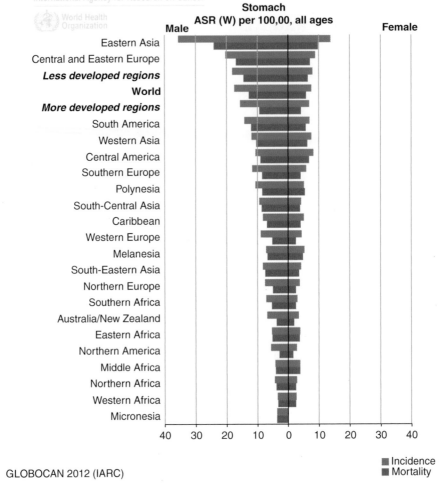

Fig. 3.1 The incidence of gastric cancer in the world [2]. Reproduced from http://globocan.iarc. fr. Accessed on 10/11/2017

Low or Decreasing Incidence in Caucasian Populations

Overall, gastric cancer is uncommon in the West and ranks 15th in frequency in the United States [3, 5–7, 12]. In a population-based epidemiology study from the US National Cancer Institute, the incidence of gastric cardiac cancer was 2.4 cases per 100,000 individuals in 1977–1981 and had slightly increased to 2.9 cases per 100,000 individuals in 2001–2006 among Caucasians [6]. However, the most recent data now show a low but stable incidence of 1.94 cases per 100,000 individuals between 2003 and 2008. Meanwhile, the data from the Surveillance, Epidemiology, and End Results (SEER) Program from 1973–2009 has similarly shown that the incidence of gastric cardiac cancer initially increased from 1.8% in 1978–1983 to 2.2% in 1996–2000, then decreased to 2.1%, and has since remained at a plateaued low level. In contrast, the incidence of esophageal adenocarcinoma has continually increased during this period and surpassed gastric cardiac cancer incidence in 1996 [5–7, 12]. In other Western countries with a predominant Caucasian population, gastric cardiac cancer incidence remains low and shows a decreasing incidence in the United Kingdom (using the data from the National Cancer Data Repository) from 5.7 per 100,000 in 1998 to 4.2 per 100,000 in 2007 in men, which is a decrease of more than 26% [13]. Similar trends have also been present in the Netherlands (National Cancer Registry) for both men and women [14] and in Central Switzerland in men [15]. In Norway, a population-based epidemiology report of the Norway Cancer Registry for the period between 1958 and 1992 showed that the incidence of gastric cardiac cancer remained relatively stable in men and somewhat decreased in women [16]. Remarkably, esophageal adenocarcinoma incidence is continuously rising in those countries. In Italy, the data from the Italian Association of Cancer Registries suggest a slight increase in gastric cardiac cancer incidence in both men and women over the period from 1986 to 1997, but the difference was statistically significant only for women [17]. The authors also acknowledged that "approximately 50% of the tumors were classified as unspecified or of overlapping origin" between esophageal adenocarcinoma and gastric cardiac cancer [17].

Rising Incidence in East Asian Populations

In contrast to Caucasian populations, the incidence of gastric cardiac cancer has been rising in East Asian populations. According to the International Agency for Research on Cancer, gastric cardiac cancer incidence in 1998–2002 among men varied from a high rate of 3.4 per 100,000 individuals in China and Belarus to 2.7 in the United States [4]. Remarkably, gastric cardiac cancer incidence in female patients worldwide is the highest (1.2 per 100,000 individuals) in China [4]. In China, gastric cancer is the third most common cancer, accounting for over 42% of gastric cancer cases in the world (Fig. 3.2), whereas in Europe, this cancer accounts for only 15% of the global burden [2, 3]. Epidemiology data from the cancer registry of the Cixian County in the Henan Province in China show an overall gastric cardiac cancer incidence of 25.6 per 100,000 in 1988–2003 [18], which is more than tenfold higher than that in the United States. In that county, gastric cardiac cancer incidence in 2003 significantly increased by 107% for men and 81% for women, compared to that in 1988 [18]. A similar rising gastric cardiac cancer incidence trend has also been reported by several recent single-center studies in Nanjing, China, [19] and also in Korea [20]. The data from the cancer registries of Singapore

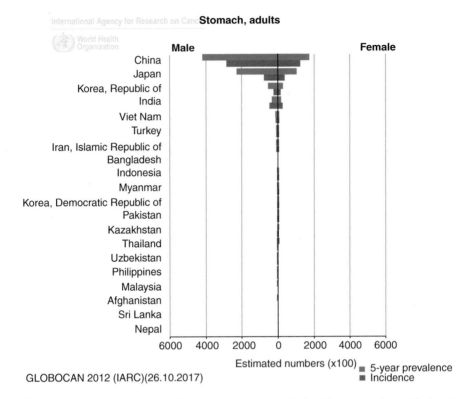

Fig. 3.2 Graph shows the estimated gastric cancer age-standardized 5-year prevalence (blue) and incidence (red) per 100,000 (reproduced from http://globocan.iarc.fr/) [2]

[21], the British Columbia of Canada (with a large East Asian population) [22], and Japan [23] recorded a parallel rising gastric cardiac cancer incidence trend by 20–207%. In Japan, the data from the Japanese National Cancer Registry over a 28-year period from 1963 to 1990 reveal a significant increase in gastric cardiac carcinoma incidence by 41.8% between 1963 and 1990 [23]. This increased gastric cardiac cancer incidence was found in another study only in Japanese men between 1975 and 1989 [24]. Unfortunately, the pathologic classification of gastric cardiac cancer is sometimes difficult to accurately distinguish it from distal esophageal adenocarcinoma. Although this can potentially lead to a falsely increased incidence of esophageal adenocarcinoma in the Caucasian population [25], the rising gastric cardiac cancer incidence data from East Asian countries, such as China, Korea, and Japan, are substantial because of the rarity of esophageal adenocarcinoma in those countries (Table 3.1) [8–11, 23, 26, 27].

The striking worldwide ethnic and geographic heterogeneity in gastric cardiac cancer incidence underscores fundamental differences in pathogenesis mechanisms between gastric cardiac cancer and esophageal adenocarcinoma in that "these two malignancies are separate entities …" [28].

Table 3.1 Differences in changes of prevalence of esophageal adenocarcinoma (EAC) and gastric cardiac carcinoma between the Western and East Asian countries

Country	Data source	Period	Change in EAC (%)	Change in GCC (%)	References
Western					
USA	SEER	1980–2010	600	Decreased by 15	[12]
UK	National	1998–2007	125	Decreased by 28	[13]
Netherlands	National	1990–2008	320	Decreased by 30	[14]
Central Switzerland	Regional	1986–2006	200	Decreased by 56	[15]
East Asian					
Japan	National	1963–1987	na	42	[23]
Japan	Regional	2008–2010	0	na	[11]
Singapore	National	1982–2005	na	319	[21]
Korea	Single center	2000–2005	na	120	[20]
Korea	Single center	1970–1999	Decreased by 22	na	[8]
China	Single center	2004–2011	0	90	[32]
Hong Kong	Regional	1984–2003	Decreased by 55	na	[9]

Note: *na* not available, *USA* United States of America, *UK* United Kingdom

Table 3.2 Comparison of possible risk factors among gastric cardiac carcinoma (GCC), esophageal adenocarcinoma (EAC), and distal gastric carcinoma (DGC)

Risk factor	GCC	EAC	DGC
Advancing age older than 50 years	++	+++	+
Male/female gender ratio	++	+++	+
Gastroesophageal reflux disease	+/−	++	0
Barrett's esophagus	+	+++	0
Obesity	+	++	0
Dietary factors	+	++	++
Environmental toxin/pollution	++	+	+
Tobacco use	++	++	++
Helicobacter pylori infection	+	0	+++
Predominant race	East Asians	Caucasian	East Asians
Family history of esophageal cancer	+	0	0

Note: 0, minimal/no effect; +, mild; ++, moderate; +++, severe

Aging, Male Gender, Environmental Toxins

Despite worldwide intense efforts to study risk factors for cancer in the gastro-esophageal junction region, the data are extremely limited, and no single definitive risk factor has been identified for gastric cardiac carcinoma. The cause is likely multifactorial, and the available scientific evidence highlights a few similarities and differences between gastric cardiac carcinoma, esophageal adenocarcinoma, and distal gastric carcinoma (Table 3.2).

Gastric cardiac carcinoma occurs primarily in elderly populations older than 50 years [14, 15, 24, 28–33]. A recent Chinese study on early gastric cardiac carcinoma patients fails to identify any patient younger than 40 years old [32]. However, compared to esophageal adenocarcinoma patients, the age of patients with gastric cardiac carcinoma is significantly younger [34, 35].

Similar to esophageal adenocarcinoma and distal gastric non-cardiac carcinoma, the male gender is a significant risk factor for the development of gastric cardiac carcinoma [31, 33, 35–37]. However, the male-to-female ratio in gastric cardiac carcinoma is much lower than that in esophageal adenocarcinoma, but higher than that in distal gastric non-cardiac carcinoma, and also varies among different ethnic populations [35, 37, 38]. For instance, the male-to-female ratio of gastric cardiac carcinoma in the United States [28], based on the SEER data, is about twice as higher as that in Korea [20, 39]. The overwhelming evidence indicates a predominance of esophageal adenocarcinoma, but not gastric cardiac carcinoma, in the elderly Caucasian male population [37, 40].

A number of environmental exposures to toxins may play a role in gastric cardiac carcinoma pathogenesis [37]. The most important is tobacco smoking, which is an established risk factor for esophageal adenocarcinoma and gastric cardiac and non-cardiac carcinomas. For example, a US population-based, case-control study revealed an odds ratio of 2.1 for smoking in risk of gastric cardiac carcinoma [41]. According to a meta-analysis of 42 eligible studies from the United States, Europe, and Asia [42], tobacco smoking has an odds ratio of 1.87-fold risk for gastric cardiac carcinoma in both men and women. This risk level is also dose dependent with an odds ratio of 2.0 for ever smokers and 4.1 for current smokers [43]. In the East, the risk odds ratio of gastric cardiac carcinoma for tobacco smoking varies from 5.38 in Koreans [31] to 1.56–1.94 in Chinese [44, 45]. In a Japanese study, tobacco smoking was found to be a significant risk factor for gastric cardiac carcinoma [29]. Other environmental toxins such as industrial pollutions have also been identified as an independent risk factor with an odds ratio of 2.31 for early gastric cardiac carcinoma in a Chinese patient population [32].

H. pylori has been declared as a definite carcinogen by the World Health Organization for gastric cancer, but primarily for distal gastric non-cardiac carcinoma, and not for gastric cardiac carcinoma, according to a meta-analysis of 12 prospective studies [46]. In a Chinese population, *H. pylori* infection remains prevalent (53%) in small (2 cm or less) gastric cardiac carcinoma but is significantly lower in frequency than that (74%) in distal gastric non-cardiac carcinoma [47]. In some studies, *H. pylori* was not found to be a risk factor for early gastric cardiac carcinoma [32], including a recent Korean study of gastric cardiac carcinoma [31].

At present, most studies suggest that consumption of alcoholic beverages is not a significant risk factor for gastric cardiac carcinoma [28, 32, 37], except for a recent Chinese population-based, case-control study carried out in the Linzhou region of the Henan Province with a large cohort of 470 gastric cardiac carcinoma cases, which shows an odds ratio of 2.36 for gastric cardiac carcinoma [44]. It is noteworthy that the common alcoholic beverage used by the residents in that particular region is frequently hard liquor with alcohol concentrations as high as 50%.

High intake of salty and preserved food and deficient fresh vegetables and fruit in diet are well-known risk factors for gastric cancer overall, but are not associated with gastric cardiac carcinoma [37, 48]. The results of a most recent single-center study on early gastric carcinoma in Chinese patients cannot confirm these dietary factors as independent risk factors for early gastric cardiac carcinoma ($n = 115$) [32]. Similarly, a population-based case-control study on risk factors of gastric cardiac carcinoma in the Linzhou region of the Henan Province in China failed to show that intake of salty foods affected the risk of gastric cardiac carcinoma [44].

Gastroesophageal Reflux Disease

Gastroesophageal reflux disease significantly increases the risk of development of esophageal adenocarcinoma [3] but is only weakly associated with gastric cardiac carcinoma [48]. In a seminal publication of a nationwide, population-based, case-control study in Sweden [49], Lagergren et al. revealed that up to 71% of gastric cardiac carcinoma patients did not have reflux symptoms; even in gastric cardiac carcinoma patients with reflux disease, the odds ratio for the risk (2.0) was much smaller than that (7.7) in esophageal adenocarcinoma. In patients with severe reflux disease, the odds ratio is also considerably smaller in gastric cardiac carcinoma (4.4) than in esophageal adenocarcinoma (43.5). Based on the study data, the authors established a probable causal relationship only between reflux disease and esophageal adenocarcinoma, but not gastric cardiac carcinoma [49]. In fact, reflux disease has not been found to be an independent risk factor for gastric cardiac carcinoma in Korean [31], Chinese [32], and Japanese [30] patients. The obvious racial disparity on roles of gastroesophageal reflux disease in pathogenesis of gastric cardiac carcinoma and esophageal adenocarcinoma has also been confirmed in studies from the United States [28, 48].

Obesity

Obesity has been shown to be a significant risk factor for gastric cardiac carcinoma in the Caucasian population in Europe and North America with an odds ratio of 1.5 in a meta-analysis of 14 studies with 2509 qualified cases [50], but the risk appears to be smaller in gastric cardiac carcinoma (1.46) than in esophageal adenocarcinoma (1.67), according to a nested case-control study carried out in the United Kingdom [51]. For gastric carcinoma, a meta-analysis of 16 qualified cases on risk of obesity shows a significant risk of 1.6-folds for gastric cardiac carcinoma [52]. A recent case-series study in China shows a similar finding with a risk odds ratio of 2.12 for early gastric cardiac carcinoma [32]. Furthermore, racial diversity on the risk of obesity in gastric cardiac carcinoma is exemplified by the conflicting findings of the higher prevalence of obesity among African Americans but with a much lower and stable incidence of both gastric cardiac carcinoma and esophageal adeno-carcinoma [38]. Based on the 13-year US 7-center Gastric Cancer Collaborative database, researchers also did not find obesity as a major characteristic of gastric cardiac carcinoma patients [33]. In a Japanese population, no significant differences in body mass index have been identified between gastric cardiac and non-cardiac carcinomas [29].

Insufficient Intake of Nutrients

Insufficient antioxidant intake has been suspected to increase the risk of gastric cardiac carcinoma and esophageal adenocarcinoma [37, 53, 54]. A recent meta-analysis with 16 qualified publications investigated the effects of vitamins A, C, and E, selenium, and beta-carotene on prevention of gastric cardiac carcinoma and esophageal adenocarcinoma. The authors reported that most antioxidants did have protective effects on esophageal adenocarcinoma, but not on gastric cardiac carcinoma, except beta-carotene [55]. In early gastric cardiac carcinoma patients, dietary habits with less vegetable/fruit intake were found not to be independent risk factors for this carcinoma [32].

Hereditary Risk Factors

Family history of esophageal squamous cell carcinoma has been recognized as a significant risk factor for gastric cardiac carcinoma. In a population-based, case-control study of newly diagnosed gastric cardiac carcinoma between 1992 and 1997 registered with the Los Angeles County Cancer Surveillance Program in the United States, researchers reported a strong association of gastric cardiac carcinoma ($n = 182$) with a family history of esophageal cancer with an odds ratio of 5.18 [56]. A similar Chinese study reported an odds ratio of 2.83 [44], which is slightly higher than that (1.75) reported in Japanese gastric cardiac carcinoma patients with a positive maternal, but not paternal, family history of gastric cancer [57]. However, a recent histopathology study of gastric carcinoma in 190 twins from the Henan Province in China reveals a very low and inconsistent prevalence in precancerous and cancerous diseases of the stomach [58], suggesting a predominant role of environmental, rather than hereditary, factors in the pathogenesis of gastric carcinoma.

Summary

In brief, most recent study results suggest, but do not conclude, several potential risk factors for gastric cardiac carcinoma, including advanced age, male gender, history of esophageal cancer, environmental toxins, and tobacco abuse, among others. The evidence is not strong, and those factors are only partially overlapped by those of esophageal adenocarcinoma, but not gastric non-cardiac carcinoma, suggesting different pathogenesis mechanisms for gastric cardiac carcinoma.

References

1. Torre LA, Bray F, Siegel RL, Ferlay J, Lortet-Tieulent J, Jemal A. Global cancer statistics, 2012. CA Cancer J Clin. 2015;65(2):87–108.
2. Ferlay J, Shin HR, Bray F, et al. GLOBOCAN 2008 v2.0, Cancer Incidence and Mortality Worldwide: IARC Cancer Base No. 10 [Online]. http://globocan.iarc.fr. Accessed on 11/18/2016.
3. Crew KD, Neugut AI. Epidemiology of upper gastrointestinal malignancy. Semin Oncol. 2004;31:450–64.
4. Chen W, Zheng R, Zhang S, et al. Report of incidence and mortality in China cancer registries, 2009. Chin J Cancer Res. 2013;25:10–21.
5. de Martel C, Forman D, Plummer M. Gastric cancer: epidemiology and risk factors. Gastroenterol Clin North Am. 2013;42:219–40.
6. National Cancer Institute. http://www.cancer.gov/types/stomach/hp/stomach-treatment-pdq#link/_163_toc. Accessed on 6/7/2015.
7. Wu H, Rusiecki JA, Zhu K, Potter J, Devesa SS. Stomach carcinoma incidence patterns in the United States by histologic type and anatomic site. Cancer Epidemiol Biomarkers Prev. 2009;18:1945–52.
8. Son JI, Park HJ, Song KS, et al. A single center's 30 years' experience of esophageal adeno-carcinoma. Korean J Intern Med. 2001;16:250–3.
9. Yee YK, Cheung TK, Chan AO, Yuen MF, Wong BC. Decreasing trend of esophageal adeno-carcinoma in Hong Kong. Cancer Epidemiol Biomarkers Prev. 2007;16:2637–40.
10. Fang WL, Wu CW, Chen JH, et al. Esophagogastric junction adenocarcinoma according to Siewert classification in Taiwan. Ann Surg Oncol. 2009;16:3237–44.
11. Matsueda K, Manabe N, Sato Y, et al. Adenocarcinoma of the esophagogastric junction is still low in Japan—multicenter epidemiological study in Kurashiki, Japan. Gastroenterology. 2015;148(4 Suppl 1):S-764.
12. Dubecz A, Solymosi N, Stadlhuber RJ, Schweigert M, Stein HJ, Peters JH. Does the incidence of adenocarcinoma of the esophagus and gastric cardia continue to rise in the twenty-first century?—a SEER database analysis. J Gastrointest Surg. 2014;18:124–9.
13. Coupland VH, Lagergren J, Konfortion J, et al. Ethnicity in relation to incidence of oesopha-geal and gastric cancer in England. Br J Cancer. 2012;107:1908–14.
14. Dikken JL, Lemmens VE, Wouters MW, et al. Increased incidence and survival for oesophageal cancer but not for gastric cardia cancer in the Netherlands. Eur J Cancer. 2012;48:1624–32.
15. Schmassmann A, Oldendorf MG, Gebbers JO. Changing incidence of gastric and oesoph-ageal cancer subtypes in central Switzerland between 1982 and 2007. Eur J Epidemiol. 2009;24:603–9.
16. Hansen S, Wiig JN, Giercksky KE, Tretli S. Esophageal and gastric carcinoma in Norway 1958-1992: incidence time trend variability according to morphological subtypes and organ subsites. Int J Cancer. 1997;71:340–4.
17. Orengo MA, Casella C, Fontana V, et al. Trends in incidence rates of oesophagus and gas-tric cancer in Italy by subsite and histology, 1986-1997. Eur J Gastroenterol Hepatol. 2006;18:739–46.
18. He YT, Hou J, Chen ZF, et al. Trends in incidence of esophageal and gastric cardia cancer in high-risk areas in China. Eur J Cancer Prev. 2008;17:71–6.
19. Shi J, Sun Q, Xu BY, et al. Changing trends in proportions of small (≤ 2 cm) proximal and non-proximal gastric carcinomas treated at a high-volume tertiary medical center in China. J Dig Dis. 2014;15:359–66.

20. Park JC, Lee YC, Kim JH, et al. Clinicopathological features and prognostic factors of proximal gastric carcinoma in a population with high Helicobacter pylori prevalence: a single-center, large-volume study in Korea. Ann Surg Oncol. 2010;17:829–37.
21. Deans C, Yeo MS, Soe MY, Shabbir A, Ti TK, So JB. Cancer of the gastric cardia is rising in incidence in an Asian population and is associated with adverse outcome. World J Surg. 2011;35:617–24.
22. Bashash M, Shah A, Hislop G, Brooks-Wilson A, Le N, Bajdik C. Incidence and survival for gastric and esophageal cancer diagnosed in British Columbia, 1990 to 1999. Can J Gastroenterol. 2008;22:143–8.
23. Blaser MJ, Saito D. Trends in reported adenocarcinomas of the oesophagus and gastric cardia in Japan. Eur J Gastroenterol Hepatol. 2002;14:107–13.
24. Liu Y, Kaneko S, Sobue T. Trends in reported incidences of gastric cancer by tumour location, from 1975 to 1989 in Japan. Int J Epidemiol. 2004;33:808–15.
25. Ekström AM, Signorello LB, Hansson LE, et al. Evaluating gastric cancer misclassification: a potential explanation for the rise in cardia cancer incidence. J Natl Cancer Inst. 1999;91:786–90.
26. Huang Q, Shi J, Sun Q, et al. Distal esophageal carcinomas in Chinese patients vary widely in histopathology, but adenocarcinomas remain rare. Hum Pathol. 2012;43:2138–48.
27. Suh YS, Han DS, Kong SH, et al. Should adenocarcinoma of the esophagogastric junction be classified as esophageal cancer? A comparative analysis according to the seventh AJCC TNM classification. Ann Surg. 2012;255(5):908–15.
28. El-Serag HB, Mason AC, Petersen N, Key CR. Epidemiological differences between adenocarcinoma of the oesophagus and adenocarcinoma of the gastric cardia in the USA. Gut. 2002;50:368–72.
29. Maeda H, Okabayashi T, Nishimori I, et al. Clinicopathologic features of adenocarcinoma at the gastric cardia: is it different from distal cancer of the stomach? J Am Coll Surg. 2008;206:306–10.
30. Okabayashi T, Gotoda T, Kondo H, et al. Early carcinoma of the gastric cardia in Japan: is it different from that in the West? Cancer. 2000;89:2555–9.
31. Kim JY, Lee HS, Kim N, et al. Prevalence and clinicopathologic characteristics of gastric cardia cancer in South Korea. Helicobacter. 2012;17:358–68.
32. Fang C, Lu L, Shi J, et al. Risk factors of early proximal gastric carcinoma in Chinese diagnosed with the WHO criteria. J Dig Dis. 2015;16:327–36.
33. Amini N, Spolverato G, Kim Y, et al. Clinicopathological features and prognosis of gastric cardia adenocarcinoma: a multi-institutional US study. J Surg Oncol. 2015;111:285–92.
34. Huang Q, Fan XS, Agoston AT, et al. Comparison of gastroesophageal junction carcinomas in Chinese versus American patients. Histopathology. 2011;59:188–97.
35. Carneiro F, Moutinho C, Pera G, et al. Pathology findings and validation of gastric and esophageal cancer cases in a European cohort (EPIC/EUR-GAST). Scand J Gastroenterol. 2007;42:618–27.
36. Bytzer P, Christensen PB, Damkier P, Vinding K, Seersholm N. Adenocarcinoma of the esophagus and Barrett's esophagus: a population-based study. Am J Gastroenterol. 1999;94:86–91.
37. Crew KD, Neugut AI. Epidemiology of gastric cancer. World J Gastroenterol. 2006;12:354–62.
38. Kubo A, Corley DA. Marked multi-ethnic variation of esophageal and gastric cardia carcinomas within the United States. Am J Gastroenterol. 2004;99:582–8.
39. Shim JH, Song KY, Jeon HM, et al. Is gastric cancer different in Korea and the United States? Impact of tumor location on prognosis. Ann Surg Oncol. 2014;21:2332–9.
40. Rogers EL, Goldkind SF, Iseri OA, et al. Adenocarcinoma of the lower esophagus. A disease primarily of white men with Barrett's esophagus. J Clin Gastroenterol. 1986;8:613–8.
41. Wu AH, Wan P, Bernstein L. A multiethnic population-based study of smoking, alcohol and body size and risk of adenocarcinomas of the stomach and esophagus (United States). Cancer Causes Control. 2001;12:721–32.

42. Ladeiras-Lopes R, Pereira AK, Nogueira A, et al. Smoking and gastric cancer: systematic review and meta-analysis of cohort studies. Cancer Causes Control. 2008;19:689–701.
43. González CA, Pera G, Agudo A, et al. Smoking and the risk of gastric cancer in the European Prospective Investigation Into Cancer and Nutrition (EPIC). Int J Cancer. 2003;107:629–34.
44. Sun CQ, Chang YB, Cui LL, et al. A population-based case-control study on risk factors for gastric cardia cancer in rural areas of Linzhou. Asian Pac J Cancer Prev. 2013;14:2897–901.
45. Tong GX, Liang H, Chai J, et al. Association of risk of gastric cancer and consumption of tobacco, alcohol and tea in the Chinese population. Asian Pac J Cancer Prev. 2014;15:8765–74.
46. Helicobacter and Cancer Collaborative Group. Gastric cancer and Helicobacter pylori: a combined analysis of 12 case control studies nested within prospective cohorts. Gut. 2001;49:347–53.
47. Huang Q, Shi J, Sun Q, et al. Clinicopathologic characterization of small (≤ 2 cm) proximal and distal gastric carcinomas in a Chinese population. Pathology. 2015;47(6):526–32.
48. Carr JS, Zafar SF, Saba N, Khuri FR, El-Rayes BF. Risk factors for rising incidence of esophageal and gastric cardia adenocarcinoma. J Gastrointest Cancer. 2013;44:143–51.
49. Lagergren J, Bergstrom R, Lindgren A, Nyrén O. Symptomatic gastroesophageal reflux as a risk factor for esophageal adenocarcinoma. N Engl J Med. 1999;340:825–31.
50. Nguyen TH, Thrift AP, Ramsey D, et al. Risk factors for Barrett's esophagus compared between African Americans and non-Hispanic Whites. Am J Gastroenterol. 2014;109:1870–80.
51. Kubo A, Corley DA. Body mass index and adenocarcinomas of the esophagus or gastric cardia: a systematic review and meta-analysis. Cancer Epidemiol Biomarkers Prev. 2006;15:872–8.
52. Lindblad M, Rodriguez LA, Lagergren J. Body mass, tobacco and alcohol and risk of esophageal, gastric cardia, and gastric non-cardia adenocarcinoma among men and women in a nested case-control study. Cancer Causes Control. 2005;16:285–94.
53. Lin XJ, Wang CP, Liu XD, et al. Body mass index and risk of gastric cancer: a meta-analysis. Jpn J Clin Oncol. 2014;44(9):783–91.
54. Guggenheim DE, Shah MA. Gastric cancer epidemiology and risk factors. J Surg Oncol. 2013;107:230–6.
55. Kubo A, Corley DA. Meta-analysis of antioxidant intake and the risk of esophageal and gastric cardia adenocarcinoma. Am J Gastroenterol. 2007;102:2323–30.
56. Jiang X, Tseng CC, Bernstein L, Wu AH. Family history of cancer and gastroesophageal disorders and risk of esophageal and gastric adenocarcinomas: a case-control study. BMC Cancer. 2014;14:60.
57. Inoue M, Tajima K, Yamamura Y, et al. Family history and subsite of gastric cancer: data from a case-referent study in Japan. Int J Cancer. 1998;76:801–5.
58. Chen J, Li XM, Zhou FY, et al. Comparative analysis on histopathological changes at gastric body and antrum of monozygotic and dizygotic twins from esophageal and cardiac cancer high-incidence area in Henan. J Zhengzhou Univ (Med Sci). 2012;47:619–21. (In Chinese).

Chapter 4
Natural History

Qin Huang and Lily Huang

Natural History

If left untreated, early gastric carcinoma will progress, metastasize, and become invasive, advanced, and fatal. Although published studies on the natural history of gastric cancer, particularly gastric cardiac carcinoma, remain scarce, almost all studies demonstrate a slow-progressive process with a 5-year survival rate higher than 60% for patients with early gastric carcinoma.

In 2000, Tsukuma et al. reported the long-term outcome of 38 Japanese patients in Osaka, who were diagnosed with early gastric cancer before 1988. Their tumors were not immediately resected because of advanced age, poor health, or patient refusal [1]. During the follow-up period (mean: 6 years; range: 1.1–17.2), 2 (5.3%) were lost to follow-up, 1 (2.6%) remained alive, 3 (7.9%) deceased with unknown diseases, 9 (23.7%) passed away with other known diseases, and 23 (60.5%) died of gastric carcinoma. Therefore, the censored and corrected 5-year natural survival rate was 67.8% [1]. Of note, the site of cancer and demographic data were not provided in that report. The diagnostic criteria might not be the same as those of the World Health Organization. A recent case report also from Japan illustrates a very slow natural history for early gastric cardiac carcinoma. The patient was an 87-year-old Japanese man who presented with a superficial early gastric cardiac carcinoma in 1999, which could not be resected because of his advanced heart disease [2]. This

Q. Huang
Pathology and Laboratory Medicine, Veterans Affairs Boston Healthcare System,
West Roxbury, MA, USA

Harvard Medical School and Brigham and Women's Hospital,
Boston, MA, USA

L. Huang (✉)
Beth Israel Deaconess Medical Center, Boston, MA, USA

© Springer International Publishing AG, part of Springer Nature 2018
Q. Huang (ed.), *Gastric Cardiac Cancer*, https://doi.org/10.1007/978-3-319-79114-2_4

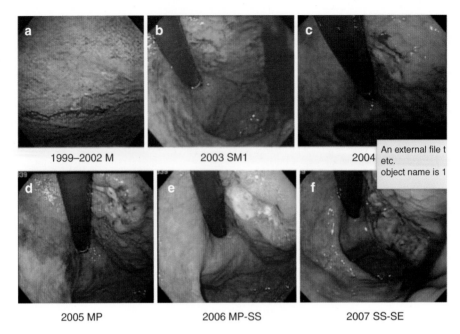

1999–2002 M   2003 SM1   2004

An external file t
etc.
object name is 1

2005 MP   2006 MP-SS   2007 SS-SE

Fig. 4.1 Natural history of gastric cardiac carcinoma diagnosed in 1999 at the intramucosal stage (M) in this 87-year-old Japanese man with severe heart disease. Over the 7-year endoscopic follow-up period, the tumor infiltrated gradually from the intramucosal stage (M) to the superficial (SM1)/deep (SM2) submucosal layer, to the muscularis propria (MP) in 2005, then to the subserosal layer (SS) in 2006, and beyond in 2007. Copyright © 2012, the Author(s) [2]. This is an open-access article distributed under the terms of the Creative Commons Attribution License, which permits unrestricted use, distribution, and reproduction in any medium, provided the original work is properly cited

patient was, therefore, followed up semiannually with upper endoscopy, and the tumor was found to progress slowly into deeply invasive carcinoma with the maximum size of 6 cm over the 7-year period. This patient eventually died of congestive heart failure, but not gastric cardiac carcinoma (Fig. 4.1).

Based on the endoscopic findings, the authors estimated the tumor progressed through the initial intramucosal phase over 4 years. Time to invasion into the deep gastric wall was 3 additional years [2].

Gastric cardiac carcinoma is uncommon in Japan but much more frequently diagnosed in China. Two small case-series studies published by Chinese investigators in patients from the high-risk regions of Henan Province have documented an unusually slow progression and insidious clinical presentation of this cancer. These patients were diagnosed with early gastric cardiac carcinoma by cytology and/or upper endoscopy by medical specialists from the Tumor Hospital of the Chinese Academy of Medical Sciences. All patients refused surgical treatment or chemoradiation therapy for a variety of reasons but agreed to be followed up endoscopically and roentgenologically. In the first report, published in 1988, investigators followed

Table 4.1 Natural history of early gastric cardiac carcinoma

Stage (pT)	Estimated time (year)	References
Intramucosal (pT0)	2–6	[2–4]
Superficial submucosal (SM1, pT1)	1–2	[2]
Deep submucosal (SM2, pT1)	1	[2]
Muscularis propria (MP, pT2)	1	[2]
Subserosa (pT3)	<1	[2]

21 early gastric cardiac carcinoma cases discovered at mass screenings for up to 6.5 years after diagnosis [3]. At the last follow-up, 8 (38.1%) patients remained alive with a stable superficial tumor, 6 (28.6%) cases progressed to advanced cancer, 2 (9.5%) patients died of other diseases, and 11 (40.7%) died of gastric cardiac carcinoma with an average survival of 4.4 years after the initial diagnosis. A Kaplan-Meier plot showed the likelihood of survival over 5 years to be 61.5% [3], which is slightly lower than that (62.8%) described in a Japanese series of 38 early gastric cancer cases [1]. The authors estimated the time to progression from intramucosal carcinoma to advanced gastric cardiac carcinoma was about 4–5 years [3]. In the second Chinese case-series report, the investigators described 17 untreated early gastric cardiac carcinoma cases, also discovered by the mass screening campaign. The average age of early gastric cardiac carcinoma patients was 61.5 years (range: 49–73) with a male/female ratio of 1.1. During the 14-year follow-up, 12 (70.6%) died of gastric cardiac carcinoma and 5 (29.4%) died of non-cancerous diseases. The Kaplan-Meier plot predicted an average survival of 7.1 years (range: 3–14 years). The overall natural survival rate was 76.5% at 5 years and 23.5% at 10 years after the index tissue diagnosis [4].

As summarized in Table 4.1, while observed only in Chinese and Japanese patients in small numbers, the natural history of gastric cardiac carcinoma appears to be slowly progressing with 5-year survival rates over 60%, which is much higher than that of esophageal adenocarcinoma.

Summary

The findings on natural history of early gastric cardiac carcinoma presented in the aforementioned reports, although small in number, are very important in at least three aspects:

1. Published studies on the natural history of early gastric cardiac carcinoma are exceedingly rare, and repeating these studies in the future will be extremely difficult due to the widespread use of upper endoscopy to detect and resect early gastric cardiac carcinoma.
2. The data on natural history of early gastric cardiac carcinoma may be useful to guide clinicians on how to optimally manage patients. As presented in the previous chapter, gastric cardiac carcinoma is primarily a disease of elderly

populations. At the time of diagnosis, the overall health and advanced age of those patients may not allow for major invasive endoscopic/surgical resection procedures. However, without any treatment, these elderly patients may die from something other than cancer. Parallels can be drawn with well-differentiated low-grade papillary thyroid carcinoma, breast ductal carcinoma in situ, uterine cervix squamous cell carcinoma in situ, skin melanoma in situ, prostate gland Gleason 3 Group 1 adenocarcinoma, etc. At present, an overwhelming body of evidence suggests that early cancers take a longer time to progress in a high proportion of cases. Thus, the best clinical management strategy should be tailored to the condition of individual patients.

3. The direction of translational research may need to focus on identifying risk factors that cause early gastric cardiac carcinoma to progress from an intramucosal disease to a submucosal carcinoma. The results acquired from this line of investigation may help develop effective and efficient strategies to prevent disease progression.

References

1. Tsukuma H, Oshima A, Narahara H, Morii T. Natural history of early gastric cancer: a non-concurrent long term follow up study. Gut. 2000;47:618–21.
2. Fujisaki J, Nakajima T, Hirasawa T, et al. Natural history of gastric cancer—a case followed up for eight years: early to advanced gastric cancer. Clin J Gastroenterol. 2012;5:351–4.
3. Guanrei Y, Songliang Q, He H, Guizen F. Natural history of earsly esophageal squamous carcinoma and early adenocarcinoma of the gastric cardia in the People's Republic of China. Endoscopy. 1988;20:95–8.
4. Wang GQ, Wei WQ, Zhang JH. Natural progression of early stage adenocarcinoma of gastric cardia: a report of seventeen cases. Ai Zheng. 2007;26:1153–6. (In Chinese).

Chapter 5
Clinical Molecular Pathology

Xiangshan Fan and Qin Huang

Introduction

Gastric cardiac carcinoma (GCC) exhibits a wide histopathologic spectrum and heterogeneous post-resection patient survival characteristics [1]. The inter- and intra-patient heterogeneity of GCC histopathology is well known, including tubular and papillary adenocarcinomas, poorly cohesive carcinoma, mucinous, adenosquamous, neuroendocrine carcinomas, pancreatic acinar-like adenocarcinoma, hepatoid and alpha-fetoprotein-producing adenocarcinoma, carcinoma with lymphoid stroma, and many rare entities, although tubular adenocarcinoma remains most common in the gastric cardia, accounting for about 60–80% [1–9].

Despite significant improvements in surgical resections and systemic chemotherapy over the past three decades, the prognosis of patients with advanced GCC remains poor, partially due to poor understanding of GCC molecular tumorigenesis mechanisms. However, epidemiology and pathology study results have uncovered a few key characteristics of GCC, such as differences from distal non-cardiac gastric carcinoma (DGC), high risk in the elderly population, association with a history of esophageal squamous cell carcinoma, Epstein-Barr virus (EBV) infection, and genetic mutations with significant clinical implications, such as HER2 (human epidermal growth factor receptor 2) gene overexpression and amplification. In this

X. Fan (✉)
Department of Pathology, The Affiliated Drum Tower Hospital, Nanjing University Medical School, Nanjing, Jiangsu, People's Republic of China

Q. Huang
Pathology and Laboratory Medicine, Veterans Affairs Boston Healthcare System, West Roxbury, MA, USA

Harvard Medical School and Brigham and Women's Hospital, Boston, MA, USA

© Springer International Publishing AG, part of Springer Nature 2018
Q. Huang (ed.), *Gastric Cardiac Cancer*, https://doi.org/10.1007/978-3-319-79114-2_5

chapter, we will present the latest, most important information on molecular pathology of GCC with a focus on clinical relevance and practical applications in clinical practice.

Genetic and Genomic Profiles

Early studies on molecular pathology of GCC were difficult because most tumors were large and the esophagogastric junction (EGJ) line was frequently obliterated, making a confident exclusion of distal esophageal adenocarcinoma (EAC) almost impossible. To avoid that problem, Taniere et al. [10] applied strict histopathologic diagnostic criteria on GCC and compared differences on expression of p53, MDM2, CK7, and CK13 genes between GCC and EAC. They reported significantly different expression characteristics in those genes, while others showed the molecular evidence drastically similar between those two carcinomas [11]. With the cDNA gene chip technique, Shah et al. [12] compared gene expression in 36 localized gastric carcinoma biopsies among 3 histopathologic subtypes: GCC non-diffuse ($n = 12$), DGC non-diffuse ($n = 14$), and diffuse ($n = 10$) carcinoma. Although gene expression overlapped to some extent among three subtypes of carcinomas and normal controls, significantly distinct genetic profiles of GCC were identified with up-expression in three genes (prostate stem cell antigen, pepsinogen A3 genes, and TRIM32) and down-expression in four genes (MLSN, IGL, ENPP4, and PLA2G2A), supporting the classification of gastric carcinoma into GCC non-diffuse, DGC non-diffuse, and diffuse subtypes.

In a comprehensive systematic study, Mocellin et al. performed 456 primary and subgroup meta-analyses on 156 variants of gastric cancer-related genes and identified 11 variants that were significantly associated with increased risk of gastric cancers [13]. Among 11 specific genetic polymorphisms in 10 genes, 2 were significantly associated with increased risk of gastric cancer in Asians (TGFBR2 rs3087465 at 3p22 and GSTP1 rs1695 at 11q13), 1 with GCC (PLCE1 rs2274223 at 10q23), and 2 with DGC (PSCA rs2294008 at 8q24.2 and PRKAA1 rs13361707 at 5p13). The GCC-related specific high-risk gene, PLCE1 (phospholipase C epsilon 1), plays an important role in cell growth, differentiation, and tumorigenesis. Further meta-analysis of PLCE1 rs2274223 in 22 qualified studies with 13,188 patients and 14,666 controls revealed that this polymorphism was significantly associated with an increased risk of esophageal squamous cell carcinoma [14]. This finding is in line with the observations of over twofold increased risks of GCC in patients with the family history of esophageal squamous cell carcinoma in both American and Chinese patients [15, 16]. Those high-quality data clearly establish the fact for GCC as a distinct subgroup of gastric cancers.

As part of The Cancer Genome Atlas Project of the US National Cancer Institute [17], investigators characterized genomic abnormalities of 295 gastric adenocarcinomas with 6 molecular platforms, based on which they subclassified gastric adenocarcinomas into 4 molecular subtypes with the chromosomal instability subtype primarily (65%) in GCC and 3 other subtypes, i.e., microsatellite instable (MSI), genomic stable, and Epstein-Barr virus (EBV) infection-related. In GCC, chromosomal instable-subtype adenocarcinoma was most common and characterized by histopathologic intestinal differentiation, TP53 mutation, and RTK-RAS activation. In addition, EBV infection-related tumors were also predominant in GCC and exhibited unique molecular signatures, such as PIK3CA mutation, PD-L1/2 overexpression, EBV-CIMP hypermethylation, CDKN2A epigenetic silencing, etc. MSI-related gastric adenocarcinomas were most common in DGC in elderly patients but infrequent in GCC. Genomic stable adenocarcinomas showed primarily diffuse histology features, as seen in poorly cohesive carcinoma, including signet-ring cell carcinoma, most commonly in young women. This subtype was also uncommon in GCC. The findings are in keeping with the histopathology study results of GCC, in which poorly cohesive carcinoma including signet-ring cell carcinoma is indeed significantly uncommon in GCC [2, 5, 18]. In general, MSI subtype has the best overall prognosis, followed by EBV-related, TP53-positive, and TP53-negative subtypes with genomic stable subtype being the worst.

The study results on genomic alterations in GCC have been confirmed and expanded by the same group of investigators in a comprehensive integrated genomic analysis of esophageal carcinomas [19]. The investigators analyzed and compared genomic alteration signatures between esophageal squamous cell carcinoma ($N = 92$) and EAC ($N = 72$), as well as between EAC and gastric adenocarcinoma. In this landmark paper, squamous cell carcinoma of the esophagus was shown to have genomic alteration patterns similar to its counterpart in the head-neck region but distinctly different from EAC that exhibited chromosomal instability in almost all (98.6%, 71/72) EAC cases. As shown in the 2014 paper on genomic profiles of 295 gastric adenocarcinomas [17], chromosomal instability is the major common feature between gastric adenocarcinoma (50%) and EAC (98.6%). Further analysis discovered a progressively enriched gradient for chromosomal instability from the lowest proportion in the most distal pylorus (antrum) to the high level in the proximal gastric cardia and to the peak in EAC [19]. Similarly, DNA hypermethylation changes in the genome followed the similar progressive enrichment fashion from DGC, to GCC, and to EAC at the highest. There was no clear demarcation in those genomic alterations among those three groups of adenocarcinomas. In contrast, EBV infection-related and MSI gastric adenocarcinomas were not found in EAC but common in GCC/EGJ carcinoma (Table 5.1) [19].

Table 5.1 Comparison of genomic features among esophageal and gastric adenocarcinomas [17, 19]

Subtype	Esophageal adenocarcinoma	Gastric cardiac/EGJ adenocarcinoma	Gastric non-cardiac adenocarcinoma
Chromosomal instability	98.6% (71/72)	84.8% (140/165)	47.6% (141/296)
Epstein-Barr virus-related	0	9.5% (6/63)	8.1% (24/296)
Microsatellite instable	0	7.1% (7/99)	24% (71/296)
Genomic stable	1.4% (1/72)	6.7% (11/165)	20.3% (60/296)

Since almost all EAC tumors exhibit chromosomal instable features similar to the chromosomal instable-subtype gastric adenocarcinoma, EAC and the chromosomal instable-subtype gastric adenocarcinoma should be grouped as a single disease entity [19]. In this 2017 seminal paper [19], EAC showed a distinct molecular profile drastically different from esophageal squamous cell carcinoma. Since the vast majority (88.9%, 64/72) of EAC tumors were actually located on the esophageal side of the EGJ region and thus classified by the study investigators as the GEJ/GCC adenocarcinomas, only seven tumors (11.1%, 7/72) were genuine EACs located in the distal esophagus. The single EAC tumor with genomic stable features was actually a GEJ (GCC) tumor, and none of the seven true EAC tumors demonstrated genomic stable characteristics that are the primary molecular features of signet-ring cell carcinoma. These results are in keeping with the reported observational findings on the absence of signet-ring cell carcinoma in the distal esophagus [18]. This game-changing paper should have profound impact on tumor classification, biomarker investigation, patient management, and design of clinical trials on the following major issues.

First, squamous cell carcinoma of the esophagus in the West Caucasian population is reestablished as the primary carcinoma in the esophagus with the molecular signatures similar to its equivalent in the head-neck region. This would unify the worldwide study data that the vast majority of esophageal cancer is indeed squamous cell carcinoma.

Second, genuine EAC tumors are rare in the distal esophagus, since most EAC tumors arise in the GEJ/gastric cardiac region (Fig. 5.1) and almost all EAC tumors share the same molecular signatures of chromosomal instable-subtype gastric adenocarcinoma. In that molecular term, EAC and chromosomal instable-subtype gastric adenocarcinoma belong to the same molecular disease entity.

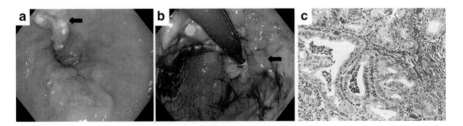

Fig. 5.1 Gastric cardiac adenocarcinoma involves the distal esophagus (**a**) in a 59-year-old previously healthy man with recent complaints of dysphagia and 10-pound body weight loss but without a history of gastroesophageal reflux disease. At upper endoscopy, the tumor extends from the gastric cardia proximally to the distal esophagus up to 37 cm from the incisors as irregularly elevated lesions (arrows in **a**). Note the characteristic absence of columnar-lined metaplastic lesions in the surrounding distal esophageal mucosal surface. With retroflex view in (**b**), the tumor is partially circumferential at the esophagogastric junction with the epicenter in the gastric cardia and spreads distally up to 45 cm from the incisor (arrow in **b**). The biopsy histology of the tumor demonstrated the features for an invasive tubular adenocarcinoma with clear cell features (**c**). The adjacent gastric cardiac mucolytic mucosa exhibited mild chronic inflammation with focal intestinal metaplasia but no evidence of *Helicobacter pylori* infection (not shown here)

Third, chromosomal instable-subtype gastric adenocarcinoma demonstrates a gradual regional crescendo gradient from the lowest proportion in the distal pylorus-antral region to the high level in the proximal gastric cardia and to the peak in EAC on the esophageal side of the GEJ region. Therefore, EAC tumors may arise in the gastric cardia/EGJ region and are actually the proximal extension of chromosomal instable-subtype gastric adenocarcinoma from the gastric cardia/GEJ to the distal esophagus with Barrett's esophagus as its precursor premalignant lesion.

Fourth, GCC/GEJ carcinoma is much more heterogeneous than EAC with all four molecular subtypes of gastric adenocarcinomas and many uncommon histopathology variants. Therefore, EAC on the esophageal side of the EGJ is not the same as, but a part of, the GCC spectrum. The molecular pathogenesis mechanism of GCC would be much more complicated than both EAC and DGC because of extreme heterogeneity.

Described in this 2017 landmark paper were considerable similarities and differences in genetic alterations among chromosomal instable adenocarcinomas in the distal esophageal (EAC), gastric cardia/EGJ (GCC) region, and gastric non-cardiac (DGC) regions in the following key molecular pathways [19]: (1) the Wnt/beta-catenin pathway, (2) genes such as FHIT or WWOX for genomic instability, (3) oncogenes such as VEGFA and MYC, (4) tumor suppressor genes such as SMAD4, and (5) epigenetic silencing genes, such as CDKN2A (Table 5.2) [19].

In contrast, DNA hypermethylation of adenocarcinoma with chromosomal instability disproportionally occurred in EAC, compared to that in gastric chromosomal

Table 5.2 Comparison of genetic alterations (%) among esophageal and gastric adenocarcinomas with chromosomal instability [17, 19]

Pathway/gene	Distal esophageal region	Gastric cardiac/EGJ region	Gastric non-cardiac region
Wnt/β-catenin pathway			
APC	6	11.5	18.5
SMARCA4	10	5	3.5
RUNX1	18	2	1.5
Tumor suppressor gene			
SMAD2	24	20	19.5
Oncogene			
MYC	31	25	22.5
VEGFA	30	17	11.5
Epigenetic silencing			
CDKN2A	48	32	5.5
Stem cell			
CD44	3	5	9.5
Genome instability			
FHIT	80	49	38
WWOX	77	47	35.5

instable adenocarcinoma. As shown in The Cancer Genome Atlas of Esophageal Carcinomas, DNA hypermethylation in cluster 1 or 2 was significantly more frequent in EAC, compared to that in gastric adenocarcinoma; on the other hand, the lowest frequency of DNA hypermethylation in cluster 4 was found in DGC, but not in EAC. These results suggest the existence of some molecular differences between DGC and EAC [19].

Asian populations are well known to be at high risk for gastric carcinoma development. Based on the database of The Cancer Genome Atlas of Gastric Carcinoma and other published gastric cancer sequencing data ($N = 473$), Jia et al. further analyzed and compared the somatic mutation rates of several driver genes responsible for gastric cancer between Asian and Caucasian patient populations [20]. They discovered significant differences in frequency of somatic mutations in five driver genes in gastric cancer patients between Asian and Caucasian descent: (1) APC (6.06% for Asian versus 14.4% for Caucasian, $p < 0.01$), (2) ARIDIA (20.7% versus 32.1%, $p = 0.01$), (3) KMT2A (4.04% versus 12.35%, $p < 0.01$), (4) PIK3CA (9.6% versus 18.52%, $p = 0.01$), and (5) PTEN (2.52% versus 9.05%, $p < 0.01$) [20]. Although the authors did not disclose the data on GCC, differences in the somatic gene mutation patterns in all gastric cancer tumors between those two ethnic populations may offer better opportunities for targeted drug development and therapy.

HER2 Gene Aberrant Expression

The discovery of similar chromosomal instable genomic profiles in both EAC and GCC tumors as one disease entity is also supported by similarly increased HER2 gene expression and amplification with the breakthrough precision HER2 target therapy for gastric and GCC/EGJ adenocarcinomas for the first time [21]. HER2 is a member of the epidermal growth factor receptor (EGFR) family of tyrosine kinases that are involved in tumor proliferation, apoptosis, adhesion, migration, differentiation, and survival. HER2 has been shown to be overexpressed through HER2 gene amplification in 32% of EACs [19] and 6–35% of gastric adenocarcinomas [21–24]. In the landmark ToGA clinical trial on trastuzumab against HER2 in gastric cancer target therapy in 2010 [21], HER2 overexpression/amplification was identified in a relatively greater proportion (32.2%) of GCC/EGJ tumors, compared with DGC tumors (21.4%) [25]. Most recently in a large, multinational HER-EAGLE study with a total of 4949 gastric cancer patients, investigators reported that 14.2% of 4920 tumor samples were HER2-positive by immunohistochemistry, in which HER2 expression in EGJ/GCC tumors was again found to be significantly higher (22.1%) than that (12.9%) of DGC tumors [26]. For gastric adenocarcinomas in the Lauren classification, HER2 overexpression in GCC/EGJ and DGC tumors has been found significantly higher in intestinal (89%) than in diffuse (11%) or mixed (0%) types of gastric cancers [27]. The data from almost all high-quality studies suggest that the intestinal-type GCC/DGC adenocarcinoma with well-moderate differentiation predicts HER2 immunopositivity, in contrast to signet-ring cell carcinoma and poorly differentiated adenocarcinoma with a minimum or absence of HER2 expression/amplification. In GCC and associated intestinal metaplasia, HER2 expression is also associated with a high frequency of Das-1 and Ki67-positive staining [28]. Interestingly, gene amplification or protein expression of EGFR, which is a molecule related to HER2, is also relatively common in intestinal-type adenocarcinomas of DGC, GCC, and EAC and reported to be positive in 72/220 (32.7%) tumors by immunohistochemistry and in 31/220 (14.1%) by in situ hybridization. The cases with high EGFR expression or amplification were associated with significantly decreased survival [29]. Because EGFR gene amplification is rarely concurrent with HER2 gene amplification, anti-EGFR therapies might be applicable to some patients who are not eligible for anti-HER2 treatment.

As the dramatic advances in molecular pathology, a number of target agents have been developed and tried clinically in gastric cancer patients. A recent comprehensive meta-analysis of 10 randomized clinical trials results in a total of 1759 elderly patients with advanced gastric cancer, including GCC; investigators reported significant survival benefits for patients treated with anti-HER2 (hazard ratio: 0.71; 95% confidence interval: 0.62–0.99; $p < 0.05$) and angiogenesis inhibitors (hazard ratio: 0.88; 95% confidence interval: 0.79–0.99), but not for those treated with anti-EGFR agents [30]. An accumulating body of evidence suggests the anti-HER2 therapy as the current best precision target therapy for gastric carcinoma, GCC/EAC in particular. Therefore, accurate determination with high precision tests for HER2 expression in GCC is crucial for GCC patient chemotherapy.

Key Practice Guidelines on HER2 Testing

At present, HER2 testing is required by the College of American Pathologists, American Society for Clinical Pathology, the American Society of Clinical Oncology, and many other national and international professional societies for all gastric carcinomas, including GCC/EAC [31]. Among various methods for testing HER2 expression in tumor tissues, immunohistochemistry remains the most important primary test because it is simple and convenient to use, low-cost, and highly reliable. Only in cases with equivocal immunostaining results is in situ hybridization testing used for HER2 gene amplification. For HER2 testing, the clinical practice guidelines set a number of rules based on the best evidence available. The testing laboratory must validate both immunostaining and in situ hybridization methods with 20 positive tumor tissues and 20 negative specimens for a government (the Food and Drug Administration of the United States)-approved test with a good-quality control procedure. The control test also includes the use of exogenous tissues to be scored to validate the test protocol.

Indication

In almost all patients with documented, unresectable, locally advanced, recurrent, or metastatic gastric adenocarcinoma, including GCC/EGJ adenocarcinomas, at stages pII and beyond, combination chemotherapy with trastuzumab HER2-targeted therapy may prolong the patient progression-free and overall survival. Thus, the tumor should be tested for HER2 gene overexpression/amplification [31]. HER2 testing is not recommended to patients with early gastric cancer because of the absence of evidence on HER2 therapy benefits for those patients [31]. For patients with surgically resectable gastric adenocarcinoma, HER2 testing is also not recommended because the HER2 status is not helpful for prognosis prediction [31]. This test may not be required in some patients who may not tolerate systemic chemotherapy because of poor general condition and poor performance status [31].

Tumor Tissue

HER2 testing can be carried out on tumor tissues in the biopsy with over five tumor tissue fragments and resection specimens, as well as a cellblock of fine needle aspiration, from either primary or metastatic lesions in the patient without neoadjuvant therapy [31].

Fresh tumor tissues should be promptly fixed in 10% buffered neutral formalin solution within 1 h, stayed in the sufficient fixative solution for 6–72 h, and then subjected to routine histology tissue processing and paraffin embedding. Tumor tissue paraffin blocks should be cut at 4 μm in thickness, and consecutive sections should be selected for hematoxylin-eosin stain, immunohistochemistry, and possible in situ hybridization [31].

Pathologists need to select the best tumor block with the area containing well-differentiated, the lowest-grade tubular adenocarcinoma that most likely yields positive HER2 immunoreactivity for HER2 testing. In a tumor with heterogeneous histology subtypes and different grades of differentiation, it is reasonable to test different areas in more than one tumor block [31]. In cases with insufficient tumor cells in a tissue block for HER2 testing for the patients who may benefit from HER2-targeted therapy, an attempt should be made to acquire additional tumor tissues, either from a primary or from a metastatic lesion [31].

There is no evidence to support repeating HER2 testing in tumors that progress after the patients have been treated with HER2-targeted therapy combined with chemotherapy [31].

Immunohistochemistry

HER2 immunostaining should be carried out at a professionally credited laboratory that participates in the quality improvement program to ensure consistent performance in all aspects of HER2 testing and reporting process. Because most advanced

gastric cancer cases, especially GCC, are inoperable at diagnosis and rapidly progressing, immediate first-line chemotherapy is urgently needed. Therefore, HER2
testing should be carried out promptly right after a histopathologic diagnosis of
gastric carcinoma is made. There are multiple commercial anti-HER2 antibodies
with generally good concordance among antibodies. The laboratory needs to document the specific antibody used for HER2 testing on each report with appropriate
positive and negative controls. Pathologists are recommended to use the Ruschoff/
Hofmann method to score HER2 stains [23, 24, 31]. Only HER2 membranous
immunostaining is used for scoring. Cytoplasmic and luminal surface-only immunostaining is considered negative. In the report, the pathologist needs to describe
histology tumor growth patterns such as glandular or diffuse, solid, sheets or loosely
discohesive, infiltrating stroma, nuclear shape (round, oval) and size (medium,
large), as the information for possible future in situ hybridization testing [31]. On
immunohistochemistry, HER2 expression is membranous and scored as negative
with scores 0 and 1+, or equivocal with score 2+, and 3+ (positive) (Fig. 5.2 and
Table 5.3). This immunostaining test is sufficient for most gastric carcinoma cases
that need HER2 testing. Care must be taken to avoid overdiagnosis of false cytoplasmic and/or nucleus staining of cancer cells or membranous reactivity of precancerous cells staining as true HER2 immunoreactivity (Fig. 5.3). For a minority of
cases with the borderline (2+) immunostaining score, further reflex testing for
HER2 gene amplification should be carried out with in situ hybridization methods.

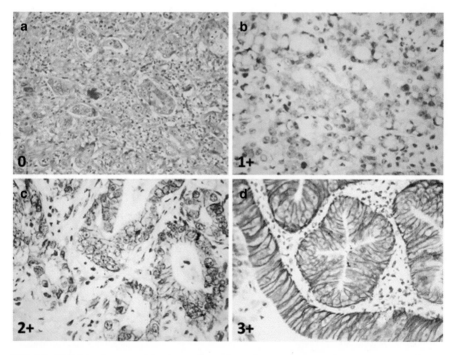

Fig. 5.2 HER2 immunoreactivity in gastric cardiac adenocarcinoma tumors was scored as 0 (**a**),
1+ (**b**), 2+ (**c**), and 3+ (**d**)

Table 5.3 Diagnostic criteria for HER2 immunostaining intensity [21, 31]

Score		0	1+	2+	3+
Criteria	Surgical resection specimens	No immunoreactivity in any viable tumor cells or in <10% of viable tumor cells	Faint membranous immunoreactivity in only part of the cell membrane in ≥10% viable tumor cells	Weak or moderate, complete, basolateral, or lateral membranous immunoreactivity in ≥10% of viable tumor cells	Strong complete, basolateral, or lateral membranous immunoreactivity in ≥10% of viable tumor cells
	Biopsy specimens	No reactivity or no membranous reactivity in any (or <5 cells) tumor cell	Tumor cell cluster with a faint or barely perceptible membranous reactivity irrespective of percentage of tumor cells stained (≥5 tumor cells)	Tumor cell cluster with a weak to moderate complete, basolateral, or lateral membranous reactivity irrespective of percentage of tumor cells stained (≥5 tumor cells)	Tumor cell cluster with a strong complete, basolateral, or lateral membranous reactivity irrespective of percentage of tumor cells stained (≥5 tumor cells)
Diagnosis		Negative	Negative	Equivocal	Positive

Fig. 5.3 False-positive cytoplasmic HER2 immunostaining should not be scored as "positive"

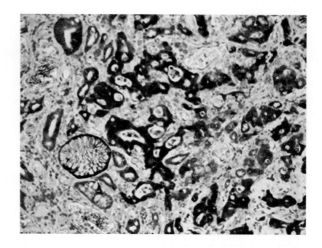

In Situ Hybridization Testing

The indications for in situ hybridization include the tumors with an equivocal immunostaining score of 2+, or borderline, or difficult to separate tumor with score 1+ from the one with score 2+. This test should not be used for tumors with scores 0, 1+ (negative), or 3+ (positive). At present, there are multiple methods for in situ hybridization to test HER2 gene overexpression/amplification. Fluorescence in situ hybridization (FISH) or silver in situ hybridization (SISH) has been proven to have good agreement for HER2 copy number testing. Extensive experience has been accumulated with FISH for this purpose. The bright-field SISH method with silver as a chromogen offers the advantages over FISH for performing the test on automated strainers, no need for fluorescence microscopy, allowing for easier identification of tumor areas and HER2-positive nuclei of neoplastic cells and a longer storage period of stained sections. However, there is no evidence for major diagnostic advantage between the two methods [31]. By using HER2 and centromere (chromosome enumeration probe 17, CEP17) probes, at least 20 individual nonoverlapping nuclei of tumor cells are needed to assess signal enumeration. To score in situ hybridization results, the HER2 immunostained slide should be scanned first to identify and mark the tumor area with the highest level of HER2 expression. Then, the same area on the adjacent tumor section with in situ hybridization testing will be scored for hybridization signals in at least 20 well-defined nuclei of tumor cells. A ratio of HER2 signal to CEP17 signal of ≥ 2.0 is defined as positive; the ratio of ≤ 2 is considered negative (Fig. 5.4) [31]. The pitfalls for in situ hybridization tests are several, such as no adequate controls, insufficient (<20) invasive viable tumor epithelial cells, poor nuclear resolution, strong autofluorescence signals, high (over 25%) unscorable weak hybridization signals, and high (>10%) cytoplasmic overlying signals (Fig. 5.5).

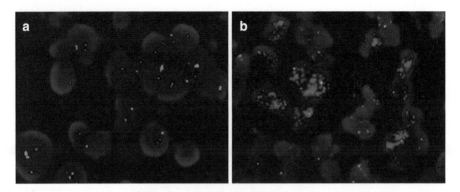

Fig. 5.4 The HER2 gene amplification FISH test in a gastric cardiac adenocarcinoma tumor. Compared to the normal control with one pair of HER2 gene (red dots) and chromosome enumeration probe 17 (CEP17, green dots) in each nucleus (**a**), neoplastic cells in gastric cardiac adenocarcinoma in (**b**) demonstrated cluster amplification of the HER2 gene (red dots) and diploid CEP 17 signal counts, diagnostic of positive HER2 gene amplification

Fig. 5.5 False-positive FISH signals because of polysomy chromosome enumeration probe 17 with more than 3 green dots per nucleus; therefore, the HER2 (red)/CDP17 (green) ratio was <2.0; the results were interpreted as negative for FISH HER2 gene amplification

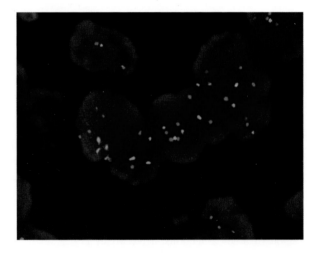

In the ToGA trial [24], extra copies of CEP17, because of intrachromosomal segmental duplication overlapping the centromere of chromosome 17, were reported in 4.1% gastric carcinomas. Thus, there are 4–6 copies of both HER2 and CEP17 signals with a ratio of <2.0 [31]. Therefore, in a tumor with three or more copies of CEP17 signals, the presence of six or more HER2 signals in the tumor is defined as positive for HER2 gene amplification, four or fewer HER2 signals as negative, and four to six as borderline, requiring scoring additional 20 nonoverlapping nuclei of different tumor cells [31].

In general, HER2 gene amplification can be evaluated by real-time or digital PCR. Because previous PCR studies demonstrated a close relationship with FISH/SISH, FISH/SISH tests have replaced PCR methods as the gold methodology for the HER2 gene amplification confirmatory molecular diagnosis [31]. According to a recent report, the droplet digital PCR method for the detection of HER2 gene overexpression was as effective as in situ hybridization methods but had the advantage of utility not only in paraffin-embedded formalin-fixed tumor tissue but also in peripheral blood samples for circulating tumor cells and DNA, which is especially appealing in gastric carcinoma cases with insufficient tumor tissues or without biopsy tissue for diagnosis [32].

The previous studies have shown that HER2 in situ hybridization positivity alone does not correlate with patient clinical responses to the trastuzumab therapy in gastric adenocarcinoma and GCC/EAC, because HER2 FISH positivity can be present in 11–24% of the cases with immunostaining score 0 or 1+ [31]. In fact, the ToGA trial demonstrated a significantly improved survival benefit only in the patients with combination of trastuzumab plus chemotherapy with high HER2 expression, defined as HER2 immunostaining score 3+ or 2+ with subsequent positive in situ hybridization results [24].

HER2 Testing Algorithm and Results Reporting

Pathologists are recommended to use the following HER2 testing algorithm in advanced gastric adenocarcinomas including GCC and EAC (Fig. 5.6). The HER2 testing turnaround time is in general 10 working days, starting from the date of the fresh specimen acquisition to the date of reporting. In the pathology report, the essential elements on HER2 test results are listed in Table 5.4.

At present, HER2 is the only clinically useful therapy-related biomarker to treat adenocarcinoma of the stomach and esophagus, and trastuzumab is the only approved HER2-targeted chemotherapy for this carcinoma with modest but statistically significantly improved survival in patients with HER2-positive adenocarci-

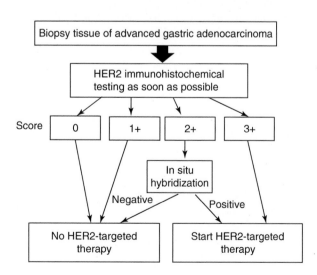

Fig. 5.6 The recommended HER2 testing algorithm for advanced gastric cancer including cardiac carcinoma

Table 5.4 Essential elements in a HER2 test report

Results	
By immunohistochemistry	Negative (score 0 or 1+)
	Equivocal (score 2+)
	Positive (score 3+)
By in situ hybridization	Negative (not amplified)
	Positive (amplified)
	Indeterminate (explain) due to…
	Number of cells counted:
	HER2 (ERBB2) to CEP17 ratio:
	Average number of HER2 signals per cell:
	Range of number of HER2 signals per cell:
Methods	
Immunohistochemistry	HER2-specific primary antibody used:
In situ hybridization	Test kit manufacturer:
	Test performer:
	Test scorer:

noma. The HER2 status should be appropriately and promptly evaluated in all patients with advanced, inoperable adenocarcinomas.

Epstein-Barr Virus Infection-Related Gastric Adenocarcinoma

EBV infection-related gastric adenocarcinoma is a distinct minor (nearly 10%) subtype of gastric adenocarcinomas [17]. This adenocarcinoma is characterized histopathologically as monoclonal proliferation of carcinoma cells with latent EBV infection (latency type I or II), which can be demonstrated by EBV-encoded small RNA (EBER) in situ hybridization. With distinct genomic profiles [17], EBV-related adenocarcinoma shows characteristic clinicopathological features, including predominance among men, the proximal location in the stomach (GCC) or in the remnant stomach, and lymphoepithelioma-like histology (also known as carcinoma with lymphoid stroma, by the WHO definition [33]). In this carcinoma, EBERs, EBNA-1, BARTs, LMP-2A, and BART miRNAs are overexpressed. Recent advances in genome-wide and comprehensive molecular analyses have demonstrated significant alterations in both genetic and epigenetic pathways in molecular pathologic carcinogenesis of this cancer. For characteristic genetic changes in EBV-related gastric carcinoma, frequent mutations have been reported in PIK3CA (80%), ARID1A (55%), and amplification of JAK2 and PD-L1/L2. Global DNA and CpG island hypermethylation leading to epigenetic silencing of tumor suppressor genes is a unique feature of this carcinoma. Because of promoter DNA hypermethylation, a number of genes are dysregulated in the cell cycle (p14ARF, p15, p16INK4A, and p73), DNA mismatch repair (hMLH1, MGMT, and GSTP1), cell adhesion and tumor metastasis (CDH1, TIMP1, and TIMP3), apoptosis (DAPK and bcl-2), and signal transduction (APC, PTEN, and RASSF1A) [7–9]. In addition to these genetic mutations in neoplastic epithelial cells for cell proliferation, apoptosis, and migration, host immune signaling is also altered with dense T-cell infiltration, which may be related to a favorable prognosis [7].

Currently, immunotherapy targeting PD-L1 and PD-1 molecules has changed the landscape of cancer treatment. This novel therapy is based on the discovery that cancerous cells use PD-L1 to defeat host antitumor immunity through interaction with programmed cell death protein 1 (PD-1) on T cells. Because recent whole-genome sequencing studies show frequent PD-L1 gene amplification in EBV-related gastric cancers, Japanese investigators analyzed the gastric cancer database of The Cancer Genome Atlas and discovered high expression of PD-L1 in EBV-related gastric cancers [34]. They reported that over 34% (33/96) tumors showed high PD-L1 expression with infiltration of PD-L1-positive cells in tumor stroma (45%, 43/96). These PD-L1-positive tumors were significantly correlated with diffuse-type histology, deeper invasion at pT1b and beyond, and poor overall and disease-specific survival, but not with tumor location [34]. This subtype of EBV-related gastric cancer may be an excellent candidate for immunotherapy targeting PD-L1/PD-1 molecules.

Expression of Programmed Death-Ligand 1 (PD-L1) Gene

Since MSI (microsatellite instable) colorectal carcinoma shows high expression of PD-L1, Jenkins et al. performed a preliminary study on PD-L1 expression in MSI gastric adenocarcinoma ($N = 52$), in which MSI was detected in 26% (10/38) of intestinal-type adenocarcinomas, 5% (2/38) of EBV-related adenocarcinomas, and none in 14 diffuse-type adenocarcinomas. They reported expression of PD-L1 was high (defined as >50% of neoplastic cells being immunopositive) in 20% (2/10) MSI intestinal-type adenocarcinomas and 50% (1/2) of EBV-related adenocarcinoma [35]. In a paired comparison study on clonality of synchronous GCC and DGC by whole-exome sequencing in 12 cases, PD1 expression was reported in all tumors, but PD-L1 expression was more common in GCC (66.7%) than in synchronous DGC (58.3%) [36]. If confirmed in future studies with larger samples, the results may have the potential for immunotherapy with PD-L1 inhibitors in patients with GCC.

Gastrointestinal stromal tumor is rare in the gastric cardia. PD-L1 expression was found in an abstract to correlate significantly with the presence of higher tumor-infiltrating lymphocytes (defined as >11 tumor-infiltrating lymphocytes per high-power field), especially in younger patients at lower stages [37]. This preliminary finding, if confirmed and validated, suggests the possibility of the use of tumor-infiltrating lymphocytes as a surrogate marker for PD-L1 expression in gastric cancers.

Summary

The advanced genomic tools provide an unprecedented opportunity to uncover the myth of GCC/EGJ carcinomas and to help identify cancer biomarkers and develop new rational targeted therapeutic strategies to treat and cure GCC as the ultimate goal. For diagnostic and therapeutic purposes, a number of biomarkers are suggested for a work-up of the biopsy-proven malignancy in the gastric cardiac region (Table 5.5). At present, there is no role for routine clinical testing on EGFR, VEGF, FGFR2, and MET to guide clinical practice, except for clinical trials. With rapid advances in effective precision target therapies, routine pathologic characterization of specific target molecules may most likely expand beyond HER2 analysis in the future.

Taken together, the most recent evidence shows distinct molecular pathologic profiles of GCC in which chromosomal instability accounts for 65% of GCC/EGJ carcinomas as well as 98.6% of EAC. As such, GCC and EAC belong to the same molecular disease entity. This concept would dramatically change the way how patients with these cancers are managed. GCC also demonstrates considerable EBV-related tumors as compared to that of DGC or EAC. At present, HER2 testing remains the priority for patient management, although PD-1 and PD-L1 testing may be required in foreseeable future. A complete understanding of GCC tumorigenesis mechanisms relies upon an illustration of its detailed genomic properties, which is on horizon.

Table 5.5 Useful biomarkers for common cancer in the gastric cardia/EGJ region

Biomarker panel	Cancer	Value
HER2, PD-L1	Adenocarcinoma, GIST	Therapy
p53, CDX2, MUC2	Adenocarcinoma	Diagnosis
CK7, CD8, EBER	EBV infection-related carcinoma	Diagnosis
Synaptophysin, chromogranin A, CD56, Ki67, p40	Neuroendocrine carcinoma	Diagnosis
p40, p63, CK5/6, synaptophysin	Adenosquamous carcinoma/squamous cell carcinoma	Diagnosis
AFP, Sall4, GPC-3, CDX2, MUC2, HerPart1,CK19	Hepatoid/AFP-producing adenocarcinoma	Diagnosis
Trypsin, alpha1-chymotrypsin	Pancreatic acinar-like adenocarcinoma	Diagnosis
CD117, DOG.1, CD34, S100, desmin, SMA, Ki67	GIST, schwannoma, leiomyoma	Diagnosis
CD45, CD3, CD20, CD79a, CD56, EBER, Ki67, AE1/AE3	Lymphoma	Diagnosis

References

1. Huang Q, Sun Q, Fan XS, et al. Recent advances in proximal gastric carcinoma. J Dig Dis. 2016;17(7):421–32.
2. Huang Q, Shi J, Sun Q, et al. Clinicopathological characterisation of small (2 cm or less) proximal and distal gastric carcinomas in a Chinese population. Pathology. 2015;47:526–32.
3. Amini N, Spolverato G, Kim Y, et al. Clinicopathological features and prognosis of gastric cardia adenocarcinoma: a multi-institutional US study. J Surg Oncol. 2015;111:285–92.
4. Carneiro F, Moutinho C, Pera G, et al. Pathology findings and validation of gastric and esophageal cancer cases in a European cohort (EPIC/EUR-GAST). Scand J Gastroenterol. 2007;42:618–27.
5. Huang Q, Zhang LH. The histopathologic spectrum of carcinomas involving the gastroesophageal junction in the Chinese. Int J Surg Pathol. 2007;15:38–52.
6. Huang Q, Gold JS, Shi J, et al. Pancreatic acinar-like adenocarcinoma of the proximal stomach invading the esophagus. Hum Pathol. 2012;43:911–20.
7. Shinozaki-Ushiku A, Kunita A, Fukayama M. Update on Epstein-Barr virus and gastric cancer (review). Int J Oncol. 2015;46:1421–34.
8. Chen JN, He D, Tang F, Shao CK. Epstein-Barr virus-associated gastric carcinoma: a newly defined entity. J Clin Gastroenterol. 2012;46:262–71.
9. Lim H, Park YS, Lee JH, et al. Features of gastric carcinoma with lymphoid stroma associated with Epstein-Barr virus. Clin Gastroenterol Hepatol. 2015;13:1738–44.e2.
10. Taniere P, Martel-Planche G, Maurici D, et al. Molecular and clinical differences between adenocarcinomas of the esophagus and of the gastric cardia. Am J Pathol. 2001;158:33–40.
11. Wijnhoven BP, Siersema PD, Hop WC, et al. Adenocarcinomas of the distal oesophagus and gastric cardia are one clinical entity. Rotterdam Esophageal Tumour Study Group. Br J Surg. 1999;86:529–35.
12. Shah MA, Khanin R, Tang L, et al. Molecular classification of gastric cancer: a new paradigm. Clin Cancer Res. 2011;17:2693–701.
13. Mocellin S, Verdi D, Pooley KA, Nitti D. Genetic variation and gastric cancer risk: a field synopsis and meta-analysis. Gut. 2015;64(8):1209–19.
14. Xue W, Zhu M, Wang Y, He J, Zheng L. Association between PLCE1 rs2274223 A > G polymorphism and cancer risk: proof from a meta-analysis. Sci Rep. 2015;5:7986.
15. Sun CQ, Chang YB, Cui LL, et al. A population-based case-control study on risk factors for gastric cardia cancer in rural areas of Linzhou. Asian Pac J Cancer Prev. 2013;14:2897–901.
16. Jiang X, Tseng CC, Bernstein L, Wu AH. Family history of cancer and gastroesophageal disorders and risk of esophageal and gastric adenocarcinomas: a case-control study. BMC Cancer. 2014;14:60.
17. Cancer Genome Atlas Research Network. Comprehensive molecular characterization of gastric adenocarcinoma. Nature. 2014;513(7517):202–9.
18. Huang Q, Fan XS, Agoston AT, et al. Comparison of gastroesophageal junction carcinomas in Chinese versus American patients. Histopathology. 2011;59(2):188–97.
19. Cancer Genome Atlas Research Network. Integrated genomic characterization of oesophageal carcinoma. Nature. 2017;541(7636):169–75.
20. Jia F, Teer JK, Knepper TC, et al. Discordance of somatic mutations between Asian and Caucasian patient populations with gastric cancer. Mol Diagn Ther. 2017;21(2):179–85. https://doi.org/10.1007/s40291-016-0250-z.

21. Bang YJ, Van Cutsem E, Feyereislova A, et al. Trastuzumab in combination with chemotherapy versus chemotherapy alone for treatment of HER2-positive advanced gastric or gastro-oesophageal junction cancer (ToGA): a phase 3, open-label, randomized controlled trial. Lancet. 2010;376(9742):687–97.
22. Gravalos C, Jimeno A. HER2 in gastric cancer: a new prognostic factor and a novel therapeutic target. Ann Oncol. 2008;19:1523–9.
23. Hofmann M, Stoss O, Shi D, et al. Assessment of a HER2 scoring system for gastric cancer: results from a validation study. Histopathology. 2008;52:797–805.
24. Bang YJ. Advances in the management of HER2-positive advanced gastric and gastroesophageal junction cancer. J Clin Gastroenterol. 2012;46:637–48.
25. Van Cutsem E, Bang YJ, Feng-Yi F, et al. HER2 screening data from ToGA: targeting HER2 in gastric and gastroesophageal junction cancer. Gastric Cancer. 2015;18:476–84.
26. Kim WH, Gomez-Izquierdo L, Vilardell F, et al. HER2 status in gastric and gastroesophageal junction cancer: results of the large, multinational HER-EAGLE Study. Appl Immunohistochem Mol Morphol. 2018;26(4):239–245.
27. Kwak H, Khor TS, Alpert L, et al. HER2 expression is predominantly negative in GEJ and gastric adenocarcinoma with signet ring cell differentiation; Study of 346 cases modern pathology. 2017;30(Suppl 2s):180A–1A.
28. Feng XS, Wang YF, Hao SG, Ru Y, Gao SG, Wang LD. Expression of Das-1, Ki67 and sulfuric proteins in gastric cardia adenocarcinoma and intestinal metaplasia lesions. Exp Ther Med. 2013;5:1555–8.
29. Birkman EM, Algars A, Lintunen M, Ristamaki R, Sundstrom J, Carpen O. EGFR gene amplification is relatively common and associates with outcome in intestinal adenocarcinoma of the stomach, gastro-oesophageal junction and distal oesophagus. BMC Cancer. 2016;16:406.
30. Wang CW, Fang XH. The role of targeted agents in the treatment of advanced gastric cancer: a meta-analysis of randomized controlled trials. Eur Rev Med Pharmacol Sci. 2016;20(9):1725–32.
31. Bartley AN, Washington MK, Colasacco C, et al. HER2 testing and clinical decision making in gastroesophageal adenocarcinoma: guideline from the College of American Pathologists, American Society for Clinical Pathology, and the American Society of Clinical Oncology. J Clin Oncol. 2017;35(4):446–64.
32. Kinugasa H, Nouso K, Tanaka T, et al. Droplet digital PCR measurement of HER2 in patients with gastric cancer. Br J Cancer. 2015;112(10):1652–5.
33. Lauwers GY, Carneiro F, Graham DY, et al. Gastric carcinoma. In: Bosman FT, Carneiro F, Hruban RH, Theise ND, editors. WHO classification of tumours of the digestive system. Lyon: IARC Press; 2010. p. 48–58.
34. Saito R, Abe H, Kunita A, Yamashita H, Seto Y, Fukayama M. Overexpression and gene amplification of PD-L1 in cancer cells and PD-L1(+) immune cells in Epstein-Barr virus-associated gastric cancer: the prognostic implications. Mod Pathol. 2017;30(3):427–39. https://doi.org/10.1038/modpathol.2016.202.
35. Jenkins TM, Tondon R, Wang LP, et al. Mismatch repair deficiency (MMR-D) and programmed death ligand (PD-L1) expression in gastric adenocarcinoma. Mod Pathol. 2017;30(Suppl 2s):178A.
36. Xing X, Jia S, Wu J, et al. Clonality analysis of synchronous gastroesophageal junction carcinoma and distal gastric cancer by whole-exome sequencing. J Pathol. 2017;243(2):165–75. https://doi.org/10.1002/path.4932.
37. Savant D, Vitkovski T, Thomas R, Rishi A. Programmed cell death ligand-1 (PD-L1) expression in gastrointestinal stromal tumors correlates significantly with presence of tumor infiltrating lymphocytes. Mod Pathol. 2017;30(Suppl 2s):199A.

Chapter 6
Pathology of Early Gastric Cardiac Cancer

Qin Huang

Introduction

The World Health Organization (WHO) defines early gastric carcinoma (EGC) as the invasive tumor confined to the mucosa, or mucosa and submucosa, regardless of the nodal status [1], as shown in Fig. 6.1.

Early gastric cardiac carcinoma (EGCC) represents an early stage of cancer development in the gastric cardia and slowly progresses, as described in the chapter of Natural History. Because of the widespread use of upper endoscopy, EGCC has been much more frequently detected and diagnosed in recent years and can be cured if diagnosed early and resected completely.

Gross Features

Gross characteristics of intraepithelial neoplasia or early carcinoma in the gastric cardia have not been well studied. The preliminary results of a few studies in Japan and China suggest that the protruding/elevated growth patterns in EGCC tumors are most common; flat and depressed patterns are infrequent; and excavated/ulcerated patterns are uncommon [2, 3]. Overall, EGCC is known to have five major gross appearances: polypoid protruding (21.4%) (Fig. 6.2), elevated-rough (40.5%) (Fig. 6.3), flat (4.6%), depressed/erosion (16.8%), and excavated/ulcerated (16.8%) (Fig. 6.4) patterns [3]. Unlike those in early gastric non-cardiac carcinoma,

Q. Huang
Pathology and Laboratory Medicine, Veterans Affairs Boston Healthcare System,
West Roxbury, MA, USA

Harvard Medical School and Brigham and Women's Hospital,
Boston, MA, USA

© Springer International Publishing AG, part of Springer Nature 2018
Q. Huang (ed.), *Gastric Cardiac Cancer*, https://doi.org/10.1007/978-3-319-79114-2_6

Fig. 6.1 Early gastric cardiac carcinoma, poorly differentiated, invading the lamina propria (M2), through the muscularis mucosae (M3), superficial submucosal (SM1, <0.5 mm), into the deep submucosal (SM2, >0.5 mm) space. The invasion front is sharp with a pushing border. Multiple lymphoid follicles are present in the tumor and overlying mucosa

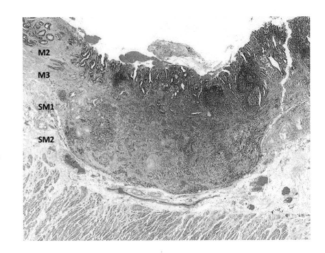

Fig. 6.2 Gross appearance of a broad-based, protruding early gastric cardiac carcinoma, corresponding to the Paris classification type I early gastric carcinoma. Note a short segment of the distal esophagus lined with benign pearl-gray squamous mucosa without salmon-red metaplastic changes

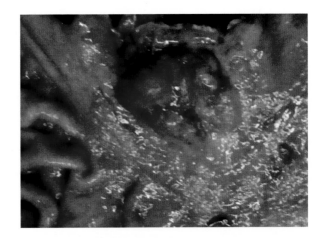

Fig. 6.3 Gross appearance of a focally elevated and partially flat early gastric cardiac carcinoma, corresponding to the Paris classification types I–II early gastric carcinoma. Note the normal distal esophageal pearl-gray squamous epithelium (arrow)

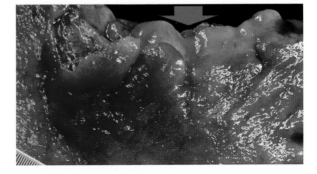

Fig. 6.4 Gross image of an ulcerated early gastric cardiac carcinoma (arrow) with the Paris classification type 0–III pattern. The tumor invades focally into the distal esophagus. Note the absence of salmon-red columnar-lined metaplastic lesions in the distal esophagus

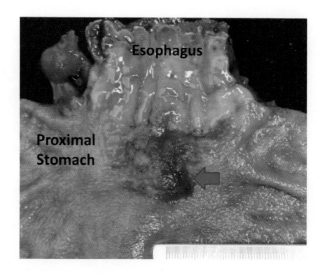

Table 6.1 Comparison of gross characteristics between early gastric cardiac and non-cardiac carcinomas [3]

WHO type	Gross feature	EGC (n = 438) (%)	Cardiac carcinoma (n = 131) (%)	Non-cardiac carcinoma (n = 307) (%)
0-I	Protruding	63 (14.4)	28 (21.4)	35 (11.4)
0-IIa	Elevated-rough	118 (26.9)	53 (40.5)	65 (21.2)
0-IIb	Flat	15 (3.4)	6 (4.6)	9 (2.9)
0-IIc	Depressed/ erosion	94 (21.5)	22 (16.8)	72 (23.5)
0-III	Excavated	148 (33.8)	22 (16.8)	126 (41.0)

Note: *EGC* early gastric carcinoma

polypoid/protruding and elevated-rough patterns are significantly more common, but excavated/ulcerated patterns are significantly lesser frequent in EGCC (Table 6.1).

As shown in Fig. 6.5, most small (≤2 cm) gastric carcinoma tumors are located in the lesser curvature region and range in size from 0.3 to 5 cm [4]. The protruding and elevated gross growth patterns (Figs. 6.2 and 6.3) are commonly seen in tubular and papillary adenocarcinomas, while poorly cohesive and signet-ring cell carcinomas show primarily depressed and ulcerated gross patterns in the gastric cardia [2–4].

Microscopic Features

By histology, EGCC consists of both epithelial and stromal components of malignancy.

Fig. 6.5 Distribution of
small gastric carcinoma in
size of 2 cm or less in the
stomach demonstrated two
concentrated regions:
about 2/3 in the antrum-
pylorus region and 1/3 in
the gastric cardia [4]

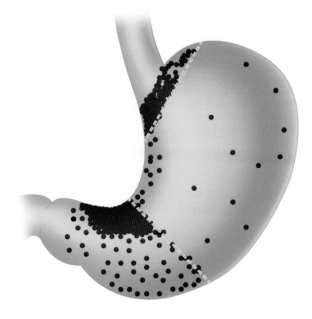

Fig. 6.6 Desmoplastic
reaction to poorly
differentiated early gastric
cardiac carcinoma invading
into the submucosal space

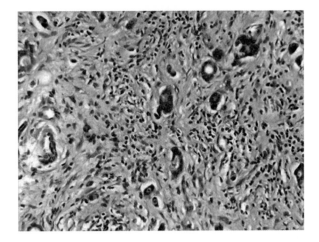

Stromal Reaction

In general, the stromal responses to EGCC are composed of five major types: desmoplasia (Fig. 6.6), lymphocytic infiltrate (Fig. 6.7), stromal eosinophilia, neutro-
philia (Fig. 6.8), and granulomatous responses. In intramucosal carcinoma, the
desmoplastic response may not be as conspicuous as that seen in submucosal carcinoma. Intraepithelial and peri-tumor lymphocytic infiltrates are associated with a
better prognosis, but scirrhous stromal reaction is most frequently seen in advanced
carcinoma, due to infiltration of poorly cohesive and signet-ring cell carcinomas,
which has a high frequency of nodal metastasis and peritoneal spread [3].

Fig. 6.7 Dense small lymphocytic infiltrate in poorly differentiated early gastric cardiac carcinoma with lymphoid stroma

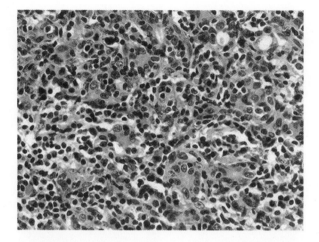

Fig. 6.8 Massive neutrophilic infiltrate is evident in the stroma of the lamina propria along with crypt microabscess in this early gastric cardiac carcinoma

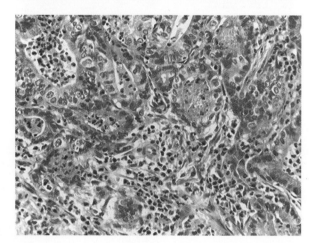

Associated Epithelial Lesions

Chronic Gastric Carditis

Almost all EGCCs are associated with chronic gastric carditis [3]. The etiology is generally considered to be related to either reflux disease or *H. pylori* infection or both [3, 5]. Autoimmune carditis is vanishingly rare. The updated Sydney chronic gastritis classification system has been widely used to grade the type, degree, and extent of inflammation and *H. pylori* infection [6]. The histologic distinction between reflux disease-induced carditis and *H. pylori*-initiated chronic inflammation is important but difficult because of the frequent presence of both conditions in the same patient. In general, reflux disease often shows focal mucosal erosion and mild lymphoplasmacytic and eosinophilic infiltrate; in contrast, lymphoid follicles and conspicuous neutrophilic and eosinophilic (>10 eosinophils/high-power field) infiltrate are rarely observed (Fig. 6.9). *H. pylori* gastric carditis is characterized with marked neutrophilic and eosinophilic infiltrate and crypt microabscess and dense lymphoplasmacytic infiltrate with lymphoid follicles (Fig. 6.10 and Table 6.2). Because of the clinical importance for patient management, *H. pylori* infection should be routinely ruled out in all patients by histology stains (such as

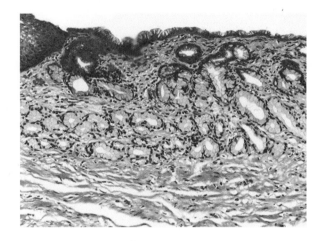

Fig. 6.9 Reflux-induced mild gastric carditis features mild mixed small lymphocytic and eosinophilic infiltrate, without lymphoid follicles, in the lamina propria of this 75-year-old male patient

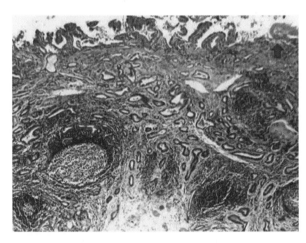

Fig. 6.10 Gastric *H. pylori* carditis with moderate chronic active inflammation, prominent lymphoid follicles, and foveolar papillary hyperplastic changes in a 61-year-old Chinese man without a history of gastroesophageal reflux disease. *H. pylori* was identified on a Giemsa stain (not shown here). An arrow at the right upper corner shows a squamous island as the landmark for the esophagogastric junction

Table 6.2 Differential diagnosis between *H. pylori* infection and reflux disease

Histology feature	*H. pylori* infection	Reflux disease
Erosion	Rare	Common
Neutrophilic infiltrate and crypt microabscess	Very common	Rare
Lymphoplasmacytic infiltrate	Severe	Mild
Lymphoid follicle	Very common	Rare
Eosinophilic infiltrate	Severe	Mild
H. pylori stain	Usually positive	Negative

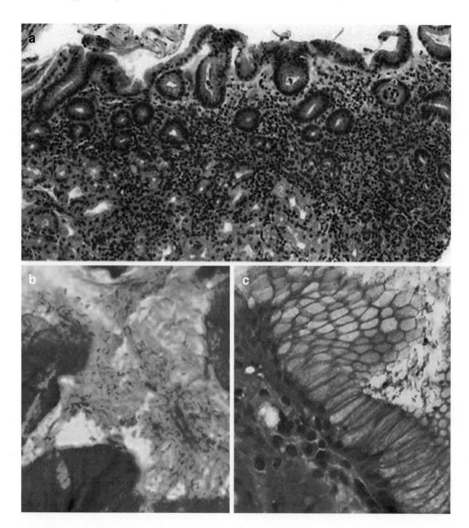

Fig. 6.11 Gastric chronic active *H. pylori* carditis (**a**) with characteristic dense lymphoplasma-cytic infiltrate and neutrophilic crypt microabscess primarily in the superficial mucosa, as con-firmed with a positive Giemsa (**b**) stain with numerous bacteria in the lumen or an immunohistochemical stain for *H. pylori* as brown-colored bacteria on the mucosal surface on the right (**c**)

hematoxylin-eosin, Giemsa, and immunohistochemistry) (Fig. 6.11) or other means, such as the ^{13}C breath test or the Meridian *H. pylori* stool antigen test. On a well-oriented histology section with a routine hematoxylin-eosin stain, *H. pylori* bacteria can be identified on the mucosal surface and within crypts, usually associated with dense chronic and acute inflammation. In that setting, a Giemsa or immunostain may not be necessary to document *H. pylori* infection. Although the WHO has declared *H. pylori* as a category I carcinogen for gastric cancer, the role of *H. pylori* infection in carcinogenesis of gastric cardiac carcinoma (GCC) remains to be illustrated.

Intestinal Metaplasia

By histology, intestinal metaplasia is defined as the presence of goblet cells replacing normal gastric crypt epithelial mucous cells and can be divided into two major categories: (1) the complete type with histology features similar to those of small intestine, also known as type I intestinal metaplasia, and (2) the incomplete type with the morphology mimicking that of the colon, also known as type IIA and type IIB intestinal metaplasia on the basis of different responses to histochemical stains. By immunohistochemistry, the epithelial cells with intestinal metaplasia are strongly immunoreactive to CDX2 and MUC2 antibodies (Fig. 6.12), indicating intestinal differentiation; the response to other gastric mucin antibodies, such as MUC1, MUC5AC, and MUC6, is little or absent for complete intestinal metaplasia but reserved for incomplete intestinal metaplasia, indicating aberrant gastric and intestinal differentiations [7]. Some studies suggested a higher risk of carcinogenesis for patients with the incomplete-type intestinal metaplasia, but others refuted that claim. In fact, many patients with intestinal metaplasia do not progress to dysplasia or cancer, also known as "stable" intestinal metaplasia with a low risk for gastric cancer development [8]. Intestinal metaplasia occurs most frequently in cardiac mucous glands and can be seen in patients with either reflux disease or *H. pylori* infection or both. In the real world, routine subtyping of intestinal metaplasia is unrealistic and does not provide clinically and pathologically useful information for patient management, partially due to the fact that both complete and incomplete intestinal metaplasia types are frequently mixed together in mucosal biopsy specimens taken from the same patient. Furthermore, the results of a recent pathologic study suggest a weak relationship between carcinomas in the esophagogastric junction region and intestinal metaplasia in cardiac mucous glands [9]. Overall, intestinal metaplasia is more frequently related to reflux disease in the West; but in the East, *H. pylori* infection in the gastric cardia appears to be the major etiology [3, 10]. The results of a retrospective pathology study from the United Kingdom with 37 cases of GCC show 35.2% of cases that are associated with background intestinal metaplasia and only 3 (8.1%) cases with *H. pylori* infection, suggesting a minimal role for *H. pylori* in GCC tumorigenesis in that population [11]. In a major prospective study conducted in the United States, chronic carditis was found to be significantly related to reflux disease, and *H. pylori* infection was detected in only

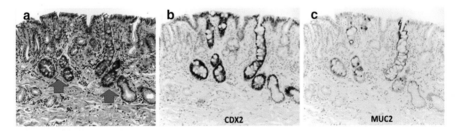

Fig. 6.12 Intestinal metaplasia, complete type (arrows in **a**), arises in two gastric units and is immunoreactive to CDX2 (a transcription factor for intestinal differentiation) in (**b**) and MUC2 (an intestinal mucin protein) in (**c**)

27.4% of cases [5]. In contrast, in a Chinese patient population with EGCC, over 92% of cases showed intestinal metaplasia in the mucosa adjacent to carcinoma, and over 51% of cases were found to have active *H. pylori* infection [3], indicating *H. pylori* indeed to be a major player in carcinogenesis of EGCC in the Chinese population. There appear different pathogenesis mechanisms for EGCC among different ethnic populations. Nevertheless, the pathologic diagnosis of intestinal metaplasia depends upon the unequivocal identification of goblet cells and should not be confused with the pseudogoblet cells (Fig. 6.13).

Atrophy

By definition, a reduction in number or function of gastric glands constitutes atrophy (Fig. 6.14). In the gastric cardia, a biopsy specimen frequently shows a reduction in the number of cardiac mucous glands. The significance is unknown. In contrast, in gastric non-cardiac carcinomas, clinical and pathologic study results

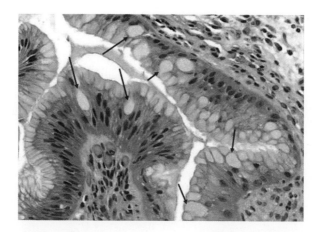

Fig. 6.13 Pseudogoblet cells (arrows) are frequently observed in the gastric cardiac mucosa with chronic inflammation and characterized by evenly distributed eosinophilic cytoplasmic mucus accumulation without the blue hue and uneven-sized cytoplasmic mucus droplets seen in true goblet cells

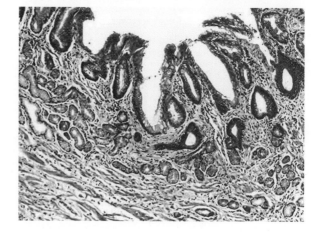

Fig. 6.14 Refluxed-induced gastric chronic atrophic carditis with markedly reduced number of cardiac glands. Metaplastic goblet cells are present in the hyperplastic foveolar epithelium in the right upper corner

suggest that the "pattern, extent, and severity of atrophy with/without intestinal metaplasia is a far more important predictor of increased cancer risk than intestinal metaplasia subtype" [12]. In the gastric cardia, however, the significance of mucosal atrophy in carcinogenesis remains poorly understood. For an optimal patient management, it is very important for endoscopists to biopsy gastric mucosa at various sites, including the antrum, angularis, and cardia for a pathologist to identify, compare, and determine the extent and severity of cardiac mucosal atrophy.

Pancreatic Acinar Metaplasia

Pancreatic acinar metaplasia in the cardia is common and characterized by dense basophilic cytoplasmic granules concentrated in the basal part of the cytoplasm with eosinophilic granules accumulated in the luminal cytoplasm, mimicking pancreatic exocrine acinar glands (Fig. 6.15). This metaplasia is most commonly observed in the gastric cardia than in any other gastric regions with unknown mechanisms and clinical significance [3, 13]. Frequently, pancreatic acinar metaplasia may extend from the cardia into the distal esophagus as superficial esophageal glands, also known as "buried gland" (Fig. 6.16). This metaplasia may be physiologic but not premalignant. The results of a prospective multicenter European upper endoscopy study revealed a prevalence of 17.2% of subjects with pancreatic metaplasia but without significant relationship between pancreatic acinar metaplasia and reflux disease or *H. pylori* infection [13]. In a recent pathology study of early GCC in Chinese patients, pancreatic acinar metaplasia was found in over 36% of patients, which was significantly higher than that of early gastric non-cardiac carcinoma [3] and also more than twice as higher as that (17.2%) of Europeans described in a recent report [13]. It is speculated that the proteolytic enzymes released from

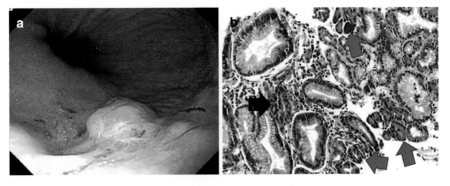

Fig. 6.15 Pancreatic acinar metaplasia arising in the gastric cardia, adjacent to an intramucosal well-differentiated tubular adenocarcinoma with a polypoid protruding growth pattern (**a**). In the tissue adjacent to adenocarcinoma, benign cardiac glands show pancreatic acinar metaplasia (blue arrows in **b**). Note, an adjacent dysplasia gland (black arrow)

Fig. 6.16 The same cardiac mucous glands are present in the gastric cardia and also underneath the esophageal squamous epithelium and termed superficial esophageal glands, also known as "buried glands." Note the focal dilation and continuality of those glands from the gastric cardia to the distal esophagus. *EGJ* esophagogastric junction (arrow)

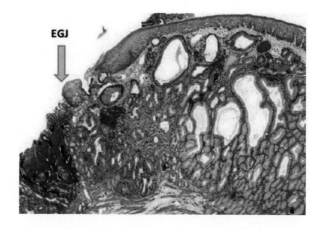

Fig. 6.17 Fibromuscular hyperplasia along with markedly atrophic cardiac glands (arrows) is frequently observed in the gastric cardia

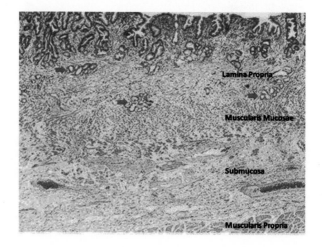

pancreatic metaplastic cardiac mucosa may help infiltration and spread of neoplastic cells of GCC and explain the reason why EGCC invades deeper than early gastric non-cardiac carcinoma [3].

Fibromuscular Hyperplasia

In the gastric cardia of elderly subjects, considerable fibromuscular hyperplasia along with atrophic cardiac glands is frequently present. As shown in Fig. 6.17, the thickness of the cardiac mucosa is markedly increased, but the number of cardiac glands is conspicuously decreased. The significance of this common change remains to be explored.

Premalignant Neoplasia

Pathologic diagnosis of premalignant neoplasia, which is also known as dysplasia primarily in the West, or intraepithelial neoplasia by the WHO, dictates clinical management of patients and must be distinguished from reactive/reparative atypia in the settings of erosion, acute inflammation, radiation, drug effects, among others (Figs. 6.18 and 6.19).

In addition, premalignant intramucosal neoplasia must be distinguished from invasive carcinoma for an optimal patient therapeutic triage, which has been proven occasionally very difficult by the histology evidence alone. Therefore, an accurate mucosal biopsy diagnosis may need the cooperation between the endoscopist and the pathologist. At present, the WHO categorizes premalignant gastric neoplasia

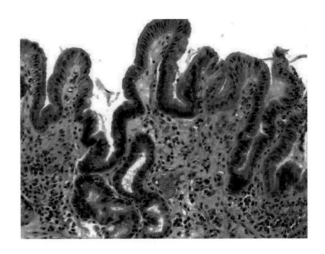

Fig. 6.18 Reparative/reactive atypia in the gastric cardia shows epithelial nuclear hyperchromasia, mimicking dysplasia. Note the uniformity of epithelial nuclei and inflammatory background

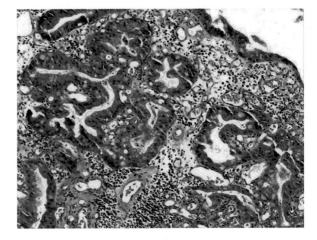

Fig. 6.19 *H. pylori* infection-associated inflammatory/hyperplastic polyp in the gastric cardia exhibits marked architectural disarray, mimicking intramucosal carcinoma. Note the bland epithelial nuclei and edematous inflammatory stroma

into three major types [1]: (1) negative for intraepithelial neoplasia, (2) indefinite for intraepithelial neoplasia, and (3) intraepithelial neoplasia.

Negative for Intraepithelial Neoplasia or Dysplasia

In this category, the histology changes include benign reactive/reparative processes in epithelial cells, primarily in response to erosion and acute inflammation (Fig. 6.20), among other physical/chemical insults. The overall mucosal architecture of biopsy tissue remains intact. Nuclei may be hyperchromatic, enlarged with prominent nucleoli. However, the nuclear changes in the epithelium are uniform. The nuclear-to-cytoplasm ratio remains small. There should be no evidence of atypical mitosis, obvious nuclear pleomorphism, and tumor necrosis. At endoscopy, the disease is limited to the mucosal surface, and there should be no evidence of a mass lesion. Differential diagnosis between reactive atypia and dysplasia is shown in Table 6.3.

Indefinite for Intraepithelial Neoplasia or Dysplasia

The category of indefinite for intraepithelial neoplasia or dysplasia is used as a descriptive interpretation of biopsy pathology in the situation in which the morphologic changes in a biopsy are ambiguous between premalignant neoplasia and benign reactive or regenerative changes, because of marked acute inflammation, erosion, ulceration, small tissue fragments, and obscured nuclear abnormality, which do not fit with the criteria for premalignant neoplasia or bizarre nuclear morphology in the setting of radiation therapy (Fig. 6.21). In those scenarios, the pathologist may want to conduct further investigation to resolve the dilemma by cutting

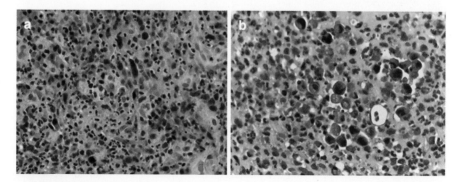

Fig. 6.20 Reactive atypia in the setting of acute inflammation and granulation tissue in the gastric cardia in (**a**), mimicking poorly cohesive carcinoma in (**b**). Note distinct nuclear dysplasia with marked pleomorphism, some with signet-ring cell features in (**b**)

Table 6.3 Differential diagnosis between reactive atypia and dysplasia

Feature	Reactive atypia	Intraepithelial neoplasia/dysplasia
Overall architecture	Intact	Distorted
Nuclear abnormality	Mild, uniform	Marked, varied
Hyperchromasia	Weak	Strong
Pleomorphism	Absent	Marked
Irregularity	Absent	Marked
Atypical mitosis	Absent	May present
Necrosis	Absent	May present
Cytoplasm	Unchanged	Reduced
Associated with:		
Erosion/ulcer	May present	May be absent
Marked neutrophilic infiltrate	Present	May be absent
Luminal necrotic debris	Absent	Present

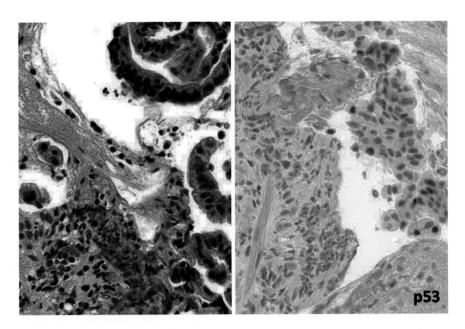

Fig. 6.21 Indefinite for dysplasia in a lesion in the gastric cardia was depicted on the left with erosion, acute inflammation, and marked epithelial nuclear atypia. The p53 immunostain of this lesion on the right showed weak, heterogeneous, wild-type staining characteristics, supporting a reactive/reparative, rather than dysplastic, process

deeper levels, performing special stains, and reviewing the endoscopy report along with the gross endoscopic images, patient medical records, and clinical notes. It is also very helpful for the responsible general pathologist to discuss the case with an experienced gastrointestinal pathologist. In the same way, the gastroenterologist may manage the patient conservatively with anti-reflux and other appropriate therapies to minimize the degree of acute inflammation and then repeat upper endoscopy for a second look with a biopsy in 3 months. In other words, this pathologic interpretation is not a definitive diagnosis and should be used only temporarily.

Intraepithelial Neoplasia or Dysplasia

Intraepithelial neoplasia or dysplasia is the diagnosis used for biopsy histology demonstrating unequivocal epithelial neoplastic proliferative features, including both cytological and architectural dysplastic characteristics without the morphologic evidence of invasion. It has been controversial over the past decades as to the definition of invasion in EGC between Western and Japanese pathologists. According to Western pathologists, invasion is defined as neoplastic cells or glands breaking through the basement membrane into the stroma. This definition is applicable easily for carcinoma invading into the submucosa but not so clear-cut for intramucosal carcinoma in the stomach, including the gastric cardia. Oftentimes, the same intramucosal neoplasia interpreted as high-grade dysplasia (Fig. 6.22) by Western pathologists is considered as intramucosal carcinoma by Japanese pathologists. To reach a common ground, two major international expert conferences have produced two consensus classification systems as the Padova and Vienna classifications with the purposes of unifying terminology of the histomorphologic spectrum of intraepithelial neoplasia from nonneoplastic changes to early invasive carcinoma [14–16]. Since then, the gap in diagnosing intraepithelial neoplasia between the West and Japanese pathologists has become smaller than before.

Microscopically, intraepithelial neoplasia or dysplasia is divided into low- and high-grade categories in order to easily manage patients clinically. Both types of premalignant lesions may be termed as "adenoma" by Western pathologists for lesions with the discrete, protruding gross appearances.

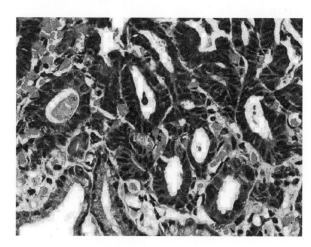

Fig. 6.22 Intraepithelial neoplasm in the stomach may be diagnosed as high-grade dysplasia by some Western pathologists but interpreted as well-differentiated intramucosal tubular adenocarcinoma by Japanese pathologists

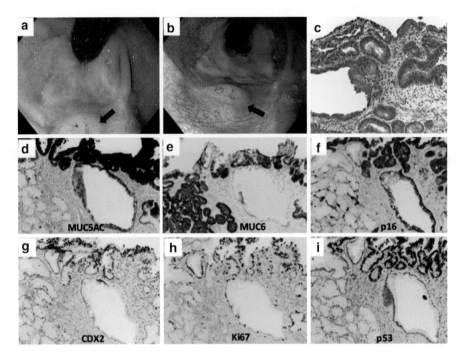

Fig. 6.23 High-grade adenoma of the foveolar type in the gastric cardia was discovered in a 79-year-old man with a history of gastroesophageal reflux disease, presented at upper endoscopy as a broad-based, elevated the Paris 0-Ip lesion (arrow in **a**), better illustrated by the narrowband imaging study (arrow in **b**). Histopathologic examination of the endoscopic mucosal resection specimen showed characteristic papillary-tubular growth patterns with enlarged, round-oval neoplastic epithelial nuclei and eosinophilic cytoplasm (**c**). By immunohistochemistry, neoplastic cells were strongly immunoreactive to MUC5AC (**d**) and negative/weakly positive to MUC6 in (**e**), negative to MUC2 and CD10 (not show) but positive to p16 in (**f**), CDX2 in (**g**), Ki67 in (**h**), and p53 in (**i**)

Adenoma

In the gastric cardia, most dysplastic or intraepithelial lesions show the foveolar features with papillary and tubular growth patterns (Fig. 6.23).

Dysplastic epithelial cells are immature with hyperchromatic, round-oval, enlarged, cuboidal, and crowded nuclei and eosinophilic cytoplasm. By immunohistochemistry, these neoplastic cells may show immunoreactivity for MUC5AC but negative to CD10, MUC2, and MUC6 [17, 18]. Those cells are also immunoreactive to p16, p53, Ki67, and CDX2 (Fig. 6.23). A minority of intraepithelial lesions in the gastric cardia may demonstrate the intestinal-type adenomatous phenotype and also the features of pyloric gland adenoma. Pyloric gland adenoma in the gastric cardia may exhibit the clear cell morphology with ground-glass-like cytoplasm and small bland but crowded nuclei and prominent nucleoli. These cells are immunoreactive to MUC6. Although rare in daily practice, pyloric gland adenoma was reported to

Table 6.4 Differential diagnosis of adenomas in the gastric cardia

Feature	Intestinal	Foveolar	Pyloric gland	Reference
Nuclei	Enlarged, cigar, pleomorphic	Enlarged, round/oval	Bland, crowded	[17, 19]
Cytoplasm	Hyperchromatic	Clear/pale eosinophilic	Clear	[17, 19]
Immunostain				
MUC5AC	Negative	Positive	Positive	[17, 19]
CD10, MUC 2	Positive	Negative	Negative	[17, 19]
CDX2	Strongly positive	Weakly positive	Negative	[17, 19]
MUC6	Negative	Negative/weakly positive	Positive	[19]
MLH1	Present	Present	Absent	[19]
Lynch syndrome	Unknown	Unknown	Present	[19]

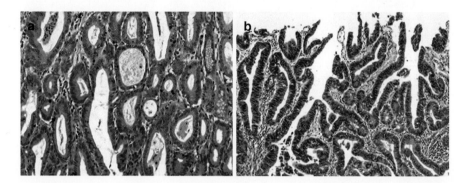

Fig. 6.24 Comparison between foveolar (**a**) and intestinal (**b**) adenomas. Nuclei in (**a**) are oval-round with vesicular chromatin patterns; cytoplasm is eosinophilic, in contrast to intestinal-type adenoma in (**b**) with cigar-shaped nuclei and basophilic cytoplasm, mimicking colorectal tubular adenoma

account for 20% of cases with Lynch syndrome in the gastric cardia [19]. Table 6.4 shows differential diagnostic features among intestinal, foveolar, and pylori gland adenomas in the gastric cardia (Fig. 6.24).

Cardiac Gland Duct Adenoma

In the gastric cardia, there exists a mucous epithelium-lined multilayered gland duct-like structure that has not been well characterized but may show hyperplastic changes, as shown in Chap. 2. This common but poorly understood structure may undergo neoplastic proliferation as demonstrated in Fig. 6.25 in a 65-year-old patient who was found at upper endoscopy, a broad-based polypoid lesion right below the gastroesophageal junction. The lesion was completely resected by endoscopic mucosal resection. The entire lesion exhibited an expansible growth pattern with proliferative gland ducts containing Alcian blue-positive mucin. The lining cells were

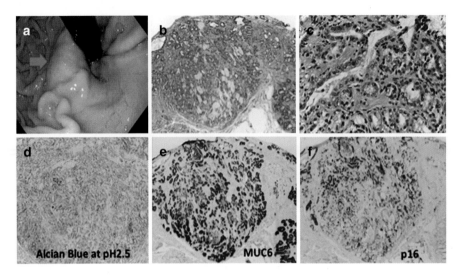

Fig. 6.25 Gastric cardiac gland duct-like adenoma presented as a broad-based polypoid lesion (0-Ip) immediately below the gastroesophageal junction at retroflex view of upper endoscopy (**a**, arrow). The resected lesion was well circumscribed with an expansible growth pattern and a pushing border above the muscularis mucosae (**b**). Neoplastic epithelial cells were uniform as a part of the duct-like network embedded in an eosinophilic stroma rich in hyperplastic smooth muscle and collagen fiber (**c**). The lumen of glands/ducts contained alkaline mucin highlighted by an Alcian blue stain at pH2.5 (**d**). By immunohistochemistry, neoplastic epithelial cells were immunoreactive to MUC6 (**e**), p16 (**f**), and also to (not shown here) CK7, rarely MUC5AC and Ki67 (about 2%); immunostains were negative for CK20, CDX2, MUC2, and p53 (not shown here)

immunoreactive to CK7, MUC6, and p16, rarely also to p63, but negative to CK20, CDX2, MUC2, p53, and Ki67. The morphologic evidence suggestive of malignancy such as atypical mitosis, necrosis, and nuclear pleomorphism was absent.

Low-Grade Intraepithelial Neoplasia or Dysplasia

At this stage of neoplastic epithelial proliferation, the overall architecture of the lesion mucosa remains intact or shows minimal changes, but the dysplastic glands are crowded, and the stroma between glands is reduced (Fig. 6.26). The lesion may be tubular or papillary and involves the mucosal surface epithelium. The dysplastic epithelial nuclei are enlarged, hyperchromatic, and pleomorphic but remain basally located with no evidence of pseudostratification. Mitosis may be frequent, and cytoplasm is immature. The nuclear-to-cytoplasm ratio is increased. Neoplastic cells usually show strong immunoreactivity to p53 with a high Ki67 index. However, in some cases, p53 immunostain is completely negative with a null expression pattern (Fig. 6.27).

For the patient with a pathologic diagnosis of low-grade intraepithelial neoplasm or dysplasia, clinical and endoscopic follow-up is required with a biopsy in

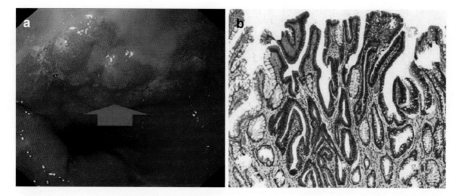

Fig. 6.26 Low-grade intraepithelial neoplasm or dysplasia presented as broad-based elevated lesion (arrow) in the gastric cardia at upper endoscopy (**a**, courtesy of Professor Shuxin Tian of Xingjian Shi-He-Zi Medical College in China). Microscopically, the lesion was characterized with a sharp transition from the adjacent nonneoplastic foveolar epithelium with extensive intestinal metaplasia in the gastric cardia (**b**)

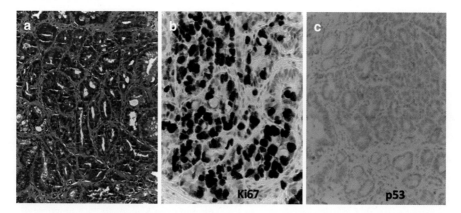

Fig. 6.27 Low-grade dysplastic lesion (**a**) showed strong and high immunoreactivity to Ki67 (**b**) but a null expression pattern for p53 (**c**)

6–12 months. Although regression of a low-grade lesion has been reported, the true incidence of such regression remains controversial because of the frequent overdiagnosis of low-grade dysplasia among general pathologists who do not have extensive experience in gastrointestinal pathology.

High-Grade Intraepithelial Neoplasia or Dysplasia

Once a low-grade dysplastic lesion progresses and demonstrates pronounced architectural disarray with nuclear pseudostratification to the luminal portion of the neoplastic epithelium, and numerous mitosis, especially in atypical forms, the lesion is

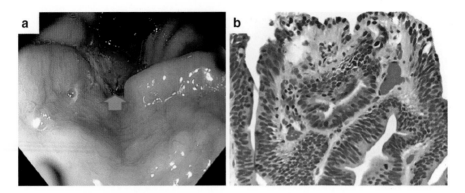

Fig. 6.28 A broad-based polypoid tumor (arrow) was located in the gastric cardia right below the gastroesophageal junction (**a**). The tumor in the endoscopic mucosal resection specimen demonstrated high-grade dysplasia (**b**) with immature neoplastic epithelium, marked nuclear dysplasia, brisk mitosis, and pseudostratification toward the surface of the epithelium

Table 6.5 Pathologic differential diagnosis between low- and high-grade intraepithelial neoplasia

Feature	Low-grade neoplasia	High-grade neoplasia
Architectural disarray	No or minimal	Marked
Nuclear dysplasia	Mild	Marked
Hyperchromasia	Present	Present
Pleomorphism	Mild	Marked
Mitosis	Present	Numerous
Atypical mitosis	Rare	Common
Apoptosis/necrosis	Rare	Common
Pseudostratification	Absent	Present
Cytoplasm reduction	Mild	Marked
Cellular immaturity	Mild	Marked

diagnosed as high-grade (Fig. 6.28). At this stage of carcinogenesis, neoplastic cells are hyperchromatic nuclei with a high nuclear-to-cytoplasmic ratio and prominent amphophilic cytoplasm. Importantly, nuclei are crowded and markedly pleomorphic. Nuclear polarity is usually lost. Although definitive invasion into the stroma is absent for a lesion with high-grade dysplasia, the patient management strategy is similar at present to that of intramucosal carcinoma. A high-grade dysplastic lesion in the stomach may be safely resected endoscopically rather than open surgically for both diagnostic and therapeutic purposes. In gastric resection specimens with a biopsy diagnosis of high-grade dysplasia, focal invasive intramucosal carcinoma is frequently identified somewhere in the same resection specimen, as also well-known for surgically resected Barrett's high-grade dysplasia that frequently shows a minute focus of an invasive component embedded in a high-grade dysplastic lesion [20]. Therefore, a pathologic distinction between low- and high-grade intraepithelial lesions becomes very important clinically and crucial for optimal patient triage (Table 6.5) but not so demanding between high-grade dysplasia and intramucosal carcinoma in the stomach.

Basal Crypt Dysplasia

Traditional teaching in anatomical pathology holds that if intraepithelial neoplasia or dysplasia maintains nuclear polarity without involvement of the surface epithelium, the lesion should not be classified as low- or high-grade dysplasia. This doctrine has been challenged recently because of the discovery of dysplastic glands involving the basal but not surface portion of a crypt(s) [21, 22]. Microscopically, gastric basal crypt dysplasia is therefore defined as the presence of epithelial nuclear dysplasia in the basal portion of a crypt without the involvement of the surface epithelium (Fig. 6.29).

The characteristics of epithelial dysplasia, such as nuclear enlargement, pleomorphism, hyperchromasia, pseudostratification, increased nuclear-to-cytoplasmic ratio, and frequent mitoses, are similar in both low- and high-grade dysplasia but more pronounced in a high-grade lesion. In the adjacent tissue, significant acute inflammation and surface regenerative atypia are usually absent or minimal. By immunohistochemistry, neoplastic basal crypt usually shows strong immunoreactivity to Ki67 and p53 (Fig. 6.29c). According to a most recent pathology study in Korean patients [22], the prevalence of basal crypt dysplasia is 21.6% (11/51) in the upper stomach including the cardia, much lower than that (78.4%) (40/51) in the distal non-cardiac region. At endoscopy, most (70.6%, 36/51) cases were elevated; flat and depressed patterns accounted for only 29.4% [22]. It must be emphasized that the diagnosis of dysplasia is primarily based on nuclear and architectural features; the interpretation of p53 immunostaining must be placed in the context of morphologic, clinical, and endoscopic features (Fig. 6.30).

Invasive Early Cardiac Carcinoma

In small GCC with the size of 2 cm or less, the location of the primary tumor can be accurately determined. According to a recent single-center study in Chinese patients, small GCC accounted for about one quarter of all small gastric cancer radical

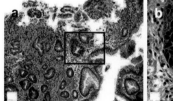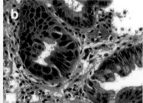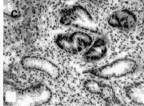

Fig. 6.29 Basal crypt dysplasia in the gastric cardia features dysplastic changes in the basal, not superficial, crypts in (**a**). The squared area in (**a**) is enlarged in (**b**) to show characteristic dysplastic changes. The dysplastic epithelial nuclei of basal glands are strongly immunoreactive to p53 compared to the wild-type expression of p53 in adjacent non-dysplastic glands in (**c**), supporting the diagnosis of basal crypt dysplasia in this case

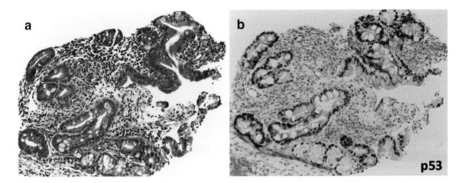

Fig. 6.30 Marked glandular reactive/reparative atypia in the gastric cardiac glands in response to acute and chronic inflammation and erosion (**a**) should not be overdiagnosed as dysplasia solely based on p53 immunoreactivity (**b**)

Fig. 6.31 Intramucosal carcinoma with extensive intraluminal necrotic debris

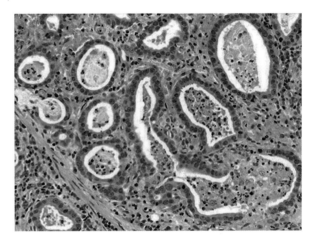

gastrectomy cases [4]. Most small GCCs were located in the lesser curvature side with the epicenter in the cardia (Fig. 6.5), in which columnar-lined esophagus was uncommon. Similar distribution patterns of early GCC have been reported [3].

Intramucosal Carcinoma

By definition, intramucosal carcinoma differs from high-grade intraepithelial neoplasia or dysplasia by the presence of the morphologic evidence of invasion such as desmoplastic reaction and marked architectural disarray. Nuclear dysplasia is much more conspicuous. The neoplastic nuclei are usually cuboidal and markedly enlarged with hyperchromasia and pleomorphism and show abundant mitosis, often in atypical forms. Intraluminal necrotic debris is also a common feature (Fig. 6.31). The nuclear-to-cytoplasmic ratio is high. Nucleoli are large and amphiphilic.

Nuclear polarity is lost with pseudostratification in the neoplastic epithelium. The risk of lymphovascular invasion is high. In EGCC, the most common histology type is tubular adenocarcinoma (50.4%), similar to that in early gastric non-cardiac carcinoma [3], according to one report in Chinese patients [3]. However, the proportion of early papillary adenocarcinoma is significantly higher in the gastric cardia (32.1%) than in gastric non-cardiac regions (12.1%) [3]. Both tubular and papillary adenocarcinomas in the stomach are grouped as the "intestinal" (versus "diffuse," according to the Lauren classification) or "differentiated" (versus "undifferentiated," based on the Japanese classification) type of gastric carcinomas [23, 24].

Tubular Adenocarcinoma

Microscopically, a pathologic diagnosis of early tubular adenocarcinoma requires two essential histology features: (1) marked nuclear dysplastic changes with hyperchromasia, nuclear enlargement in the size of 3–4 naïve small lymphocytes, high nuclear-to-cytoplasmic ratio, marked pleomorphism, increased mitotic figures, especially with atypical forms, prominent nucleoli, and cellular immaturity and (2) pronounced architectural abnormalities with a spectrum of growth patterns at low-power view, such as anastomosing (Fig. 6.32), fusing (Fig. 6.33), cribriforming

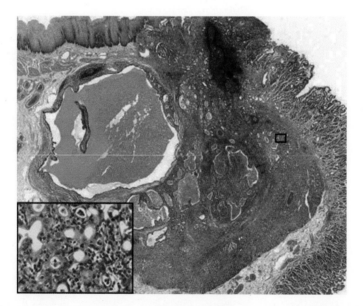

Fig. 6.32 Early gastric cardiac carcinoma in a 68-year-old Chinese man arose in the esophagogastric junctional region and invaded into the submucosa with a sharp pushing border. Microscopically, the tumor showed the predominant anastomosis pattern (insert in the left lower corner, taken from the squared area on the right). Note prominent lymphoid follicles on the right upper. Barrett's esophagus-related lesions are characteristically absent in the proximal esophageal squamous mucosa in this case [4]

96   Q. Huang

(Fig. 6.34), budding (Fig. 6.35), back-to-back crowding (Fig. 6.36), microcysts (Fig. 6.37), disunion (Fig. 6.38), clear cell changes (Fig. 6.39), solid pattern (Fig. 6.40), lacy appearance (Fig. 6.41), spiky glands with sharp projections (Fig. 6.42), single-cell clusters (Fig. 6.43), abortive glands (Fig. 6.44), and necrotic debris in the gland lumens. At the early stage, tubular adenocarcinoma in the gastric cardia may present in a pure form in the majority of cases, whereas a substantial proportion of cases show a mixed minor component(s) such as papillary, mucinous, and signet-ring cell carcinomas. Recognition of the morphologic characteristics of early tubular adenocarcinoma is essential for pathologic diagnosis in small biopsies to guide patient triage and management, as most patients with early tubular adeno-carcinoma are treated by endoscopic, rather than surgical, resection at present.

Fig. 6.33 Intramucosal carcinoma with fused neoplastic glands infiltrating into the lamina propria

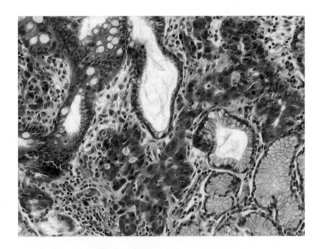

Fig. 6.34 Intramucosal carcinoma with the cribriform growth pattern

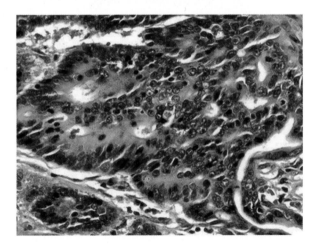

Fig. 6.35 Intramucosal
carcinoma with neoplastic
glands and cells budding
through the basement
membrane into the lamina
propria

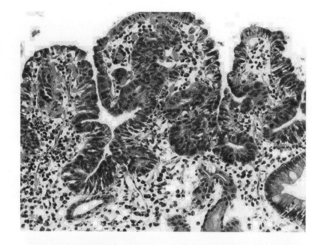

Fig. 6.36 Intramucosal
carcinoma with the
back-to-back pattern

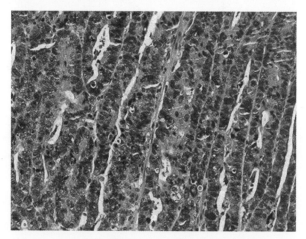

Fig. 6.37 Intramucosal
carcinoma with the
microcyst growth pattern.
Note the marked variation
of the cysts in size, nuclear
dysplasia of the epithelial
cells, and intraluminal
necrotic debris

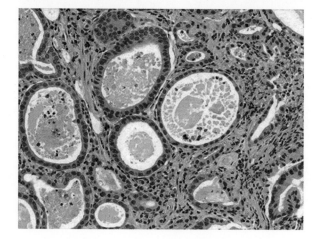

Fig. 6.38 Early gastric
cardiac carcinoma, with
the disunion growth
pattern, invaded the
superficial submucosa with
marked desmoplastic
reaction. The squared area
in (**a**) is enlarged in (**b**)

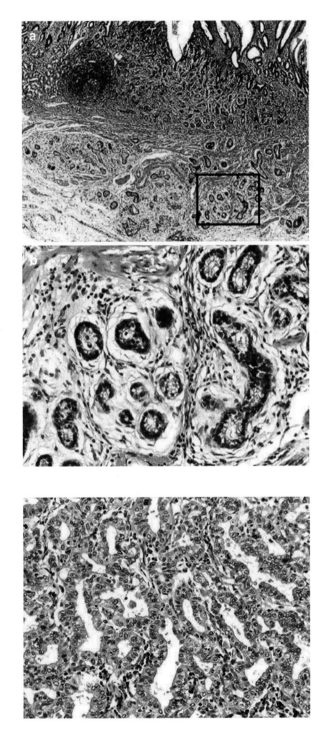

Fig. 6.39 Intramucosal
carcinoma with clear cell
changes

Fig. 6.40 Early gastric cardiac carcinoma invaded the submucosa with a solid growth pattern. Note one atypical mitotic figure

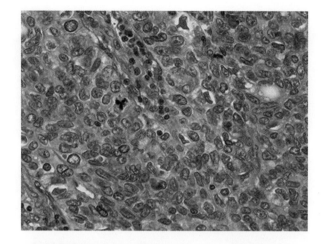

Fig. 6.41 Intramucosal carcinoma is composed of angulated, irregular, dilated glands filled with mucus and in an infiltrative lacy growth pattern

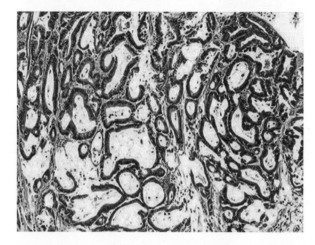

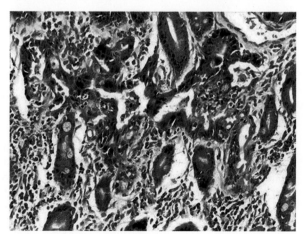

Fig. 6.42 Intramucosal carcinoma with the spiky lateral growth pattern, infiltrated the lamina propria

Fig. 6.43 Intramucosal
carcinoma was confined in
the upper lamina propria
with single dysplastic cells
and glands and invaded the
lamina propria

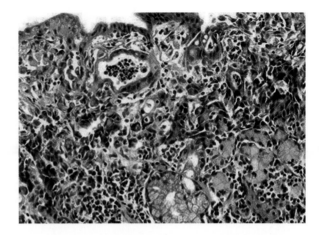

Fig. 6.44 Intramucosal
carcinoma was composed
of abortive glands in an
infiltrative growth pattern,
invading into the
muscularis mucosae

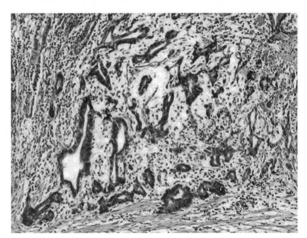

Papillary Adenocarcinoma

Papillary adenocarcinoma is characterized by finger-like projections on the mucosal surface, which is lined by neoplastic columnar cells surrounding a fibrovascular core. Oftentimes in the gastric cardia, early papillary adenocarcinoma may show villiform (Fig. 6.45) and serrated patterns (Fig. 6.46) and occasionally with a minor component of micropapillary and tubular growth patterns in some tumors. Recent studies in clinicopathology of early papillary adenocarcinoma have demonstrated the evidence for worse prognosis (Fig. 6.47) with deeper penetration and higher frequency of lymphovascular invasion and nodal metastasis, compared to early tubular adenocarcinoma [25–27]. Early study in 2000 by Yasuda et al. showed a high (14%, 9/65) rate of liver metastasis in Japanese patients with papillary adeno-carcinoma and a significantly worse 5-year survival rate (63%, versus 76% in non-papillary carcinomas) [26]. More recently, Lee et al. reported a high (18.3%, 9/49) frequency of lymph node metastasis in early papillary adenocarcinoma of Korean patients [27]. The abovementioned results have been confirmed most recently in

Fig. 6.45 Early papillary gastric cardiac carcinoma with the villiform growth pattern

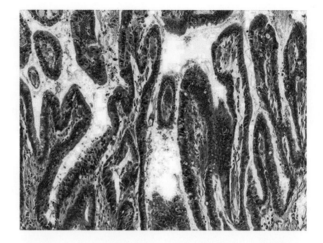

Fig. 6.46 Early papillary adenocarcinoma with an intraluminal serrated pattern

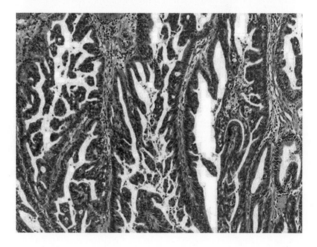

Fig. 6.47 The Kaplan-Meier survival analysis demonstrated worse prognosis for patients with early papillary adenocarcinoma than those with early tubular adenocarcinoma [25]

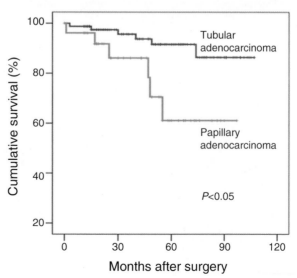

Chinese patients [3, 25, 28]. Compared to early tubular adenocarcinoma, early papillary adenocarcinoma is associated with a significantly worse 5-year survival rate (80.5%, compared to 96.8% in early tubular adenocarcinoma, $p < 0.05$), significantly more frequent submucosal invasion (64.4% versus 43.6%) ($p < 0.05$), and the micropapillary growth pattern (6.8% vs. 0) ($p < 0.003$) [25, 27]. The cases with a micropapillary growth pattern were all associated with early papillary adenocarcinoma and had a high (50%, 2/4) nodal metastasis rate, though in a small sample [3, 28]. Thus, a growing body of evidence suggests a dismal prognosis in early papillary adenocarcinoma, primarily due to deeper invasion, higher association with the micropapillary growth pattern, and more frequent lymphovascular invasion and nodal metastasis. Apparently, early papillary adenocarcinoma in the gastric cardia should be taken seriously with regard to making the decision for endoscopic resection of this early carcinoma.

Micropapillary Adenocarcinoma

Micropapillary adenocarcinoma is defined as small pseudopapillary tumor clusters in at least 5% of the estimated total tumor volume without fibrovascular cores and characteristically surrounded by empty lacuna spaces (Fig. 6.48) [3, 29]. Extensive nodal metastasis with lymphovascular invasion has been reported in up to 50% of cases ($N = 2/4$) with early micropapillary adenocarcinoma in a Chinese patient population [3]. A most recent case report demonstrated a GCC tumor composed of primarily micropapillary adenocarcinoma with a minor component of tubular and papillary growth patterns, invading into the distal esophagus in a 71-year-old Japanese man [30]. The tumor was resected with curative intent and found to arise in the cardia, centered at 2.5 cm below the esophagogastric junction, and showed widespread submucosal invasion, as shown in a Chinese patient in Fig. 6.49.

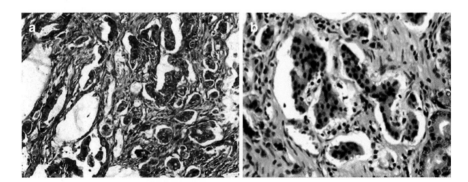

Fig. 6.48 Micropapillary early gastric cardiac carcinoma in (**a**) showed characteristic peri-micropapillary empty lacunar spaces, in contrast to physical injury-induced peri-epithelial empty spaces in (**b**), in which the nuclei of epithelial cells were pyknotic and degenerated, compared to those of reactive, benign epithelial cells in the right lower corner. Image (**b**) courtesy of Yuqing Cheng, MD, Changzhou Second Hospital in Changzhou, China

Fig. 6.49 Micropapillary gastric cardiac adenocarcinoma is associated superficial submucosal invasion

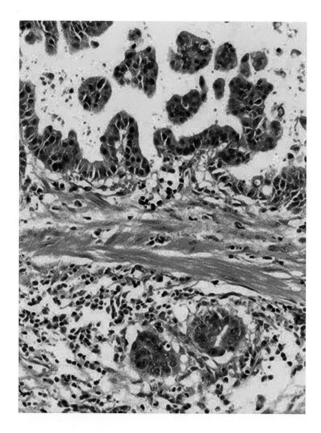

Micropapillary adenocarcinoma has been shown to have a high tendency for lymphovascular invasion and metastasis to the locoregional lymph nodes and the liver [30]. As shown in Chinese patients [10], no morphologic evidence of Barrett's esophagus is identified in this Japanese case. Those cases with micropapillary adenocarcinoma in the cardia, although in small number, illustrate the very aggressive nature of this type of carcinoma in the gastric cardia.

Poorly Cohesive and Signet-Ring Cell Carcinomas

The WHO defines poorly cohesive carcinoma as a group of tumors with discohesive, isolated, and small aggregates of neoplastic cells [1]. This group of carcinoma is uncommon in the gastric cardia and accounts for about 5.3% of EGCC, significantly fewer than that (35.8%) of EGC in the gastric non-cardiac regions [3]. By histology, poorly cohesive carcinoma includes both non-signet-ring and signet-ring cell carcinomas that are well-known for dismal prognosis with high risk of nodal and distant metastases.

By definition, signet-ring cell carcinoma is composed of predominantly neoplastic signet-ring cells with a centrally located clear, globoid droplet of cytoplasmic mucin and an eccentrically placed hyperchromatic, dysplastic nucleus (Fig. 6.50). These mucin-containing neoplastic cells originate in the upper portion of the mucosa, may grow in a lace-like glandular or trabecular pattern, and infiltrate from the top down to the muscularis mucosae; once invading into the submucosal space and beyond, it initiates prominent stromal desmoplastic reaction. These neoplastic signet-ring cells have to be distinguished from the foamy histiocytes in the lamina propria (Fig. 6.51).

Non-signet-ring cell poorly cohesive carcinoma is composed of discohesive neoplastic cells with eosinophilic or hyperchromatic nuclei, resembling histiocytes and lymphocytes, featuring irregular, bizarre, and pleomorphic dysplastic nuclei and often mixed with scattered mucin-containing signet-ring cells (Fig. 6.52).

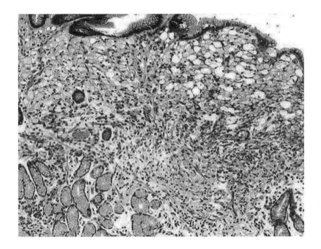

Fig. 6.50 Intramucosal signet-ring cell carcinoma confined to the upper lamina propria with characteristic cytoplasmic mucin droplets that push dysplastic nuclei to the edge of the cells. Note that signet-ring cells were present primarily in the subepithelial, upper half of the lamina propria

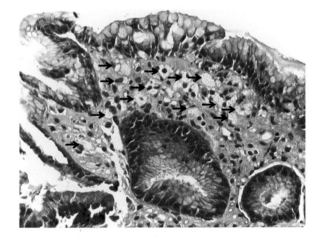

Fig. 6.51 Foamy histiocytes (arrows) in the lamina propria mimic signet-ring cells. Note the round, bland nuclei and foamy cytoplasm with uniform intracytoplasmic lipid-containing microvesicles

Fig. 6.52 Poorly cohesive carcinoma in the gastric cardia featured discohesive neoplastic cells with eosinophilic or signet-ring-like cytoplasm and pleomorphic, hyperchromatic nuclei. Note a residual benign gland in the right upper corner

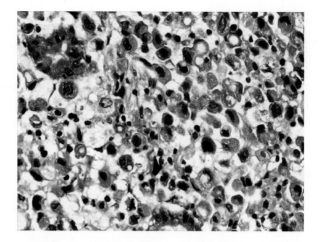

Uncommon Types of Early Gastric Cardiac Carcinoma

In the gastric cardia, uncommon types of EGC such as mucinous, adenosquamous, and neuroendocrine carcinomas, carcinoma with lymphoid stroma, hepatoid adenocarcinoma, and pancreatic acinar-like adenocarcinoma are more (11.5%) frequently encountered than those (3.6%) of EGC in the non-cardiac regions [3]. Those uncommon tumors are often discovered at advanced stages, which will be presented in Chap. 7. Although detailed molecular pathogenesis mechanisms remain unknown, the presence of residual embryonic opportunistic cells in the esophagogastric junction may be responsible for the much wider histologic spectrum of EGC in the gastric cardia, as opposed to that in the non-cardiac regions [31]. The results of a Chinese retrospective clinicopathologic study on EGC suggest no increased risk of lymph node metastasis for these uncommon types of EGC in the gastric cardia, compared to those in the gastric non-cardiac regions [3].

Important Characteristics of Early Gastric Cardiac Carcinoma

The results of clinicopathologic and endoscopic studies from Japan ($N = 49$) and China ($N = 131$) on early GCC show the following distinctly significant clinicopathologic and endoscopic characteristics [2, 3]:

1. Elderly male predominance and no patients younger than 40 years old
2. More polypoid protruded and fewer excavated macroscopic growth patterns in early GCC than those in early non-cardiac carcinomas
3. Better histological differentiation
4. A wider morphologic spectrum but fewer signet-ring cell carcinomas, compared to early non-cardiac carcinomas

5. Deeper invasion but fewer lymph node metastases (2.9%, compared to 16.7% in early non-cardiac carcinoma)
6. Lower frequency of *H. pylori* infection
7. Significant association with pancreatic metaplasia

Those findings may have significant impact upon clinical patient management strategy. Due to unique fibromuscular hyperplasia with double-layered muscularis mucosae frequently observed only in the gastric cardia, early tubular GCC is often associated with an unusually thickened submucosal layer, in which malignant neoplastic glands infiltrate deep and are surrounded by hyperplastic smooth muscle fibers, mimicking invasion into the muscularis propria. As shown in Fig. 6.53, the

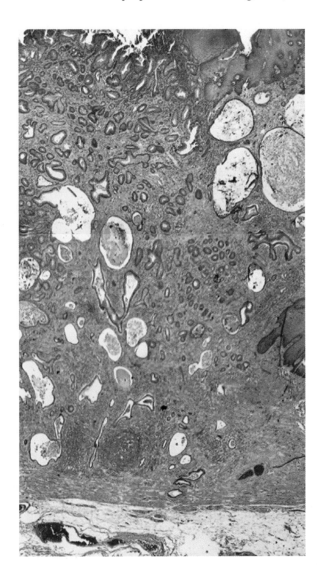

Fig. 6.53 Well-differentiated early tubular gastric cardiac carcinoma invaded into the deep submucosal layer (SM2) with a sharp invasion front and a total of 6 mm in depth from the tumor surface to the deep edge. Malignant neoplastic glands were surrounded by smooth muscle fibers and initiated desmoplastic reaction

Fig. 6.54 Invasion of well-differentiated tubular adenocarcinoma, sampled from Fig. 6.53, into the hyperplastic muscularis mucosae, not muscularis propria, in the gastric cardia. Note the interlacing hyperplastic smooth muscular fiber growth pattern. Malignant glands featured marked nuclear hyperchromasia, pleomorphism, and intraluminal necrosis

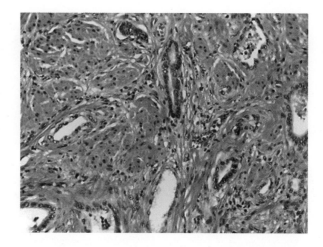

total thickness of this well-differentiated early tubular GCC is 6 mm in depth. The neoplastic glands are surrounded by smooth muscle fibers with stromal desmoplastic reaction. Therefore, one of pitfalls in the biopsy diagnosis of tumors in the gastric cardia is to accurately recognize this unique characteristic of early tubular GCC and prevent overdiagnosis of tumor invasion into the muscularis propria (Fig. 6.54).

Other Neoplastic Polyps in the Gastric Cardia

At endoscopy, many polypoid, broad-based, protruding lesions may mimic early GCC. Differential diagnosis requires a thorough understanding of underlying pathology of those polypoid lesions, including adenomatous polyp and mesenchymal tumors such as leiomyoma and gastrointestinal stromal tumor (GIST).

Adenomatous Polyp

In the gastric cardia, adenomatous polyps consist of intestinal, gastric foveolar, and pyloric gland types. The morphologic and immunophenotypical features are the same as those in non-cardiac regions.

Leiomyoma

In the gastric cardia, leiomyoma is the most common mesenchymal tumor, twice as frequent as GIST [32–34]. In the surgical resection specimens for carcinoma in the esophagogastric junction, small (<1 cm in size) leiomyomas are common incidental

Fig. 6.55 Leiomyoma of the gastric cardia was characterized with nodular proliferation of smooth muscle with the plump eosinophilic cells similar to the adjacent smooth muscle cells in the muscularis propria

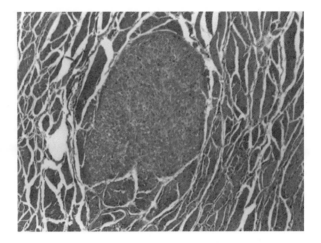

findings (Fig. 6.55). In a case-series study, incidental CD117- and CD34-negative minute leiomyomas were detected in 47% of patients with a mean of three leiomyomas per patient and a mean size of 1.7 mm (range 0.2–12 mm) [33]. Most leiomyomas are seated deep in the inner muscularis propria [33] and are endophytic [34]. In a retrospective single-center study of gastric submucosal lesions from Korea, small leiomyoma was reported most common in the gastric cardia with the frequency of 55.2–63.6%, significantly higher than that in any other gastric locations [32–34]. The histomorphologic and immunophenotypical features of leiomyoma in the cardia are straightforward for the diagnosis. Interestingly, a most recent study from Korea reported perilesional lymphadenopathy was associated only with GIST or schwannomas but not with leiomyoma [34]. The much higher incidence of small leiomyoma and GIST tumors in the cardia without clinical significance suggests different genetic and epigenetic tumorigenesis mechanisms for those common gastric mesenchymal tumors in the cardia.

Gastrointestinal Stromal Tumor (GIST)

In the gastric cardia, GIST is the second most common mesenchymal tumor [32–34], although accounts for only 8.1% (21/258) of all gastric GISTs. In that seminal paper, Abraham et al. reported about 10% (15/150) prevalence of small GIST tumors in the EGJ region with an average size of 1.3 mm (range: 0.2–2.0 mm), all of which arose in the muscularis propria [33]. By histology, all small GIST tumors featured spindle cell morphology with immunoreactivity to CD34 and CD117. There was no significant nuclear pleomorphism. These tumors were too small to be symptomatic, and most were incidental findings at diagnosis. In contrast, for symptomatic GISTs in the cardia, the tumors were large with a mean size of 5 cm and prone to occur in elderly patients without significant difference in gender [34]. By histology, the

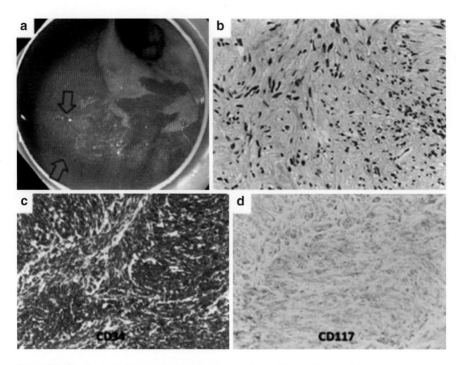

Fig. 6.56 Gastric gastrointestinal stromal tumor in the cardia in a 68-year-old man, presented at upper endoscopy as a slightly elevated protruding lesion (arrows) in the cardia below the squamo-columnar junction (**a**). Note the tongue-like columnar metaplastic lesion in the distal esophagus. The tumor was resected endoscopically, measured 0.3 × 0.3 × 0.2 cm in size, and showed the spindle cell morphology (**b**). No mitosis/necrosis was identified. By immunohistochemistry, neoplastic cells were strongly immunoreactive to CD34 (**c**) and weakly positive to CD117 (**d**). The Ki67 index was about 1%

GIST tumor in the gastric cardia was characterized by interlacing bundles of bland spindle cells without mitosis or necrosis. By immunohistochemistry, these spindle cells were reactive to both CD34 and CD117 (Fig. 6.56). In the gastric cardia, collision tumor with both tubular adenocarcinoma and a minute (0.6 cm) GIST has been described in a case report [35]. Surprisingly, the dedicated clinicopathologic studies on GIST tumors in the cardia remain rare.

Neuroendocrine Tumor of Gastric Cardia

Neuroendocrine tumors of the stomach are grouped into four types with similar location, morphology, and immunophenotypical profiles but different presentations and therapies (Table 6.6) [1, 36].

Most neuroendocrine tumors of the stomach are nonfunctional and well-differentiated, also known as typical carcinoid, and occur primarily in the gastric

Table 6.6 Four types of neuroendocrine tumors in the stomach

Type	I	II	III	IV
Prevalence (%)	80	5	Rare	Very rare
Location	Fundus/body	Fundus/body	Antrum mainly	Any location
Size	Most are small (<1 cm)	Larger, 0.6–4.5 cm	May be large, >2 cm in one third	Large, fungating
Associated disease	Marked atrophic gastritis	MEN1 and Zollinger-Ellison syndrome	Sporadic, may not have inflammation	Similar to small-cell neuroendocrine carcinoma
Serum gastrin level	High	Moderate, but high if with neuroendocrine carcinoma	May increase; increased 5-hydroxy-trypsin level	Low
Differentiation	Well	Moderate	Moderate-poor	Very poor
Mitosis	0	0–2	May be >9/hpf	>10/hpf
Grade	Low	High	High	High
Ki67 index	Low	High	90–100%	100%
Prognosis	Rely on size/Ki67 index	Moderate	Moderate–poor	Very poor, penetrate through the wall, spread to the nodes and liver
Therapy	Endoscopic, if small	Endoscopic, if small	Surgical	Systemic

NOTE: *hpf* high-power field

body-fundus or antrum-body [1] but rare in the gastric cardia. The tumor is usually well-circumscribed and small. Neoplastic cells are usually uniform with the classical "salt-pepper" chromatin pattern, mild atypia, and the absence of mitosis. Cytoplasm is generally moderate, eosinophilic, and slightly granular. There should have no evidence of tumor necrosis. Neoplastic cells grow in a variety of patterns such as organoid, solid/nested, trabecular, glandular, microcystic, and papillary. Diagnosis is in general straightforward with typical immunoreactivity of neoplastic cells to chromogranin, CD56, and synaptophysin. Most tumors are benign with excellent prognosis. The strongest prognosis predictors include tumor size >1 cm, high stage, lymphovascular invasion, high mitotic index/Ki67 activity, and sporadic occurrence [1, 36], on the basis of a 5-year review of carcinoid tumors in the US National Cancer Institute and Surveillance, Epidemiology and End Results databases performed in 2003 [36]. The most favorable prognostic factors include size <1 cm, nonfunctioning, with chronic atrophic gastritis or Zollinger-Ellison syndrome or MEN-1 disease [1].

Proliferative Lesion of Cardiac Gland Ducts

In the gastric cardia, we encountered a polypoid protruding lesion in a 58-year-old man who did not have a history of gastroesophageal reflux disease. At upper endoscopy, a broad-based polypoid protruding lesion was detected in the gastric cardia

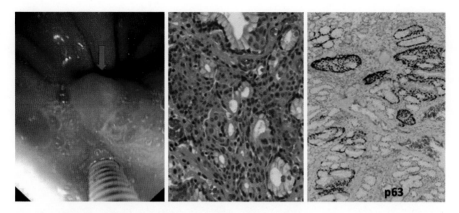

Fig. 6.57 At endoscopy (the far left), an broad-based protruding lesion was centered in the gastric cardia with smooth mucosal surface. After endoscopic resection, the lesion histology (middle) featured marked proliferation of the bland mucous gland ductal epithelium that was strongly immunoreactive to p63 (the far right), weakly reactive (wild-type expression) to p53 (not shown here). The Ki67 index was about 10% (not shown here)

below the esophagogastric junction in the maximum size of 1.5 cm. The lesion was resected endoscopically. Microscopically, the lesion was confined in the gastric cardia with proliferation of cardiac gland-ductal epithelium that was immunoreactive to p63, high molecular weight cytokeratin, and CK7 but negative to p53, CDX2, and CK20. The Ki67 index was about 10%. No nuclear dysplasia was noted. No mitosis was identified. There was no evidence of Barrett's esophagus-related lesions identified endoscopically and histopathologically. The significance of this lesion remains to be explored (Fig. 6.57).

Nonneoplastic Polyp

Hyperplastic Polyp

For gastric cardiac polyps in the American population, most (59.1%) are hyperplastic but not associated with Barrett's esophagus, gastroesophageal reflux disease, chemical gastropathy, or *H. pylori*-related gastritis [37]. These uncommon polyps are benign in nature. In the Chinese population, a hyperplastic polyp may be related to *H. pylori* infection or previous injury (Fig. 6.58).

Hamartomatous Polyposis Syndrome

This group of rare hamartomatous polyps includes Cowden polyps, juvenile polyposis syndrome, and Peutz-Jeghers polyps, as part of hereditary polyposis syndromes. Cowden polyps are small and frequently misdiagnosed as hyperplastic or inflammatory polyps. By histology, the polyp stroma may show chronic

Fig. 6.58 Hyperplastic polyp of the gastric cardia. Note the squamous epithelium of the esophagus was present on the right as the histology landmark of the esophagogastric junction

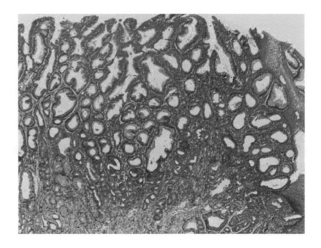

inflammation with lymphoid follicles, occasional ganglion cells, and fatty changes. Genetically, this polyp may be related to PTEN tumor suppressor gene mutation in about 80% cases [38].

Juvenile polyposis syndrome may exclusively involve the stomach and has been found to result from *smad*4 gene mutation in about 15% of cases and associated with Menetrier's disease [39]. Morphologically, the polyp features large sizes, surface erosion, stromal inflammation, and mucin-containing microcysts. The patients with juvenile polyposis syndrome are at increased (55%) risk for digestive track cancer [40].

Gastric Peutz-Jeghers polyps are extremely rare with few than 10 cases published in the English literature. A recent case report described a giant ($15 \times 7 \times 5$ cm) Peutz-Jeghers polyp located in the gastric cardia, surrounding the esophagogastric junction in a 43-year-old Caucasian woman presented with gastrointestinal bleeding and anemia. The polyp was resected and showed hyperplastic, multiple mucous microcysts along with extensive arborization of smooth muscle bundles in the mucosal and submucosal layers (Fig. 6.59) [41]. This polyp is related to the *STK11* gene mutation and has an 18-fold higher risk for malignancy. The statistically significant relative risk is found primarily in the digestive tract cancer, including 218-fold risk for gastric cancer, 57-fold for esophageal cancer, 520-fold for cancer of the small intestine, 84-fold for colorectal cancer, and 132-fold for pancreatic cancer [42]. The average age at diagnosis is 30 years old, and early diagnosis is crucial for optimal patient management [39, 42, 43]. Table 6.7 compares major clinicopathologic characteristics among those three major hamartomatous syndromic polyps.

In the McCune-Albright syndrome, a circumferential gastric cardiac polypoid adenoma with high-grade dysplasia has been described in a recent report. Multiple phenotypic features are present in the same tumor as a mixture of pyloric-, foveolar-, and intestinal-type adenomas [44].

Fig. 6.59 Giant Peutz-Jeghers polyp surrounded the esophagogastric junction and was centered in the gastric cardia [41]

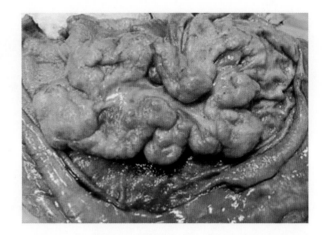

Table 6.7 Comparison in clinicopathology among Cowden syndrome (CS), juvenile polyposis syndrome (JP), and Peutz-Jeghers syndrome (PJS) [43]

Feature	CS ($n = 127$)	JP ($n = 88$)	PJS ($n = 103$)
Frequency in the stomach	12%	22%	18%
Mean size (cm)	0.35	1.06	0.54
Exophytic	12%	47%	44%
Surface erosion	3%	68%	4%
Chronic inflammation	41%	92%	88%
Stroma edema	24%	55%	54%
Mucin microcyst	36%	97%	90%
Stromal ganglion cells and fat	10–14%	0%	0%
Lymphoid follicle	50%	30%	21%
Marked smooth muscle proliferation	18%	8%	64%
Low-grade dysplasia	10%	14%	1%
Genetic mutation	PTEN	smad4	STK11/LKB1
Cancer risk	Low	Moderate	High

Gastritis Cystica Profunda

By definition, gastritis cystica profunda or polyposa is an irregular hyperplastic polyp characterized by misplaced foveolar or glandular epithelium beyond the lamina propria into deeper layers of the gastric wall, such as the muscularis mucosae, submucosa, and even muscularis propria (Fig. 6.60). The lesion has been frequently found in patients after partial gastrectomy and believed to result from the misplaced gastric glands at the anastomosis site [45]. However, in Korean and Chinese populations [3, 46, 47], this disease is often found in nonsurgical patients and most frequently in the gastric cardia, accounting for 9.1% (40/438) of all EGC resection

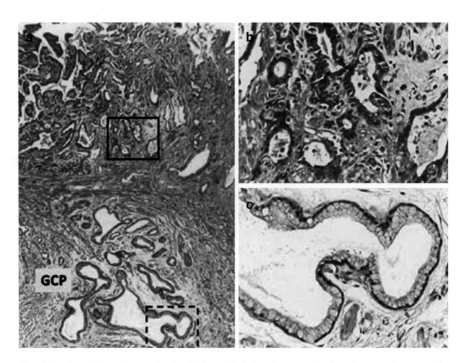

Fig. 6.60 Gastritis cystica profunda (GCP) on the left was located in the submucosal space without direct connection to the above intramucosal tubulopapillary adenocarcinoma in (**a**). The area outlined with a solid square in (**a**) was enlarged in (**b**) and showed tubular adenocarcinoma with markedly dysplastic nuclei, abortive and infiltrative glands. The GCP area outlined with the dashed square in (**a**) at the bottom was enlarged in (**c**) to illustrate benign, flat mucous epithelium without dysplastic changes. The stroma surrounding GCP was edematous. This patient did not have a history of gastric trauma or surgery

cases [3], and significantly more common in the gastric cardia (80%, 32/40) than in the non-cardiac region (20%, 8/40) [47]. The underlying pathogenesis mechanisms are unknown. According to a case-series study in a nonsurgical cohort [47], the lesion, under conventional white light upper endoscopy, is sessile, protruded with defined borders and eroded surface in 88.2% (15/17) cases, which is similar to hyperplastic polyps. By endoscopic ultrasonography, the lesion mean maximal dimension is 2.9 cm (range 0.5–8.5 cm) in the basal mucosa and the submucosal space. Microscopically, all 34 cohort cases exhibited similar morphology with characteristically ecstatically dilated glands lined by bland foveolar epithelium without nuclear dysplasia or mitosis. The lesion stroma is edematous with mild mixed mononuclear and some neutrophilic and eosinophilic infiltrate (Fig. 6.60). The dilated benign glands and microcysts appear originating in the basal mucosa and extending through the muscularis mucosae into the submucosal space but not into the muscularis propria in patients without prior gastrectomy history. Adjacent and overlying gastric mucosa shows chronic gastritis in all cases. In one study in Chinese patients, associated upper epithelial dysplasia was identified in 44.1% (15/34) cases

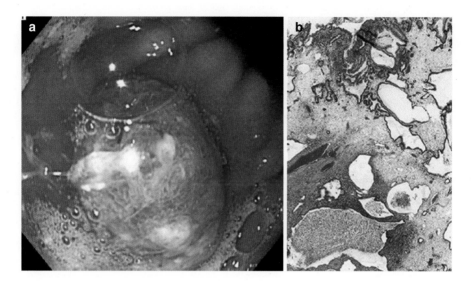

Fig. 6.61 A 77-year-old male patient with a history of gastroesophageal reflux disease treated with proton pump inhibitors for over 40 years presented with heartburn and anemia. At upper endoscopy, a well-circumscribed nodule was discovered in the gastric cardia (**a**) and endoscopically resected. Histology on the right showed an inflammation polyp with marked edema and abscess formation in microcysts (**b**)

with low- or high-grade dysplasia and intramucosal carcinoma in five cases for each disease [47]. Those features differ to some extent from the reported cases with prior gastrectomy history [45]. Whether or not gastritis cystica profunda is a premalignant lesion or associated with Epstein-Barr virus infection remains to be thoroughly worked out [48].

Inflammatory Polyp

In the gastric cardia, inflammatory polyp is uncommon, usually related to *H. pylori* infection. At endoscopy, the polyp is sessile, protruding with smooth surface and defined borders (Fig. 6.61). By histology, the stroma is frequently edematous with prominent neutrophilic and mononuclear cell infiltrate. Mucous glands are usually ecstatic to form microcysts that are often filled with neutrophils (Fig. 6.61).

Summary

EGCC occurs primarily in elderly male patients and most frequently demonstrates protruding polypoid appearances at upper endoscopy. Ulcerative lesions are uncommon. By histology, most EGCC tumors are tubular and papillary with a variety of growth patterns, such as anastomosing, budding, disunion, microcyst, lacy, back-to-back, solid, cribriforming, clear cells, spiky, and abortive glands, single-cell infiltration, villiform, serrated, and micropapillary patterns, among others. The most important histopathologic feature of EGCC is nuclear dysplasia with hyperchromasia, pleomorphism, high nuclear-to-cytoplasmic ratio, necrosis, and atypical mitosis. These changes have to be distinguished from reactive/reparative changes. Poorly cohesive carcinoma including signet-ring cell carcinoma is uncommon in EGCC. Although the preliminary study results from a handful of single-center studies suggest a lower risk for nodal metastasis in EGCC, compared to those in early distal non-cardiac carcinoma, the true risk factors for nodal metastasis in EGCC remain to be further investigated by multicenter studies to guide the optimal patient management decision-making process.

References

1. Lauwers GY, Carneiro F, Graham DY, et al. Gastric carcinoma. In: Bosman FT, Carneiro F, Hruban RH, Theise ND, editors. WHO classification of tumours of the digestive system. Lyon: IARC Press; 2010. p. 48–58.
2. Tajima Y, Nakanishi Y, Yoshino T, et al. Clinicopathologic study of early adenocarcinoma of the gastric cardia: comparison with early adenocarcinoma of the distal stomach and esophagus. Oncology. 2001;61:1–9.
3. Huang Q, Fang C, Shi J, et al. Differences in clinicopathology of early gastric carcinoma between proximal and distal location in 438 Chinese patients. Sci Rep. 2015;5:13439. https://doi.org/10.1038/srep13439.
4. Huang Q, Shi J, Sun Q, et al. Clinicopathologic characterization of small (≤ 2 cm) proximal and distal gastric carcinomas in a Chinese population. Pathology. 2015;47:526–32.
5. Cestari R, Villanacci V, Bassotti G, et al. The pathology of gastric cardia: a prospective, endoscopic, and morphologic study. Am J Surg Pathol. 2007;31(5):706–10.
6. Dixon MF, Genta RM, Yardley JH, Correa P. Classification and grading of gastritis. The updated Sydney System. International Workshop on the Histopathology of Gastritis, Houston 1994. Am J Surg Pathol. 1996;20(10):1161–81.
7. Reis CA, David L, Correa P, et al. Intestinal metaplasia of human stomach displays distinct patterns of mucin (MUC1, MUC2, MUC5AC, and MUC6) expression. Cancer Res. 1999;59(5):1003–7.
8. Abadir A, Streutker C, Brezden-Masley C, Grin A, Kim YI. Intestinal metaplasia and the risk of gastric cancer in an immigrant Asian population. Clin Med Insights Gastroenterol. 2012;5:43–50.
9. Aida J, Vieth M, Shepherd NA, et al. Is carcinoma in columnar-lined esophagus always located adjacent to intestinal metaplasia?: a histopathologic assessment. Am J Surg Pathol. 2015;39(2):188–96.
10. Huang Q, Fan X, Agoston AT, et al. Comparison of gastro-oesophageal junction carcinomas in Chinese versus American patients. Histopathology. 2011;59(2):188–97.
11. Al-Haddad S, Chang AC, De Hertogh G, et al. Adenocarcinoma at the gastroesophageal junction. Ann N Y Acad Sci. 2014;1325:211–25.
12. El-Zimaity HM, Ramchatesingh J, Saeed MA, Graham DY. Gastric intestinal metaplasia: subtypes and natural history. J Clin Pathol. 2001;54(9):679–83.

13. Schneider NI, Plieschnegger W, Geppert M, et al. Pancreatic acinar cells—a normal finding at the gastroesophageal junction? Data from a prospective Central European multicenter study. Virchows Arch. 2013;463(5):643–50.
14. Rugge M, Correa P, Dixon MF, et al. Gastric dysplasia: the Padova international classification. Am J Surg Pathol. 2000;24(2):167–76.
15. Schlemper RJ, et al. The Vienna classification of gastrointestinal epithelial neoplasia. Gut. 2000;47:251–5.
16. Schlemper RJ, Kato Y, Stolte M. Review of histological classifications of gastrointestinal epithelial neoplasia: differences in diagnosis of early carcinomas between Japanese and Western pathologists. J Gastroenterol. 2001;36(7):445–56.
17. Park DY, Srivastava A, Kim GH, et al. Adenomatous and foveolar gastric dysplasia: distinct patterns of mucin expression and background intestinal metaplasia. Am J Surg Pathol. 2008;32(4):524–33.
18. Park DY, Srivastava A, Kim GH, et al. CDX2 expression in the intestinal-type gastric epithelial neoplasia: frequency and significance. Mod Pathol. 2010;23(1):54–61.
19. Lee SE, Kang SY, Cho J, et al. Pyloric gland adenoma in Lynch syndrome. Am J Surg Pathol. 2014;38(6):784–92.
20. Cameron AJ, Carpenter HA. Barrett's esophagus, high-grade dysplasia, and early adenocarcinoma: a pathological study. Am J Gastroenterol. 1997;92(4):586–91.
21. Zhang XQ, Huang Q, Goyal K, Odze R. DNA Ploidy Abnormalities in basal and superficial regions of the crypts in Barrett's esophagus and associated neoplastic lesions. Am J Surg Pathol. 2008;32(9):1327–35.
22. Kim A, Ahn SJ, Park DY, et al. Gastric crypt dysplasia: a distinct subtype of gastric dysplasia with characteristic endoscopic features and immunophenotypic and biological anomalies. Histopathology. 2016;68(6):843–9.
23. Lauren P. The two histological main types of gastric carcinoma: diffuse and so-called intestinal-type carcinoma. An attempt at a histo-clinical classification. Acta Pathol Microbiol Scand. 1965;64:31–49.
24. Japanese Gastric Cancer Association. Japanese classification of gastric carcinoma: 3rd English edition. Gastric Cancer. 2011;14:101–12.
25. Yu HP, Fang C, Chen L, et al. Worse prognosis in papillary, compared to tubular, early gastric carcinoma. J Cancer. 2017;8(1):117–23.
26. Yasuda K, Adachi Y, Shiraishi N, Maeo S, Kitano S. Papillary adenocarcinoma of the stomach. Gastric Cancer. 2000;3:33–8.
27. Lee HJ, Kim GH, Park DY, et al. Is endoscopic submucosal dissection safe for papillary adenocarcinoma of the stomach? World J Gastroenterol. 2015;21:3944–52.
28. Fang C, Shi J, Sun Q, et al. Risk factors of lymph node metastasis in early gastric carcinomas diagnosed with WHO criteria in 379 Chinese patients. J Dig Dis. 2016;17(8):526–37.
29. Roh JH, Srivastava A, Lauwers GY, et al. Micropapillary carcinoma of stomach: a clinicopathologic and immunohistochemical study of 11 cases. Am J Surg Pathol. 2010;34(8):1139–46.
30. Hattori T, Sentani K, Hattori Y, Oue N, Yasui W. Pure invasive micropapillary carcinoma of the esophagogastric junction with lymph nodes and liver metastasis. Pathol Int. 2016;66(10):583–6.
31. Wang X, Ouyang H, Yamamoto Y, et al. Residual embryonic cells as precursors of a Barrett's-like metaplasia. Cell. 2011;145(7):1023–35.
32. Lee HH, Hur H, Jung H, Jeon HM, Park CH, Song KY. Analysis of 151 consecutive gastric submucosal tumors according to tumor location. J Surg Oncol. 2011;104(1):72–5.
33. Abraham SC, Krasinskas AM, Hofstetter WL, Swisher SG, Wu TT. "Seedling" mesenchymal tumors (gastrointestinal stromal tumors and leiomyomas) are common incidental tumors of the esophagogastric junction. Am J Surg Pathol. 2007;31(11):1629–35.
34. Min YW, Park HN, Min BH, Choi D, Kim KM, Kim S. Preoperative predictive factors for gastrointestinal stromal tumors: analysis of 375 surgically resected gastric subepithelial tumors. J Gastrointest Surg. 2015;19(4):631–8.

35. Idema DL, Daryanani D, Sterk LM, Klaase JM. Collision tumor of the stomach: a case of an adenocarcinoma and a gastrointestinal stromal tumor. Case Rep Gastroenterol. 2008;2(3):456–60.
36. Grin A, Streutker CJ. Neuroendocrine tumors of the luminal gastrointestinal tract. Arch Pathol Lab Med. 2015;139:750–6.
37. Melton SD, Genta RM. Gastric cardiac polyps: a clinicopathologic study of 330 cases. Am J Surg Pathol. 2010;34(12):1792–7.
38. Zbuk KM, Eng C. Hamartomatous polyposis syndromes. Nat Clin Pract Gastroenterol Hepatol. 2007;4:492–502.
39. Howe JR, Mitros FA, Summers RW. The risk of gastrointestinal carcinoma in familial juvenile polyposis. Ann Surg Oncol. 1998;5:751–6.
40. Burmester JK, Bell LN, Cross D, Meyer P, Yale SH. A *SMAD*4 mutation indicative of juvenile polyposis syndrome in a family previously diagnosed with Menetrier's disease. Dig Liver Dis. 2016;48(10):1255–9.
41. Lunca S, Porumb V, Velenciuc N, Ferariu D, Dimofte G. Giant solitary gastric Peutz-Jeghers polyp mimicking a malignant gastric tumor: the largest described in literature. J Gastrointestin Liver Dis. 2014;23(3):321–4.
42. Giardiello FM, Brensinger JD, Tersmette AC, et al. Very high risk of cancer in familial Peutz-Jeghers syndrome. Gastroenterology. 2000;119:1447–53.
43. Shaco-Levy R, Jasperson KW, Martin K, et al. Morphologic characterization of hamartomatous gastrointestinal polyps in Cowden syndrome, Peutz-Jeghers syndrome, and juvenile polyposis syndrome. Hum Pathol. 2016;49:39–48.
44. Wood LD, Noë M, Hackeng W, et al. Patients with McCune-Albright syndrome have a broad spectrum of abnormalities in the gastrointestinal tract and pancreas. Virchows Arch. 2017;470(4):391–400.
45. Franzin G, Novelli P. Gastritis cystica profunda. Histopathology. 1981;5:535–47.
46. Lee HJ, Lee TH, Lee JU, et al. Clinical features of gastritis cystica profunda in patients without history of gastric surgery. Gastric cancer patients vs. non-cancerous patients. Korean J Med. 2006;71:511–7.
47. Xu G, Peng C, Li X, et al. Endoscopic resection of gastritis cystica profunda: preliminary experience with 34 patients from a single center in China. Gastrointest Endosc. 2015;81(6):1493–8.
48. Choi MG, Jeong JY, Kim KM, et al. Clinical significance of gastritis cystica profunda and its association with Epstein-Barr virus in gastric cancer. Cancer. 2012;118(21):5227–33.

Chapter 7
Pathology of Advanced Gastric Cardiac Carcinoma Cancer

Qin Huang

Introduction

Once invading into the muscularis propria (pT2) and beyond, gastric cardiac carcinoma (GCC) becomes much more aggressive and is classified as advanced cancer. At this stage, GCC in some cases may invade the distal esophagus as a minor component (Fig. 7.1) [1, 2], also known as carcinoma of the gastroesophageal junction (GEJ).

Microscopically, GCC usually shows heterogeneous morphology, especially in large tumors with the size over 5 cm [1–3]. Compared to early GCC, most advanced GCC tumors are staged at pT3 and display a much wider histopathologic spectrum, characterized by the much more frequent presence of uncommon histologic subtypes than typical intestinal, diffuse, or mixed histology subtypes. Unlike GEJ carcinoma in Caucasian patients, the metaplastic Barrett's mucosa with goblet cells present in columnar-lined esophagus is rare or absent in most cases of GCC in Chinese patients [1]. In contrast to typical distal esophageal Barrett's adenocarcinoma with a tubular or papillary adenocarcinoma growth pattern in almost all cases [3–5], conventional intestinal tubular/papillary adenocarcinomas have been found in only 77% of advanced GCC in Chinese patients (Table 7.1) [1]. In earlier reports in American Caucasian patients [3–5], the epicenters of "esophageal adenocarcinomas" with uncommon histology subtypes, such as adenosquamous carcinoma, signet-ring cell carcinoma, mucinous carcinoma, etc., were mainly located below or straddling the GEJ; sometimes, the tumor was too large in size and completely obliterated the landmark of the GEJ, making a confident classification of esophageal or

Q. Huang (✉)
Pathology and Laboratory Medicine, Veterans Affairs Boston Healthcare System, West Roxbury, MA, USA

Harvard Medical School and Brigham and Women's Hospital, Boston, MA, USA

© Springer International Publishing AG, part of Springer Nature 2018   119
Q. Huang (ed.), *Gastric Cardiac Cancer*, https://doi.org/10.1007/978-3-319-79114-2_7

Fig. 7.1 Advanced gastric cardiac carcinoma with a large ulcerated surface invades, in a small component, into the distal esophagus where, however, no evidence of Barrett's esophagus can be identified in this Chinese patient. *GEJ* gastroesophageal junction

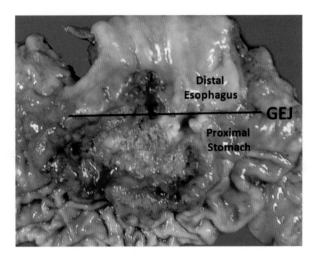

Table 7.1 Comparison of pathology between advanced gastric cardiac carcinoma in Chinese patients and distal esophageal adenocarcinoma in American patients [1]

Pathology		Americans (%)	Chinese (%)	P
Tumor epicenter				0.001
	Proximal stomach	11	100	
	Distal esophagus	89	0	
Tumor histology type				
	Adenocarcinoma	100	77	0.001
	Uncommon variants	0	23	0.018
Chronic proximal gastritis				
	Helicobacter pylori infection	15	35	0.012
	Intestinal metaplasia	19	47	0.009
	Dysplasia	58	5	0.001
Columnar-lined esophagus		81	14	0.001
	Presence of goblet cells	87	0	0.001
	Dysplasia	80	0	0.001

gastric origin almost impossible. In this situation, some authorities have speculated that the absence of typical Barrett's metaplastic epithelium in the adjacent esophageal mucosa of large tumors straddling the GEJ may be explained with the "overgrown" phenomenon of typical Barrett's epithelium by large esophageal adenocarcinomas in the distal esophagus. Alternatively, however, those large tumors in the GEJ without the evidence of Barrett's esophagus may not be genuine Barrett's adenocarcinomas, but instead, represent large advanced GCC invading into the distal esophagus from the gastric cardia below the GEJ line. In fact, the incorrect classification of large advanced GCC tumors in the GEJ region as esophageal ade-

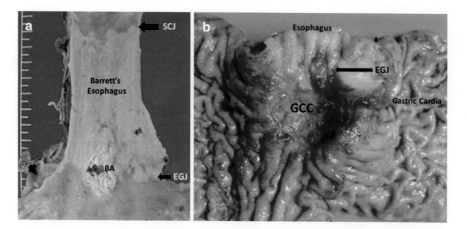

Fig. 7.2 Comparison of cancers involving the esophagogastric junction (EGJ) between American Caucasian (**a**) and Chinese (**b**) patients. In (**a**), Barrett's adenocarcinoma (BA) arises in a long segment of Barrett's esophagus (SCJ: squamocolumnar junction). In contrast in (**b**), a giant ulcerated gastric cardiac carcinoma (GCC) originated in the gastric cardia but invaded the distal esophagus without the evidence of Barrett's esophagus. Modified from [1]

nocarcinoma has been shown to result in an inflated high incidence of esophageal adenocarcinoma reported in some Western countries [6]. Complexity also stems from the controversial anatomic definition of the gastric cardia, as discussed in Chap. 2. Some investigators hypothesized that cardiac mucosa was an acquired, metaplastic lesion, generated in response to reflux disease [1, 7, 8]. As such, GCC has been considered as esophageal, not gastric, carcinoma in origin [8, 9]. The implication of this concept is clinically very significant and critical on how to optimally manage patients with this group of cancer. In Chinese patients, almost all large advanced GCC tumors do not have the clinical, endoscopic, and histomorphologic evidence of Barrett's esophagus (Fig. 7.2) [1]. Therefore, it is not appropriate to classify GCC as esophageal carcinoma. In fact, GCC demonstrates prognostic and lymphatic invasion patterns similar to non-cardiac gastric carcinoma, representing the same gastric tumor category, according to a German study [10]. Nevertheless, an accurate classification of tumors arising in the gastric cardiac region is not of a purely academic interest but truly of great clinical importance. In order to clarify the confusion and misunderstanding on GCC pathology, a most recent histopathology study carried out in Chinese patients specifically restricted pathology investigation to small GCC tumors in size up to 2 cm to allow a better preservation of histological landmarks of the GEJ and to eliminate any misclassification of GCC as an esophageal origin [11]. In that study, the pathology data clearly demonstrated unique histopathologic characteristics of this carcinoma, which were distinctly different from those of either distal esophageal Barrett's adenocarcinoma or gastric non-cardiac carcinoma (Table 7.2) [11–14]. In this chapter, we share with the readers major pathologic features of advanced GCC tumors.

Table 7.2 Comparison of histology types of cancer among gastric cardiac, non-cardiac, and esophageal adenocarcinoma

Morphology type	Gastric cardiac carcinoma	Esophageal adenocarcinoma	Gastric non-cardiac carcinoma	Reference
Tubular, papillary adenocarcinoma	77%	95–100%	57%	[1, 3, 5, 11]
Signet-ring cell carcinoma	6–9%	0–6%	16–35%	[13, 11, 12]
Mucinous carcinoma	1–2%	0–7%	0–1%	[1, 2, 11, 12]
Adenosquamous carcinoma	2%	0	0	[1, 3, 12]
Carcinoma with lymphoid stroma	2%	0	0.5%	[11]
Neuroendocrine tumor	2–5%	0	Rare (1.5%)	[1, 2, 11]
Carcinosarcoma	Rare (6–10 cases)	0	Rare (4–10 cases)	[13]
Choriocarcinoma	Rare (12–53)	0	Rare (41–53)	[14]

Gross Features

The exact anatomic location of GCC is important to define because of cancer staging requirements and patient management. Once a fresh gastric cancer radical resection specimen arrives at a pathology laboratory, the pathologist has to clearly identify and confirm the GEJ and then inspect the surface of the pearl-gray distal esophageal squamous mucosa for any salmon-red-colored columnar metaplastic lesion. If such a columnar lesion is present, the pattern, the circumferential, and longitudinal lengths of the lesion should be measured, recorded, and photographed. Advanced GCC may exhibit several gross appearances that can be grouped with Borrmann's types. For advanced GCC, Borrmann's type I (polypoid) tumors account for about 11–15% (Fig. 7.3a), type II (fungating) in 13–33% (Fig. 7.3b), type III (ulcerated) in 36–51% (Fig. 7.3c), and type IV (diffusely infiltrating) in 18–19% (Fig. 7.3d) [1, 2]. Unlike in esophageal adenocarcinoma and gastric non-cardiac carcinoma, the Borrmann's type III ulcerated growth pattern is most common in advanced GCC (Fig. 7.3c) [1, 2].

Microscopic Features

In the literature, the Lauran histology classification of gastric carcinoma is followed most frequently in the world because of the simplicity for clinicians to use. This classification includes primarily two key types: intestinal and diffuse and a minor indeterminate type. This has been slightly modified in the Japanese classification, in which the intestinal type is grouped as "differentiated" and the diffuse type as

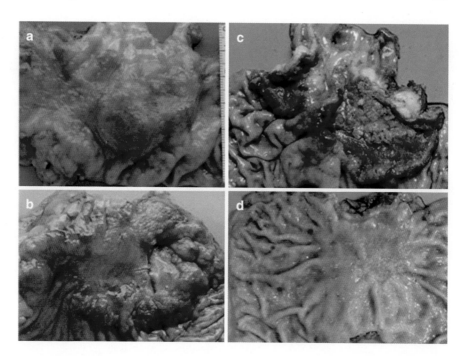

Fig. 7.3 Gross Borrmann's types of advanced gastric cardiac carcinoma in Chinese patients [2]: (**a**), type I, polypoid; (**b**), type II, fungating; (**c**), type III, ulcerated; and (**d**), type IV, flat. Note the characteristic absence of Barrett esophagus-related lesions in the distal esophagus

Table 7.3 Most commonly used gastric carcinoma classification schemes

WHO	Lauren	Japan
Tubular/papillary adenocarcinoma	Intestinal	Differentiated
Poorly cohesive, signet-ring, mucinous carcinoma	Diffuse	Undifferentiated
Undifferentiated (adenosquamous, small-cell carcinoma, carcinoma with lymphoid stroma, and others rare entities)	Indeterminate	Undifferentiated

"undifferentiated" in general. In contrast, the World Health Organization (WHO) uses a strict descriptive scheme to group gastric carcinomas into five main types of adenocarcinoma and uncommon entities [15]. According to the WHO system, which is followed worldwide except in Japan, the majority of advanced GCC are adenocarcinoma (Table 7.3).

In advanced GCC, marked histologic heterogeneity has been described in tumor growth pattern, differentiation, histology type, and cytological and architectural characteristic. Oftentimes, foveolar or intestinal or ciliated carcinoma cells can be found in the same tumor [2]. By immunohistochemistry, gastric- (MUC5AC+, MUC6+, MUC2-), intestinal- (MUC2+, CDX2+, CD10+, MUC5AC-, MUC6-), or mixed phenotypic carcinoma is distinguishable. In GCC, however, only MUC2 (50%) expression is significantly higher than that in gastric non-cardiac carcinoma (about 20%) [16], suggesting the predominance of intestinal differentiation in

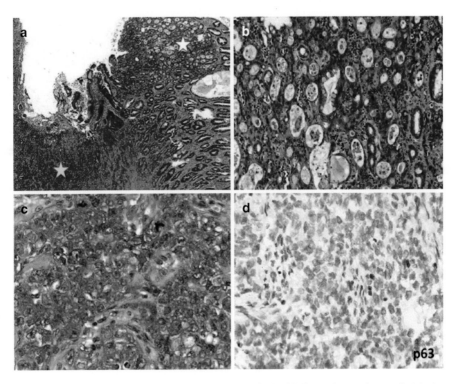

Fig. 7.4 Adenosquamous carcinoma of the gastric cardia. In this large ulcerated tumor in (**a**), the glandular component (white star in the right upper corner) was enlarged in (**b**) and admixed with benign glands with goblet cells. The solid component of poorly differentiated squamous cell carcinoma (yellow star in the left lower corner in **a**) was enlarged in (**c**) with an atypical mitosis in the upper right quadrant. In (**d**), neoplastic cells in (**c**) demonstrated focal immunoreactivity to p63, a marker for squamous differentiation

GCC. In addition, well-formed malignant tubules or papillae may be mixed with a minor component of poorly cohesive carcinoma, including signet-ring cell, squamous cell, or neuroendocrine carcinomas (Fig. 7.4).

By the WHO definition [15], tubular and papillary adenocarcinomas are composed of invasive tubules, glands, or papillae. The differentiation of adenocarcinomas can be subgrouped as well, moderate and poorly differentiated, defined by the estimated percentage of discernible malignant glands/papillae in the overall tumor volume on a histology tumor section. Well-differentiated adenocarcinoma is composed of well-formed malignant glands in over 95% of a tumor, while poorly differentiated adenocarcinoma features the difficulty for a pathologist to recognize well-formed glands at low-power view, because less than 50% of the tumor volume show recognizable glands/papillae on a tumor section. Thus, moderately differentiated adenocarcinoma exhibits an intermediate proportion of well-formed glands/papillae between well and poorly differentiated tumors. Poorly differentiated carcinoma often invades deep and shows a marked desmoplastic fibrotic reaction to make the tissue firm on touch (Fig. 7.5). Clinically, well and moderately differentiated adenocarcinomas are frequently considered as low-grade, while the poorly differentiated adenocarcinoma is high-grade.

Fig. 7.5 Poorly
differentiated tubular
adenocarcinoma often
shows marked stromal
malignant desmoplastic
reaction with hyaline
fibrosis to harden the
tumor tissue

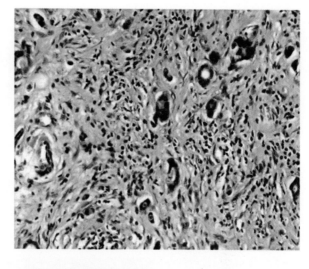

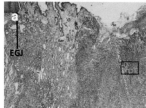
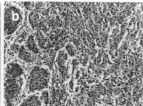
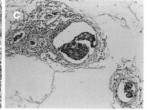

Fig. 7.6 Poorly differentiated tubular adenocarcinoma in a nest growth pattern. In (**a**), low-power view shows poorly differentiated tubular adenocarcinoma arose in the gastric cardia on the right of the esophagogastric junction (EGJ). The squared area is enlarged in (**b**) and highlights solid nests in various sizes and loosely arranged aggregates of neoplastic cells with ample eosinophilic cytoplasm, a few mitoses but no necrosis. The tumor invades the subserosal layer with extensive lymphovascular invasion as shown in (**c**)

In advanced GCC, tubular adenocarcinoma may show uncommon growth patterns such as nests (Fig. 7.6), solids (Fig. 7.7), and discohesive (Fig. 7.8) patterns. For the unknown reasons, those tumors are often loosely formed with extensive infiltration through the gastric wall into the subserosal layer with lymphovascular (Fig. 7.5) and intraneural (Fig. 7.9) invasion.

In general, pure tubular adenocarcinoma in advanced GCC is uncommon. Instead, most tubular adenocarcinoma tumors are associated with a small component of papillary (Fig. 7.10), mucinous and signet-ring cell (Fig. 7.11), and poorly cohesive carcinomas. In small GCC in size of 2 cm or less, tubular adenocarcinoma remains the most common type [11], accounting for about 45%. In contrast, the papillary type is significantly more (30%) common in the gastric cardia than in the non-cardiac (5%) region, often shows villiform (Fig. 7.12), nodular (Fig. 7.13), and free-floating papillary (Fig. 7.14) growth patterns. In advanced GCC, micropapillary adenocarcinoma is sometimes present as a small (5%) component of the major papillary or tubular adenocarcinoma (Fig. 7.15). This adenocarcinoma has a propensity for nodal and liver metastases [16–20] and worse prognosis [17, 19].

Fig. 7.7 Poorly differentiated adenocarcinoma with a solid growth pattern, infiltrating the muscularis propria

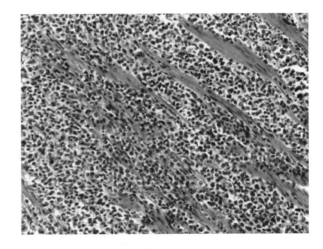

Fig. 7.8 Poorly differentiated adenocarcinoma with solid, discohesive growth patterns. Note the uniform neoplastic cells with ample eosinophilic cytoplasm, dysplastic nuclei, in a loose growth fashion without signet-ring cells

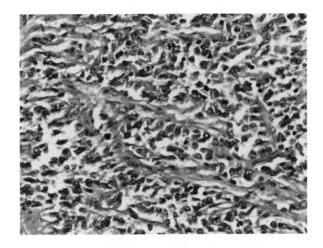

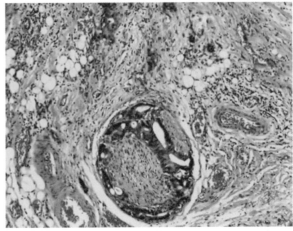

Fig. 7.9 Poorly differentiated tubular adenocarcinoma invades into the subserosa and nerve

Fig. 7.10 Tubulopapillary adenocarcinoma with both tubular (on the left) and papillary (on the right) components

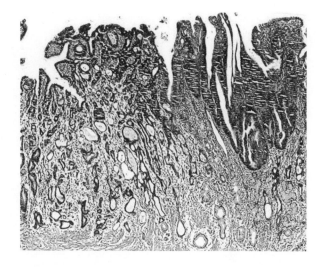

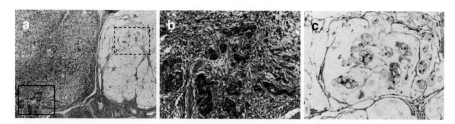

Fig. 7.11 An advanced gastric cardiac carcinoma shows tubular, signet-ring, and mucinous carcinoma components in (**a**). The area with solid lines in (**a**) is enlarged in (**b**), showing tubular adenocarcinoma. The area with dashed lines in (**a**) is enlarged in (**c**), exhibiting mucinous carcinoma with free-floating signet-ring cell carcinoma

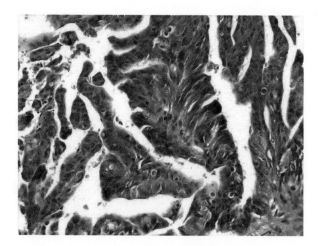

Fig. 7.12 Papillary gastric cardiac carcinoma with a villiform growth pattern

Fig. 7.13 Papillary cardiac adenocarcinoma occasionally shows a nodular growth pattern with intraluminal serrated papillary proliferation

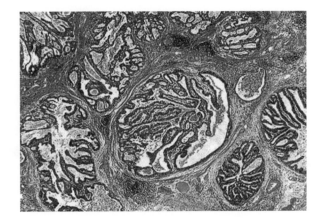

Fig. 7.14 Papillary adenocarcinoma with free-floating papillae overlies poorly differentiated carcinoma in the gastric cardia. Note the well-formed fibrovascular core in surface papillae

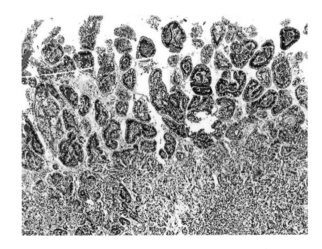

Fig. 7.15 Micropapillary adenocarcinoma features neoplastic nests surrounded by empty lacunar spaces. Note the characteristic absence of a fibrovascular core in each tumor micropapillary nest

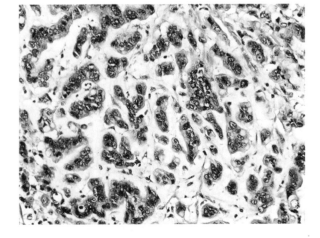

Table 7.4 Definition of histologic subtypes of major gastric cardiac carcinomas

Histologic subtype		Description
Tubular adenocarcinoma		Predominant tubular, acinar, cribriform, microcystic, anastomosing, focal solid nests
Papillary adenocarcinoma		Predominant papillary, serrated, villiform
Mixed adenocarcinoma		Predominant conventional adenocarcinoma (>50%) with a minor component of the following
	Signet-ring cell	<50% of the total estimated tumor volume
	Mucinous	<50% of the total estimated tumor volume
	Neuroendocrine	<50% of the total estimated tumor volume
Poorly cohesive carcinoma	Signet-ring cell	Discohesive mucin-containing signet-ring cells in microtrabecular or lacy patterns or nests and sheet but no glands
	Variants	Predominant discohesive histiocytic, lymphoid, deeply eosinophilic cytoplasm, pleomorphic bizarre nuclei, a few signet-ring cells
Mucinous carcinoma		>50% extracellular mucin pool with signet-ring cells and glands floating in the pool
Carcinoma with lymphoid stroma		Tubular adenocarcinoma with dense small lymphocytic stroma, positive for Epstein-Barr virus
Neuroendocrine tumor		>50% tumors, enlarged nuclei, vesicular chromatin, indistinct nucleoli, slim cytoplasm in solid nests or rosette, peripheral palisading patterns, positive for synaptophysin, CD56, or chromogranin A
Pancreatic acinar-like adenocarcinoma		Adenocarcinoma with round-oval nuclei, thickened nuclear membrane, prominent nucleoli and dark eosinophilic, fine granular cytoplasm, immunoreactive to the α1-chymotrypsin in >10% of a tumor

Micropapillary adenocarcinoma demonstrates pseudopapillary tumor clusters surrounded by empty lacuna spaces without fibrovascular cores in at least 5% of the estimated total tumor volume [19, 20].

In advanced GCC, there exists a considerably wide morphologic spectrum with many uncommon histology types (Table 7.4).

Undifferentiated Carcinoma with Ciliated Microcysts

Unlike distal non-cardiac gastric carcinoma and esophageal adenocarcinoma, some advanced GCC tumors are composed of primarily solid, organoid nests, nodules, and sheets of undifferentiated carcinoma that contains ciliated microcysts in some cases (Fig. 7.16) [2]. Some tumors are admixed with mucinous carcinoma, signet-ring cell carcinomas, and poorly differentiated carcinoma with ciliated microcysts (Fig. 7.17). Tumor nests are often floating in a mucin pool with signet-ring cells. Neoplastic cells in the nests may show the signet-ring cell morphology and become discohesive (Fig. 7.18).

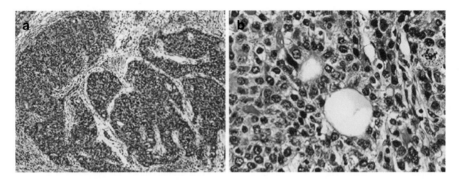

Fig. 7.16 Undifferentiated gastric cardiac carcinoma with solid nests and nodules (**a**), in which there are a few ciliated microcysts (**b**)

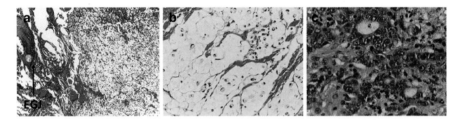

Fig. 7.17 Mixed carcinoma is composed of mucinous carcinoma with signet-ring cell carcinoma (**a**, **b**) and undifferentiated carcinoma with ciliated microcysts (**c**). EGJ in (**a**): esophagogastric junction

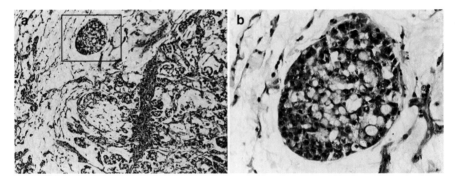

Fig. 7.18 Tumor nests are floating in a mucin pool. Neoplastic cells in some nests, squared area in (**a**), show the signet-ring cell morphology in (**b**)

Poorly Cohesive Carcinoma

By the WHO definition [15], poorly cohesive carcinoma consists of signet-ring cell carcinoma and other variants with discohesive malignant cells (Fig. 7.19). The tumor may arise in the deep layer of the gastric mucosa. In contrast, conventional

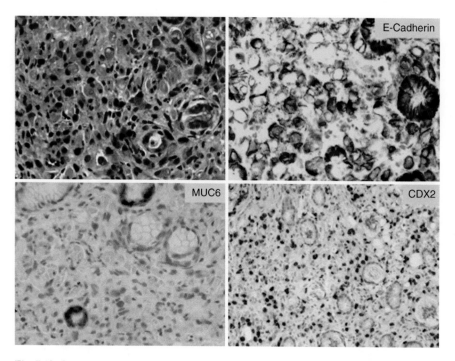

Fig. 7.19 Representative poorly cohesive carcinoma in the gastric cardia on the left upper shows neoplastic cells in a discohesive growth pattern with eosinophilic cytoplasm and rare signet-ring cells. By immunohistochemistry, those neoplastic cells show reduced immunoreactivity to E-cadherin, absence of immunoreactivity to MUC6, but positive nuclear staining for CDX2, suggesting intestinal differentiation

signet-ring cell carcinoma starts in the superficial lamina propria. As shown in Fig. 7.19, malignant discohesive cells in poorly cohesive carcinoma may show eosinophilic, dense, sometimes granular cytoplasm, and hyperchromatic, pleomorphic, irregular, and bizarre nuclei admixed with scattered mucin-containing signet-ring cells. Those malignant non-signet-ring cells are arranged in small aggregates, nests, or individual single cells with non-mucin containing cytoplasm. At present, this carcinoma is poorly understood and uncommon in advanced GCC. Non-mucinous poorly cohesive carcinoma in the gastric cardia often expresses CDX2 but rarely gastric markers, MUC5AC and MUC6 (Fig. 7.19). In both signet-ring and non-signet-ring cell poorly cohesive carcinomas, E-cadherin immunoreactivity is reduced (Fig. 7.19) or absent, suggesting that abnormal expression of this key cell adhesion molecule pays a key role in the pathogenesis of this aggressive carcinoma. Pure signet-ring cell carcinoma should not have well-formed glands, as defined by the WHO criteria, should occupy over 50% of the tumor volume, and is uncommon in the cardia [15, 20]. Most commonly, signet-ring cell carcinoma grows in single cells, small lace-like clusters (Fig. 7.20), cords, microtrabeculae, solid nests or sheets, and is also present as a minor component admixed with other major carcinoma types. Malignant signet-ring cells in the gastric wall are often in the

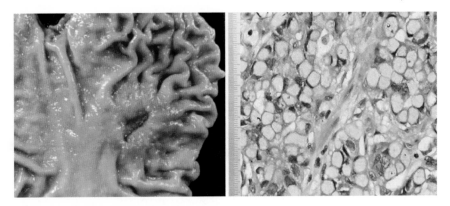

Fig. 7.20 Advanced signet-ring cell carcinoma in the gastric corpus near the antrum (Right) infiltrates deep, spreads into the entire gastric wall, and even presents at the proximal gastric cardiac resection margin (Left upper) about 8 cm proximal to the tumor epicenter

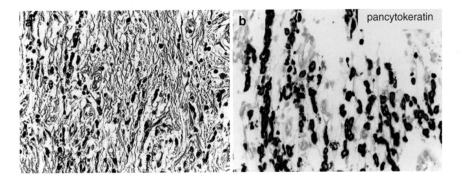

Fig. 7.21 Signet-ring cell carcinoma in the gastric cardia invades the deep gastric wall in an Indian-firing infiltrative growth pattern in (**a**), highlighted by a positive immunostain for pancytokeratin in (**b**)

Indian-firing growth pattern (Fig. 7.21) and associated with considerable desmoplastic reaction. Surprisingly, mitosis or apoptosis is uncommon, despite its very aggressive nature of growth with frequent lymphovascular invasion and widespread metastasis to the peritoneum, regional lymph nodes (Fig. 7.22), and distant organs. Oftentimes, signet-ring cells are small and difficult to be detected at the surgical margin of resection. In that scenario, a simple immunostain for cytokeratin may help visualize the infiltrating signet-ring cells (Fig. 7.23). In the gastric cardia, advanced carcinoma tumors may have a minor component of neoplastic cells with the signet-ring cell morphology.

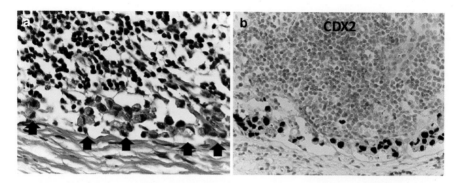

Fig. 7.22 Lymph node metastasis by signet-ring cell carcinoma occurs in the subcapsular space (arrows in **a**). Note the pale eosinophilic, mucin-distended cytoplasm pushing hyperchromatic, and pleomorphic nuclei to the edge. Those metastatic neoplastic cells are small and easily missed but can be readily highlighted by a simple but highly sensitive immunostain for CDX2 (**b**)

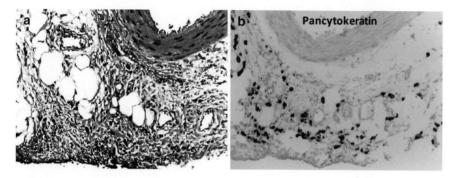

Fig. 7.23 Infiltrating signet-ring cell carcinoma is often mimicking tissue monocytes and histiocytes (**a**) but can be easily visualized by positive pancytokeratin immunostaining (**b**)

Mucinous Adenocarcinoma

By convention, mucinous adenocarcinoma is characterized by a conspicuous extracellular mucin pool in over 50% of the tumor volume with malignant mucinous cells, including signet-ring cells, which are frequently floating freely in the mucin pool (Fig. 7.24). In the cardia, this carcinoma is rare [2].

Carcinoma with Lymphoid Stroma

In the gastric cardia, carcinoma with lymphoid stroma, also known as medullary carcinoma or lymphoepithelioma-like carcinoma, is uncommon. Most cases (90%) of this carcinoma are related to Epstein-Barr virus (EBV) infection [21]. The results

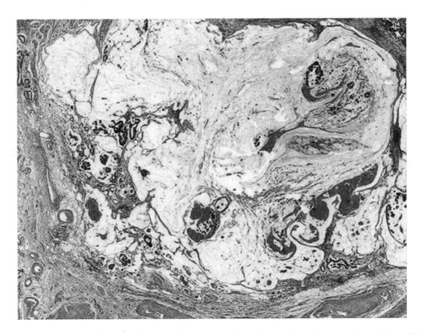

Fig. 7.24 Mucinous adenocarcinoma at low-power view shows primarily a mucin pool, in which neoplastic glands, micropapillae, or signet-ring cells are freely floating. Note, by definition, over 50% of the tumor volume should consist of mucin, to be qualified as mucinous adenocarcinoma

of a recent meta-analysis of 70 in situ hybridization studies for EBV-encoded small RNA in 15,952 patients showed a worldwide similar prevalence in Asia (8.3%), Europe (9.2%), and America (9.9%) but revealed a significantly higher frequency in men (11.1% versus 5.2% in women), gastric cardia (13.6% versus 5.2% in the antrum), remnant stomach (35.1%), and also other proximal gastric regions [21]. By in situ hybridization, intranuclear expression of EBV-encoded non-polyadenylated RNA-1 can be visualized as a diagnostic finding. Although detailed pathogenesis mechanisms for this EBV-related carcinoma remain elusive, the data from recent genome-wide comprehensive molecular analysis show an involvement of both genetic and epigenetic changes in EBV-induced gastric carcinogenesis, including mutations in PIK3CA and ARID1A genes, amplification of JAK2 and PD-L1/L2 genes, and global CpG island hypermethylation with epigenetic silencing of tumor suppressor genes, leading to significant gene expression alterations on cell proliferation, apoptosis, migration, and immune signaling pathways [22]. Grossly, the tumor is most commonly ulcerated with sharp borders (Fig. 7.25).

Microscopically, this poorly differentiated carcinoma is characterized by poorly formed tubular adenocarcinoma or poorly cohesive carcinoma embedded in a prominent lymphoid stroma with a pushing border (Fig. 7.25). Neoplastic epithelioid cells are large with prominent nucleoli and grow in irregular sheets, tubules, or

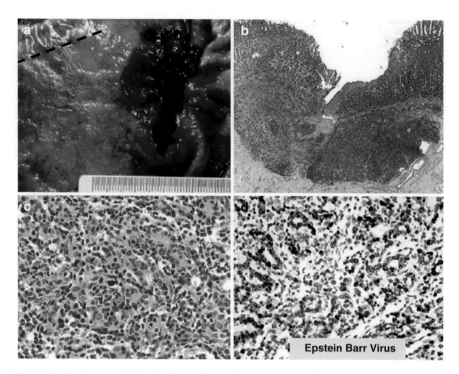

Fig. 7.25 Carcinoma with lymphoid stroma most frequently occurs in the gastric cardia, as shown in this case in (**a**). The dashed line refers to the esophagogastric junction. Note the ulcerated tumor with sharp borders. Microscopically, the tumor is well circumscribed with a pushing border at the invasion frond in the deep submucosa in (**b**). At high-power view in (**c**), dense tumor-infiltrating small lymphocytes obscure neoplastic, poorly differentiate tubular adenocarcinoma. In situ hybridization for Epstein-Barr virus highlights the viral infected nuclei of neoplastic cells in (**d**) (Modified from [11])

syncytia. These neoplastic epithelial cells are often obscured by prominent small lymphoid cells that are composed of predominantly CD8-positive T cells, some B cells, rare plasmacytes, and histiocytes. Based on the pattern of host inflammatory immune responses, described in a case-series study with 123 EBV-infected gastric carcinomas and 405 controls from Korea, EBV-related gastric carcinoma can be divided into three histologic subtypes: typical carcinoma with lymphoid stroma ($n = 53$, 43.1%), carcinoma with Crohn's disease-like lymphocytic reaction ($n = 52$, 42.3%), and conventional adenocarcinoma ($n = 18$, 14.6%) [23]. Overall, patients with carcinoma with lymphoid stroma or Crohn-like responses have significantly lower pN and pT stages, a higher 5-year survival rate of 71.4%, and a disease-free survival rate of 67.5% [23]. Interestingly, the 5-year disease-specific survival rate for patients with early gastric carcinoma with lymphoid stroma is over 98%, and the risk for lymph node metastasis is zero for mucosal involvement and 10% for submucosal invasion [24].

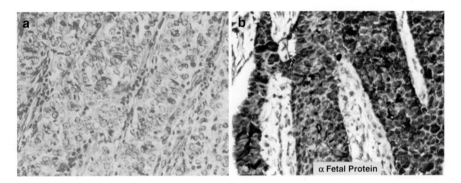

Fig. 7.26 Hepatoid and alpha-fetoprotein-producing adenocarcinoma of the gastric cardia in a 61-year-old Chinese woman. The tumor measured 2.9 × 2.3 × 0.5 cm, infiltrated the muscularis propria only, without lymph node metastasis and lymphovascular invasion. By histology, the tumor is poorly differentiated with trabecular and solid sheet growth patterns. Neoplastic cells were strongly immunoreactive to alpha-fetal protein

Hepatoid and Alpha-Fetoprotein-Producing Carcinoma

This uncommon primary gastric carcinoma is defined as a poorly differentiated adenocarcinoma with hepatoid differentiation and expression of alpha-fetoprotein (AFP). The gastric cardia is the most common (46.7%) location for this carcinoma, as described in a Chinese cohort with 31 cases [25]. The median age of patients at diagnosis was 51.2 years (rang 32–87) with a male-to-female ratio of 2.1:1. Serum AFP levels were markedly elevated in almost all patients [25, 26]. The resected tumor was usually large and fungating (Borrmann type II). Microscopically, the tumor is composed of large, polygonal cells with conspicuous eosinophilic, fine granular cytoplasm and arranged in frequent trabecular and nest growth patterns (Fig. 7.26). In some tumors, neoplastic cells are clear and presented as well-differentiated tubular adenocarcinoma. By immunohistochemistry, neoplastic cells may be immunoreactive to AFP (50–100%), arginase-1, alpha1-chymotrypsin, alpha1-trypsin, CK19, CK20, and Hep-Par 1 (0–100%), which makes it difficult separating from metastatic hepatocellular carcinoma [26, 27]. Therefore, it is prudent for pathologists to investigate the patient's past medical history for the possibility of primary hepatocellular carcinoma before making a diagnostic decision on primary gastric hepatoid adenocarcinoma. This is a fatal cancer, and the patient with this carcinoma usually has a dismal prognosis with frequent nodal (77.4%) and hepatic (41.9–50%) metastases [25, 26]; the median survival is only 6–7.2 months, and the 3- and 5-year survival rates are only 22.6% [25] and 20% [26], respectively.

Pancreatic Acinar-Like Adenocarcinoma

In advanced GCC, pancreatic acinar-like adenocarcinoma is not uncommon in the Chinese population [1, 2, 11, 28]. In a case-series study of 137 eligible advanced GCC cases, pancreatic acinar-like adenocarcinoma was identified in 31% [28]. The patient

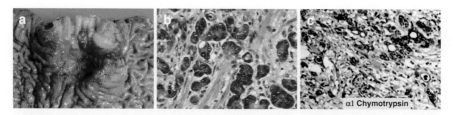

Fig. 7.27 Pancreatic acinar-like adenocarcinoma of the gastric cardia. The tumor is large and deeply ulcerated with a giant crater and invades focally into the distal esophagus (**a**). Note the absence of Barrett's esophagus-related diseases in the distal esophagus. By histology, neoplastic cells are infiltrative and show characteristic purplish and granular cytoplasm and a single giant nucleus with prominent nucleolus (**b**). By immunohistochemistry, neoplastic cells are strongly reactive to alpha1-chymotrypsin (**c**) (Modified from [1, 28])

mean age was 66-year old (range: 56–91) with a significant 7.6-fold male predominance. Grossly, the tumors were large with a mean size of 5.5 cm (range: 2–10.5), primarily in Borrmann's type III (67%), and all invading the distal esophagus minimally without the evidence of Barrett's esophagus (Fig. 7.27). Microscopically, neoplastic cells demonstrated predominant acinar (78%) and other minor growth patterns such as micropapillary, microcystic, solid, trabecular, and mixed neuroendocrine or signet-ring cell elements. Diagnostic criteria of this carcinoma consist of histologic characteristic "dense basophilic-eosinophilic cytoplasm rich in fine granules that were diffusely immunoreactive to the α1-chymotrypsin antibody" (Fig. 7.27) [28]. Neoplastic nuclei are round-to-oval in shape with stippled chromatin and single conspicuous nucleolus. Nuclear membrane is thickened. Mitotic figures are variable. Frank necrosis or hemorrhage is rare or absent. Tumor stroma is vascular, delicate, and non-desmoplastic. Lymphovascular and perineural invasion and nodal metastasis are significantly more common than those of control counterparts. Therefore, the prognosis is significantly poorer, especially for those older than 75-year old and at advanced stages [28].

High-Grade Primary Neuroendocrine Carcinoma

Primary high-grade (G3/3, WHO) neuroendocrine carcinoma of the stomach is rare and present frequently as large advanced carcinoma at diagnosis. A high proportion of such carcinomas occur in the gastric cardia, ranging from 27.6% (8/29) [29] to 40.2% (35/87) [30], as reported from China, and 40% (20/51) in the upper part of the stomach from Japan [31]. The tumor usually presents as a single large solitary protruding, fungating mass in size of over 2 cm (mean: >5 cm), and frequently invades into the distal esophagus [1, 2]. Neoplastic cells are not gastrin-dependent [29], but aggressive, invading into the muscularis propria and deeper gastric wall mainly in solid, medullary, or sheet-like, trabecular, and rosette-forming infiltrative growth patterns. Peripheral palisading, brisk mitosis, comedo necrosis, and punctate apoptosis are common. Tumor cells are small- or medium-sized; nuclei are pleomorphic, hyperchromatic with typical salt-pepper chromatin patterns, indistinct nucleoli, and scant cytoplasm (Fig. 7.28). Nuclear molding is conspicuous. By

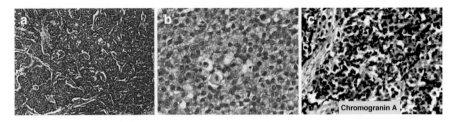

Fig. 7.28 High-grade neuroendocrine carcinoma of the gastric cardia. The tumor grows in solid sheets and nests (**a, b**). Neoplastic cells show vesicular nuclei with ample cytoplasm. Mitosis is frequent. Neoplastic cells are strongly immunoreactive to chromogranin A (**c**)

immunohistochemistry, neoplastic cells are immunoreactive to synaptophysin, CD56, and chromogranin A; the Ki67 index is over 10–20% [29–31]. In the gastric cardia, mixed high-grade neuroendocrine carcinoma and adenocarcinoma occurs commonly in about 50% of cases in a most recent Chinese cohort [32]. Overall, the prognosis of patients with this carcinoma is poor with a 5-year survival rate of 44.7%, regardless of histologic types (small or large cell) or the presence/absence of the adenocarcinoma component [31]. Importantly, HER2 expression is consistently absent, irrespective of the HER2 amplification status or mixed with a HER2-positive adenocarcinoma component [33].

Adenosquamous Carcinoma

Squamous differentiation is common in advanced GCC [1, 2], but adenosquamous carcinoma of the stomach is rare (0.25%); most reported cases are from Asian countries [34]. By definition, adenosquamous carcinoma consists of both major adenocarcinoma and minor squamous cell carcinoma components (Fig. 7.29). The proportion of the minor squamous cell carcinoma component is arbitrarily set at 25% for this diagnosis by the WHO criteria [15]. The significance of the large proportion of adenocarcinoma, but not squamous cell carcinoma, has been suspected recently as a poor prognostic indicator with more frequent nodal and distant organ metastases [34]. In a recent small case-series study in seven Chinese patients, most (57.1%) adenosquamous carcinomas occurred in the gastric cardia. The mean patient age was 62.5 years (range: 49–75), and the male-to-female ratio was 2.5. The mean tumor size was 8.1 cm (range: 4.3–11 cm). All studied tumors were deeply penetrating as advanced stage III or IV tumors with extensive nodal and distant organ metastases [34]. Microscopically, both adenocarcinoma and squamous cell carcinoma components were present in one tumor, and most were moderately to poorly differentiated with cytoplasmic keratin pearls and conspicuous intercellular bridges. Occasionally, ciliated neoplastic cells were discernable in the tumor microcytic luminal surface [1, 2]. In general, the overall prognosis is poor.

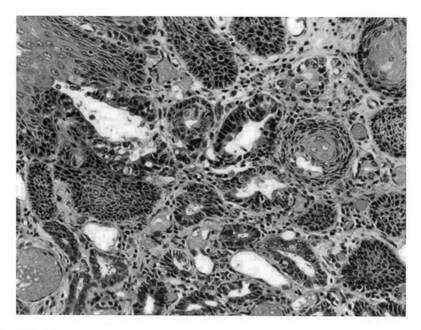

Fig. 7.29 Adenosquamous carcinoma of the gastric cardia. The tumor is composed of both tubular adenocarcinoma and keratinizing squamous cell carcinoma components

Choriocarcinoma

In the stomach, choriocarcinoma is vanishingly rare and descried only in case reports. The gastric cardia is the least (11.5%, 6/52) common site for this cancer in the early Japanese literature [35]. Elevated levels of human chorionic gonadotropin are diagnostically important and can be detected serologically, immunohistochemically, and also in urine [35]. Grossly, the tumor is large, exophytic, hemorrhagic, and necrotic. By histology, the tumor is composed of both syncytiotrophoblast and cytotrophoblast elements (Fig. 7.30). Most cases (68.4%, 54/79) show coexistence of both choriocarcinoma and conventional adenocarcinoma. Although prognosis is poor because of extensive nodal, hematogenous, and distant organ metastases at diagnosis, a standard chemotherapy regimen, consisting of etoposide, methotrexate, actinomycin D, cyclophosphamide, and vincristine, has been reported in the recent literature with a complete response, good tolerability, and long-term (10 years) disease-free survival [36, 37].

In a most recent case report in an 84-year-old Japanese man, a large (9 cm in maximum dimension) choriocarcinoma tumor was discovered in the gastric cardia along with a small-cell carcinoma component [38]. The rare collision of two exceedingly scarce malignancies in the gastric cardia illustrates the versatile nature of underlying tumorigenic cancer stem cells.

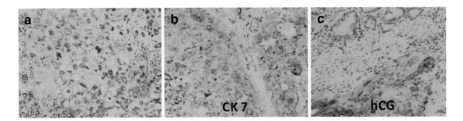

Fig. 7.30 Choriocarcinoma of the gastric cardia in a 65-year-old Chinese woman without a history of gonadal tumors or other primary sites of choriocarcinoma. The tumor measured 2.4 × 2.2 × 1.2 cm and infiltrated deeply into the gastric wall in a nodular fashion with a pushing boarder without lymphovascular invasion or nodal metastasis. By histology, the tumor was composed of both cytotrophoblasts and syncytiotrophoblastic cells and showed necrosis and hemorrhage (**a**). By immunohistochemistry, neoplastic cells were immunoreactive to CK7 (**b**) and hCG (**c**). Note the absence of hCG immunoreactivity of the adjacent well-differentiated tubular adenocarcinoma in the left upper corner in (**c**)

Carcinosarcoma

By definition, carcinosarcoma consists of both epithelial and mesenchymal elements and is diagnosed rarely in the stomach. However, gastric carcinosarcoma is prevalent in East Asian populations and described in case reports [39, 40]. In general, the proportion of two malignant components in a tumor varies widely, ranging from adenocarcinoma and neuroendocrine carcinoma in the carcinoma component, and spindle cells, round cells, and specific mesenchymal cells in the sarcoma component [41]. Gastric carcinosarcoma with a definite chondrosarcoma component is extremely rare. In a most recent case report, a large carcinosarcoma tumor confined in the gastric cardia was discovered in a 71-year-old Chinese man [42]. The resected tumor was centered in the gastric cardia, well-circumscribed, ulcerated (Borrmann type III), and large in overall size of 5 × 4 × 1 cm. The tumor invaded focally into the distal esophagus up to 1.5 cm above the GEJ. No Barrett's epithelium was identified in the distal esophagus. In histology, the major (about 90%) adenocarcinoma component consisted of moderately to poorly differentiated tubular adenocarcinoma. Admixed with adenocarcinoma was the minor (10%) chondrosarcoma component in multiple foci featuring neoplastic cartilage that was immunoreactive to S100 but negative to CK18 (Fig. 7.31).

Extensive lymphovascular and perineural invasion was also detected. Both components were present in metastasis of 13 perigastric lymph nodes. The adjacent gastric mucosa showed chronic active gastritis with intestinal metaplasia and atrophy without dysplasia. *H. pylori*-like organism was detected on both hematoxylin-eosin and Giemsa stains. The final pathologic stage of this tumor was pT3, pN3, and cM0. The patient did well at the last follow-up interview 12 months after radical resection with curative intend. In another case report [42], a large carcinosarcoma was discovered in the gastric cardia of a 73-year-old gentleman and composed of osteosarcoma in 90% and adenocarcinoma in 10%. A review of the English literature reveals a predominance of the gastric cardiac location in 6/10 reported cases of

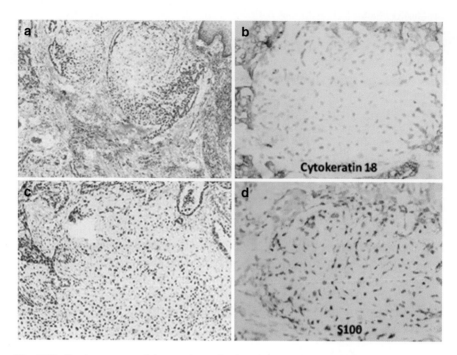

Fig. 7.31 Carcinosarcoma of the gastric cardia demonstrates both tubular adenocarcinoma and chondrosarcoma components. The tumor arose in the gastric cardia in a 71-year-old Chinese man, invaded through the gastric wall, and metastasized to 13–of 20 perigastric lymph nodes. By histology, the chondrosarcoma component grew in a nodular fashion (**a, b**), was immunoreactive to S100 (**d**) but negative to CK18 (**c**), and was surrounded by tubular adenocarcinoma that was immunoreactive to CK18 but negative to S100 in (**c**)

gastric carcinosarcoma with chondrosarcoma [13]. The findings raise the possibility of malignant transformation of multipotential differentiation of stem cells or residual embryonic progenitor cells in the cardiac region for this rare entity.

Gastric Stump Carcinoma

Gastric stump carcinoma occurs in patients with a prior history of partial gastrectomy for benign or malignant gastric disease. In general, patients with Billroth II reconstruction develops gastric stump carcinoma at the anastomotic site more frequently than those with Billroth I reconstruction [43, 44]. The latency between the first partial gastrectomy and the discovery of gastric stump carcinoma is much longer for patients with primary benign disease (34.3 years) than those with primary gastric cancer (9.9 years) [44]. However, overall survival is not significantly related to primary disease, anastomosis type, and the time interval between the primary and second surgeries [44]. The patient prognosis after resection of gastric stump carcinoma is also similar to that with conventional gastric cancer. The worse prognosis factors include older age, advanced T stage, nodal involvement, blood transfusion, multi-organ resection, and any surgical complication [43]. However, the 5-year survival rate was reported to be significantly poorer for patients with gastric stump carcinoma (53.6%, $N = 167$) than those with proximal gastric carcinoma including cardiac carcinomas (78.3%, $N = 755$), according to a multicenter study in Japan [45].

Gastric Carcinoma in Young (<40 Years Old) Patients

Early-onset gastric carcinoma in patients younger than 40 years is uncommon (3.2%), on the basis of a large single center study with consecutive 152 cases (152/4671) over an 11-year period in China [46]. In that study, no significant changes in the trend for this group of gastric cancers were demonstrated. As expected, the incidence of gastric cardiac carcinoma was significantly lower (5.3%, 8/152) in young (<40 years) patients than that (30%, 75/250) in older (>41 years) patients [45]. A female predominance, positive family cancer history, diffuse histology type, and advanced pathology stage (53.3% in pIII and pIV) were characteristic findings. Surprisingly, no significant differences in clinicopathologic characteristics were shown between familiar ($N = 38$) and sporadic ($N = 114$) groups in this Chinese patient population [46].

Gastric Adenocarcinoma with Proximal Polyposis of the Stomach

This is the most recently discovered hereditary gastric adenocarcinoma in Caucasian patients in 2012 [47]. At present, there are only six cases reported in the English literature, and involvement of the gastric cardia remains unknown. The most important clinicopathologic characteristics include: (1) more than 100 fundic gland polyps confined in the fundus and corpus without involving the antrum, regardless of the presence or absence of colorectal and duodenal polyps, (2) the existence of both hyperplastic and adenomatous polyps in the same patient, (3) development of intestinal-type gastric adenocarcinoma, (4) an autosomal dominant mode of inheritance, and (5) point mutations in exon 1B of the APC gene as a variant of familiar adenomatous polyposis [47, 48]. Because of the rarity, the detailed information on this hereditary gastric adenocarcinoma is not available at present.

Mesenchymal Tumor in the Gastric Cardia

Non-epithelial mesenchymal tumors in the gastric cardia are rarely discovered and poorly studied. The lesion is usually deeply seated in the submucosal space and beyond. A recent single center study on submucosal lesions revealed an incidence of 3% as mesenchymal tumors in a Chinese cohort [49]. The available study results on mesenchymal tumors in the cardia include gastrointestinal stromal tumor and leiomyoma.

Gastrointestinal Stromal Tumor (GIST)

GIST is the most common mesenchymal tumor in the stomach, as a result of genetic mutations of KIT or platelet-derived growth factor receptor alpha (PDGFRA) genes. GIST behaves in a wide clinical spectrum from benign to malignant. Most gastric leiomyoma, leiomyosarcoma, and leiomyoblastoma reported previously in the literature are actually GISTs. The tumor has been discovered in any part of the stomach but infrequently in the cardia where GIST accounts for only 3.8% in a recent report from China [49], 12% from Korea [50], and 10% from the USA [51]. Grossly, GIST is significantly smaller in size in the cardia than in other parts of the stomach [52] and may show an endophytic, deeply seated growth pattern. Microscopically, gastric GISTs show a broad morphologic spectrum with primarily spindle cells, some epithelioid cells, and some mixed. The epithelioid GIST tumors may exhibit hypercellularity, sclerosing fibrosis, discohesive growth, and sarcomatoid changes with conspicuous nuclear atypia and brisk mitosis. By immunohistochemistry, gastric GIST shows strong cytoplasmic and membranous immunoreactivity for KIT (CD117) in most cases (>95%) and negativity in a minority of tumors (<5%) that are frequently associated with PDGRA gene mutations. A CD34 immunostain often highlights spindle cell GISTs. The CD117-negative, PDGRA-mutated GISTs are often immunoreactive to the DOG1 antibody [52]. Usually, immunostains are positive infrequently for smooth muscle actin in some tumors and rarely for desmin. It has been reported that sporadic small GIST lesions are common in the cardia in patients older than 50 years. Those small GIST tumors were composed of neoplastic spindle cells with c-kit gene mutation in 46% of cases and PDGFRA mutations in 4%. Conspicuous hyalinization and calcification were found in over half cases, which were suspected to limit proliferation of small GIST lesions in the cardia with minimal clinical significance [53].

Leiomyosarcoma

In contrast to GIST, leiomyoscarcoma is vanishingly rare in the gastric cardia. A search of the PubMed for the past 30 years identified only a few case reports and small series before 2000 [54, 55]. Most reports were based on histology study results and did not use molecular tests to further phenotyping of the tumors. Because of the extreme similarity between GIST and leiomyosarcoma, the accuracy of the prior study results is questionable.

Other Tumors

In the gastric cardia, other mesenchymal tumors such as schwannoma, malignant melanoma, Kaposi's sarcoma, glomus tumor, hemangioma, inflammatory pseudotumor, etc., are extremely rare in the recent English literature [55].

Summary

Once invading the muscularis propria and beyond, gastric cardiac carcinoma becomes much more aggressive with extensive locoregional invasion and distant metastasis. Unlike distal esophageal Barrett's adenocarcinoma with pure tubular/papillary growth patterns, advanced gastric cardiac carcinoma demonstrates a much broader histopathologic spectrum with a substantial proportion of cases showing uncommon histologic types and rare entities, which is also more common than gastric non-cardiac carcinoma, suggesting different pathogenesis mechanisms.

References

1. Huang Q, Fan XS, Agoston AT, et al. Comparison of gastroesophageal junction carcinomas in Chinese versus American patients. Histopathology. 2011;59:188–97.
2. Huang Q, Zhang LH. The histopathologic spectrum of carcinomas involving the gastroesophageal junction in the Chinese. Int J Surg Pathol. 2007;15(1):38–52.
3. Wang HH, Antonioli DA, Goldman H. Comparative features of esophageal and gastric adenocarcinomas: recent changes in type and frequency. Hum Pathol. 1986;17:482–7.
4. Smith RR, Hamilton SR, Boitnott JK, et al. The spectrum of carcinoma arising in Barrett's esophagus. A clinicopathologic study of 26 patients. Am J Surg Pathol. 1984;8:563–73.
5. Cameron AJ, Lomboy CT, Pera M, Carpenter HA. Adenocarcinoma of the esophagogastric junction and Barrett's esophagus. Gastroenterology. 1995;109(5):1541–6.
6. Ekström AM, Signorello LB, Hansson LE, et al. Evaluating gastric cancer misclassification: a potential explanation for the rise in cardia cancer incidence. J Natl Cancer Inst. 1999;91:786–90.
7. Chandrasoma P, Makarewicz K, Wickramasinghe K, et al. A proposal for a new validated histological definition of the gastroesophageal junction. Hum Pathol. 2006;37:40–7.
8. Chandrasoma P, Wickramasinghe K, Ma Y, et al. Adenocarcinomas of the distal oesophagus and "gastric cardia" are predominantly esophageal carcinomas. Am J Surg Pathol. 2007;31:569–75.
9. American Joint Committee on Cancer Staging Manual. Chapter 10: Esophagus and esophagogastric junction. In: AJCC cancer staging manual. 7th ed. New York: Springer; 2007. p. 129–44.
10. Piso P, Werner U, Lang H, et al. Proximal versus distal gastric carcinoma—what are the differences? Ann Surg Oncol. 2000;7:520–5.
11. Huang Q, Shi J, Sun Q, et al. Clinicopathological characterisation of small (2 cm or less) proximal and distal gastric carcinomas in a Chinese population. Pathology. 2015;47(6):526–32.
12. Paraf F, Flejou JF, Pignon JP, et al. Surgical pathology of adenocarcinoma arising in Barrett's esophagus: analysis of 67 cases. Am J Surg Pathol. 1995;19:183–91.

13. Nie L, Yao F, Chen TT, Fan XS, Huang Q. Proximal gastric carcinosarcoma with chondro-sarcoma differentiation: a case report and review of the literature. Arch Pathol Lab Med. 2017;141:e11.
14. Kobayashi A, Hasebe T, Endo Y, et al. Primary gastric choriocarcinoma: two case reports and a pooled analysis of 53 cases. Gastric Cancer. 2005;8(3):178–85.
15. Lauwers GY, Carneiro F, Graham DY, et al. Gastric carcinoma. In: Bosman FT, Carneiro F, Hruban RH, Theise ND, editors. WHO classification of tumours of the digestive system. Lyon: IARC Press; 2010. p. 48–58.
16. Pinto-de-Sousa J, David L, Reis CA, Gomes R, Silva L, Pimenta A. Mucins MUC1, MUC2, MUC5AC and MUC6 expression in the evaluation of differentiation and clinico-biological behaviour of gastric carcinoma. Virchows Arch. 2002;440(3):304–10.
17. Yasuda K, Adachi Y, Shiraishi N, Maeo S, Kitano S. Papillary adenocarcinoma of the stomach. Gastric Cancer. 2000;3(1):33–8.
18. Kang HJ, Kim DH, Jeon TY, et al. Lymph node metastasis from intestinal-type early gastric cancer: experience in a single institution and reassessment of the extended criteria for endo-scopic submucosal dissection. Gastrointest Endosc. 2010;72(3):508–15.
19. Yu HP, Fang C, Chen L, et al. Worse prognosis in papillary, compared to tubular, early gastric carcinoma. J Cancer. 2017;8(1):117–23.
20. Huang Q, Fang C, Shi J, et al. Differences in clinicopathology of early gastric carcinoma between proximal and distal location in 438 Chinese patients. Sci Rep. 2015;5:13439.
21. Murphy G, Pfeiffer R, Camargo MC, Rabkin CS. Meta-analysis shows that prevalence of Epstein-Barr virus-positive gastric cancer differs based on sex and anatomic location. Gastroenterology. 2009;137(3):824–33.
22. Shinozaki-Ushiku A, Kunita A, Fukayama M. Update on Epstein-Barr virus and gastric cancer. Int J Oncol. 2015;46(4):1421–34.
23. Song HJ, Kim KM. Pathology of Epstein-Barr virus-associated gastric carcinoma and its rela-tionship to prognosis. Gut Liver. 2011;5(2):143–8.
24. Lim H, Lee IS, Lee JH, et al. Clinical application of early gastric carcinoma with lymphoid stroma based on lymph node metastasis status. Gastric Cancer. 2017;20(5):793–801. https://doi.org/10.1007/s10120-017-0703-z.
25. Yang J, Wang R, Zhang W, et al. Clinicopathological and prognostic characteristics of hepa-toid adenocarcinoma of the stomach. Gastroenterol Res Pract. 2014;2014:140587. https://doi.org/10.1155/2014/140587.
26. Lin CY, Yeh HC, Hsu CM, Lin WR, Chiu CT. Clinicopathological features of gastric hepatoid adenocarcinoma. Biomed J. 2015;38(1):65–9.
27. Chandan VS, Shah SS, Torbenson MS, Wu TT. Arginase-1 is frequently positive in hepatoid adenocarcinomas. Hum Pathol. 2016;55:11–6.
28. Huang Q, Gold JS, Shi J, et al. Pancreatic acinar-like adenocarcinoma of the proximal stomach involving the esophagus. Hum Pathol. 2012;43(6):911–20.
29. Xu TM, Wang CS, Jia CW, et al. Clinicopathological features of primary gastric neuroendo-crine neoplasms: a single-center analysis. J Dig Dis. 2016;17(3):162–8.
30. Zhang P, Zhang Y, Zhang C, et al. Subtype classification and clinicopathological characteris-tics of gastric neuroendocrine neoplasms: an analysis of 241 cases. Zhonghua Wei Chang Wai Ke Za Zhi. 2016;19(11):1241–6. (in Chinese).
31. Ishida M, Sekine S, Fukagawa T, et al. Neuroendocrine carcinoma of the stomach: mor-phologic and immunohistochemical characteristics and prognosis. Am J Surg Pathol. 2013;37(7):949–59.
32. Nie L, Li M, He X, et al. Gastric mixed adenoneuroendocrine carcinoma: correlation of histo-logic characteristics with prognosis. Ann Diagn Pathol. 2016;25:48–53.
33. Ishida M, Sekine S, Taniguchi H, et al. Consistent absence of HER2 expression, regardless of HER2 amplification status, in neuroendocrine carcinomas of the stomach. Histopathology. 2014;64(7):1027–31.
34. Chen YY, Li AF, Huang KH, et al. Adenosquamous carcinoma of the stomach and review of the literature. Pathol Oncol Res. 2015;21(3):547–51.

35. Imai Y, Kawabe T, Takahashi M, et al. A case of primary gastric choriocarcinoma and a review of the Japanese literature. J Gastroenterol. 1994;29(5):642–6.
36. Takahashi K, Tsukamoto S, Saito K, Ohkohchi N, Hirayama K. Complete response to multidisciplinary therapy in a patient with primary gastric choriocarcinoma. World J Gastroenterol. 2013;19(31):5187–94.
37. Baraka BA, Al Kharusi SS, Al Bahrani BJ, Bhathagar G. Primary gastric chorioadenocarcinoma. Oman Med J. 2016;31(5):381–3.
38. Fukuda S, Fujiwara Y, Wakasa T, et al. Collision tumor of choriocarcinoma and small cell carcinoma of the stomach: a case report. Int J Surg Case Rep. 2017;37:216–20.
39. Tanimura H, Furuta M. Carcinosarcoma of the stomach. Am J Surg. 1967;113:702–9.
40. Ikeda Y, Kosugi S, Nishikura K, et al. Gastric carcinosarcoma presenting as a huge epigastric mass. Gastric Cancer. 2007;10(1):63–8.
41. Siegal A, Freund U, Gal R. Carcinosarcoma of the stomach. Histopathology. 1988;13:350–3.
42. Selcukbiricik F, Tural D, Senel EF, Dervisoglu S, Serdengectia S. Gastric carcinoma with osteoblastic differentiation. Int J Surg Case Rep. 2012;3(11):516–9.
43. Tran TB, Hatzaras I, Worhunsky DJ, et al. Gastric remnant cancer: a distinct entity or simply another proximal gastric cancer? J Surg Oncol. 2015;112(8):877–82.
44. Irino T, Hiki N, Ohashi M, et al. Characteristics of gastric stump cancer: a single hospital retrospective analysis of 262 patients. Surgery. 2016;159(6):1539–47.
45. Tokunaga M, Sano T, Ohyama S, et al. Clinicopathological characteristics and survival difference between gastric stump carcinoma and primary upper third gastric cancer. J Gastrointest Surg. 2013;17(2):313–8.
46. Zhou F, Shi J, Fang C, Zou XP, Huang Q. Gastric carcinomas in young (younger than 40 years) Chinese patients: clinicopathology, family history, and post-resection survival. Medicine (Baltimore). 2016;95(9):e2873.
47. Worthley DL, Phillips KD, Wayte N, et al. Gastric adenocarcinoma and proximal polyposis of the stomach (GAPPS): a new autosomal dominant syndrome. Gut. 2012;61:774–9.
48. Li J, Woods SL, Healey S, et al. Point mutations in exon 1B of APC reveal gastric adenocarcinoma and proximal polyposis of the stomach as a familial adenomatous polyposis variant. Am J Hum Genet. 2016;98(5):830–42.
49. Kang WM, Yu JC, Ma ZQ, et al. Laparoscopic-endoscopic cooperative surgery for gastric submucosal tumors. World J Gastroenterol. 2013;19(34):5720–6.
50. Miettinen M, Wang ZF, Lasota J. DOG1 antibody in the differential diagnosis of gastrointestinal stromal tumors: a study of 1840 cases. Am J Surg Pathol. 2009;33(9):1401–8.
51. Abraham SC, Krasinskas AM, Hofstetter WL, Swisher SG, Wu TT. "Seedling" mesenchymal tumors (gastrointestinal stromal tumors and leiomyomas) are common incidental tumors of the esophagogastric junction. Am J Surg Pathol. 2007;31(11):1629–35.
52. Lee HH, Hur H, Jung H, Jeon HM, Park CH, Song KY. Analysis of 151 consecutive gastric submucosal tumors according to tumor location. J Surg Oncol. 2011;104(1):72–5.
53. Agaimy A, Wünsch PH, Hofstaedter F, et al. Minute gastric sclerosing stromal tumors (GIST tumorlets) are common in adults and frequently show c-KIT mutations. Am J Surg Pathol. 2007;31(1):113–20.
54. Aagaard MT, Kristensen IB, Lund O, Hasenkam JM, Kimose HH. Primary malignant non-epithelial tumours of the thoracic oesophagus and cardia in a 25-year surgical material. Scand J Gastroenterol. 1990;25(9):876–82.
55. Hsieh CC, Shih CS, Wu YC, et al. Leiomyosarcoma of the gastric cardia and fundus. Zhonghua Yi Xue Za Zhi (Taipei). 1999;62(7):418–24.

Chapter 8
Gastric Lymphoma

Hongbo Yu and Xiangshan Fan

Introduction

The gastrointestinal (GI) tract is the predominant site of extranodal lymphoma involvement. Primary lymphomas of the GI tract are rare, while secondary GI involvement is relatively common. Despite their rarity, primary lymphomas of the GI tract are important since their evaluation, diagnosis, management, and prognosis are distinct from that of lymphoma at other sites and other cancers of the GI tract. The GI tract is the predominant site of extranodal non-Hodgkin lymphomas.

Epidemiology

The stomach is the most common extranodal site of lymphoma and accounts for 68–75% of GI lymphomas [1, 2]. Primary gastric lymphoma accounts for 3% of gastric neoplasms and 10% of lymphomas [3]. Gastric lymphoma reaches its peak incidence between the ages of 50 and 60 years. There is a slight male predominance.

H. Yu (✉)
Department of Pathology and Laboratory Medicine, VA Boston Healthcare System,
West Roxbury, MA, USA

Harvard Medical School, Brigham and Women's Hospital, Boston, MA, USA
e-mail: hongbo.yu@va.gov

X. Fan
Department of Pathology, The Affiliated Drum Tower Hospital,
Nanjing University Medical School, Nanjing, Jiangsu, People's Republic of China

© Springer International Publishing AG, part of Springer Nature 2018   147
Q. Huang (ed.), *Gastric Cardiac Cancer*, https://doi.org/10.1007/978-3-319-79114-2_8

Clinical Features

Patients with gastric lymphoma typically present with nonspecific symptoms frequently seen with more common gastric conditions, such as peptic ulcer disease, gastric adenocarcinoma, and non-ulcer dyspepsia. The most common presenting symptoms include epigastric pain or discomfort (78–93%), loss of appetite (47%), weight loss (25%), nausea and/or vomiting (18%), bleeding (19%), and early satiety [1, 4–7].

Systemic B symptoms (fever, night sweats) are seen in 12% of patients. Weight loss is frequently due to local compromise of GI structures and is not always considered as a B symptom in this setting. Hematemesis and melena are uncommon. The duration of symptoms preceding the diagnosis is quite variable, ranging from a few days to 6 years.

The physical examination is often normal but may reveal a palpable mass and/or peripheral lymphadenopathy when the disease is advanced. Laboratory studies also tend to be normal at presentation. Anemia or an elevated erythrocyte sedimentation rate may be present in selected cases [4, 8, 9].

Diagnostic Evaluation

The diagnosis of gastric lymphoma is usually established during upper endoscopy with biopsy. Laparotomy and laparoscopy are typically reserved for patients with complications such as perforation or obstruction. Findings on upper endoscopy are diverse and may include mucosal erythema, a mass or polypoid lesion with or without ulceration, benign-appearing gastric ulcer, nodularity, and thickened, cerebroid gastric mucosal folds [10]. Multiple biopsies should be obtained from the stomach, duodenum, gastroesophageal junction, and from abnormal appearing lesions. An endoscopic ultrasound may help determine the depth of invasion and the presence of enlarged perigastric nodes [11–15]. The pattern seen on endoscopic ultrasound (EUS) may correlate with the type of lymphoma that is present. In one series, for example, superficial spreading or diffuse infiltrating lesions on EUS were seen with mucosa-associated lymphoid tissue lymphoma (MALT), while mass-forming lesions were typical of diffuse large B-cell lymphoma [14]. Pathologic evaluation is required for the determination of lymph node involvement. EUS alone has suboptimal accuracy in distinguishing benign from malignant lymph nodes [11–15]. When combined with endoscopic biopsy, however, overall accuracy approaches 90% (versus 66% for EUS alone). Even higher accuracy rates may be achievable if flow cytometry is performed [16]. Thus, caution is warranted in the interpretation of findings using EUS or CT alone.

Pathology

The diagnosis of gastric lymphoma may be suggested by endoscopic and imaging findings but must be confirmed by biopsy. Both suspicious appearing lesions and normal appearing mucosa should be biopsied since gastric lymphoma can occasionally present as multifocal disease with involvement of tissue that appears to be unaffected on initial visualization [17].

Endoscopists should aim to attain the largest biopsy specimen possible. Conventional pinch biopsies may miss the diagnosis, since gastric lymphoma can infiltrate the submucosa without affecting the mucosa; this problem is most likely to occur when no obvious mass is present. Jumbo biopsies, snare biopsies, biopsies within biopsies ("well technique"), and needle aspiration can all serve to increase the diagnostic yield in such cases. EUS-guided fine-needle aspiration biopsy (FNAB) [18–20] or endoscopic submucosal dissection [21] may provide even greater diagnostic capability.

The vast majority (greater than 90%) of gastric lymphomas are approximately equally divided into two histologic subtypes:

1. Extranodal marginal zone B-cell lymphoma of mucosa-associated lymphoid tissue (MALT) (previously called MALToma, MALT-type lymphoma, or MALT lymphoma) (38–48%)
2. Large B-cell lymphoma, primarly diffuse large B-cell lymphoma (45–59%)

The remaining cases of gastric lymphoma may represent any histology, but the most commonly seen are mantle cell lymphoma (1%), follicular lymphoma (0.5–2%), and peripheral T-cell lymphoma (1.5–4%) [17, 22].

Extranodal Marginal Zone B-Cell Lymphoma of Mucosa-Associated Lymphoid Tissue (MALT)

Morphology

The lymphoma cells exhibit dense lymphocytic infiltrate in the lamina propria (Fig. 8.1). The lymphoma cells of marginalzone lymphoma are small to intermediate in cell size, with round to slightly irregular nuclei, condensed chromatin, indistinct nucleoli, and abundant, pale cytoplasm. The accumulation of more pale-staining cytoplasm frequently leads to a monocytoid appearance (Fig. 8.2). Plasmacytic differentiation is present in 1/3 of cases (Fig. 8.3). Extremely rarely, Russell body gastritis may resemble a neoplastic process due to the marked expansion of the lamina propria with distension of fundic glands. However, immunohistochemistry may confirm a polyclonal pattern of plasma cells as an unusual reactive lesion of the gastric mucosa

Fig. 8.1 Dense
lymphocytic infiltrate in
lamina propria

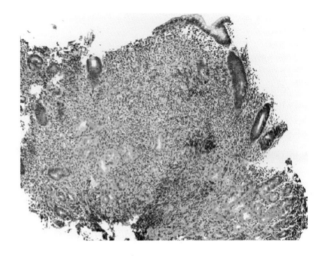

Fig. 8.2 Monocytoid
appearance of neoplastic
lymphocytes and
lymphoepithelial lesions
(arrows)

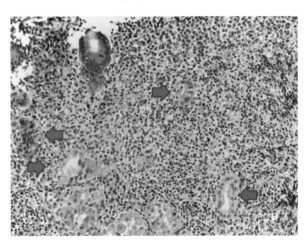

[23]. Occasional large cells resembling centroblasts or immunoblasts are usually present. Lymphoepithelial lesions (Fig. 8.2) are aggregates of three or more marginalzone lymphoid cells with distortion or destruction of the gastric epithelium, often together with eosinophilic degeneration of epithelial cells. This is a common feature in MALT lymphoma. The lymphoma cells sometimes specifically colonize the germinal centers of reactive lymphoid follicles, leading to follicular colonization.

Immunophenotype

The lymphoma cells are usually positive for CD20 and CD79a, but negative for cytokeratin, CD5, CD10, and CD23 (Fig. 8.4). CD43 stain can be positive in 50% of the cases. Staining for CD21 and CD35 shows expanded follicular dendritic

Fig. 8.3 Plasmacytic
differentiation is a
common feature

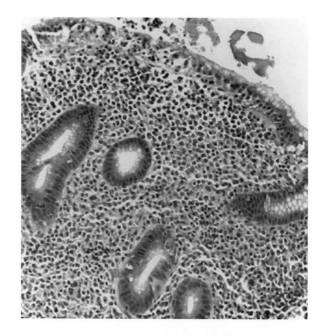

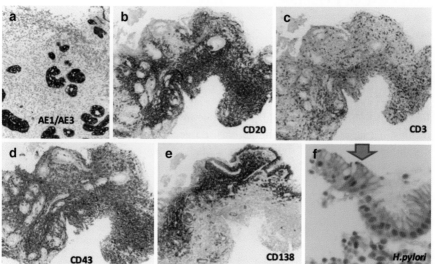

Fig. 8.4 Immunophenotypic features of gastric marginalzone lymphoma. In (**a**), pancytokeratin (AE1/AE3) highlights lymphoepithelial lesions in residual benign gastric crypts. Neoplastic lymphocytes are immunoreactive to CD20 in (**b**). CD3 stain in (**c**) exhibits mixed normal T cells. In (**d**), neoplastic B cells show aberrant expression of CD43. Increased number of plasma cells is demonstrated with CD138 in (**e**). By immunohistochemistry, *H. pylori* bacteria (arrow) are highlighted at the surface of gastric mucosa in (**f**)

meshwork. Demonstration of lightchain restriction is important in establishing the diagnosis. Molecular diagnostic studies for IgH gene rearrangements are usually necessary to confirm the diagnosis.

Cytogenetic Abnormalities

Chromosomal translocations include t (11;18)(q21;q21), t (1;14)(p22;q32), t (14;18) (q32;q21), and t (3;14)(p14.1;q32). Trisomy 3, 18, or less commonly of other chromosomes is a nonspecific but also not infrequent finding. The t (11;18) is the most common abnormality detected in gastric tumors, while others are more common at other locations.

Prognosis

MALT lymphomas have an indolent natural course and are slow to disseminate. The tumors are sensitive to radiation therapy; local treatment may be followed by prolonged disease-free intervals. Protracted remissions may be induced in *H. pylori*-associated gastric MALT lymphomas by antibiotic therapy. Cases with t (11;18) (q21;q21) appear to be resistant to *H. pylori* eradication therapy.

Large B-Cell Lymphoma

Gastric large B-cell lymphoma consists of a heterogeneous category of lymphomas and include diffuse large B-cell lymphoma (DLBCL), Epstein-Barr virus (EBV)-positive DLBCL, and plasmablastic lymphoma. Gastric DLBCL may arise de novo or as part of large-cell transformation of MALT lymphoma and other lowgrade B-cell lymphomas. The extent of the highgrade component varies in different cases. Rarely, DLBCL arising from other sites may involve the stomach, such as primary mediastinal large B-cell lymphoma [22]. Large cell transformation (Richter syndrome) of chronic lymphocytic leukemia/small lymphocytic lymphoma may manifest as gastric DLBCL [24]. Gastric DLBCL may involve any part of the stomach, including gastric cardia (Fig. 8.5).

Morphology

Gastric DLBCL usually presents as a single large ulcerated or exophytic lesion with transmural invasion and occasionally as multiple lesions. Histologically, gastric DLBCLs are indistinguishable from those found in nodal diseases. Typically, the architecture of gastric glands is almost completely effaced by tumor cells. Large neoplastic lymphoma cells infiltrate in diffuse sheets and have round, oval, irregular, or lobulated nuclei, distinct nucleoli, and moderate amount of cytoplasm, resembling centroblasts or immunoblasts (Fig. 8.6a). A few small reactive lymphocytes can be seen scattered among large tumor cells. In the cases of Epstein-Barr virus (EBV)-positive gastric DLBCL (Fig. 8.6b, c), the lesions often show large

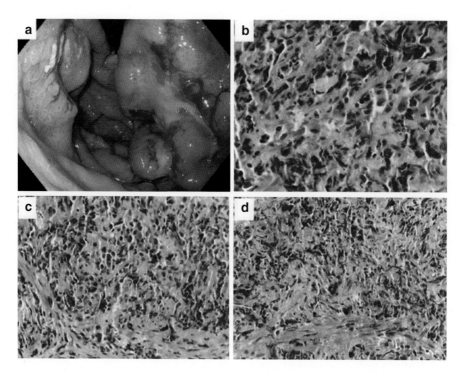

Fig. 8.5 Diffuse large B-cell lymphoma occurred in the gastric cardia of a 92-year-old man as an ulcerated mass (**a**). The biopsy of this mass demonstrated infiltrate of large neoplastic lymphocytes (**b**) with round/oval to irregular nuclei and moderate amount of cytoplasm (**c**), invading into the muscularis mucosae (**d**)

neoplastic lymphocytes, Hodgkin/Reed-Sternberg-like cells, with variable amounts of reactive small lymphocytes, plasma cells, and histiocytes. Plasmablastic lymphoma is rare, often in human immunodeficiency virus-infected patients, and composed of diffuse proliferation of large discohesive neoplastic cells (Fig. 8.6d), which resemble immunoblasts or plasmablasts. Cases with more plasmacytic differentiation are also seen. Very rarely, tumor cells may show large central artefactual vacuolar changes, displacing the nuclei to the periphery of the lymphoma cell, mimicking signet ring cells. In this and almost all gastric DLBCL, poorly differentiated carcinoma should be included in the differential diagnosis. Immunophenotyping with pancytokeratin, S100, and lymphoma markers should be routinely utilized in daily practice to help make an accurate diagnosis.

Immunophenotype

Immunohistochemically, gastric DLBCL cells are immunoreactive against pan-B-cell markers, such as CD20, CD19, CD79a, and PAX5, but negative to T-cell markers (Fig. 8.7). About half of cases are MUM1-and CD43-positive.

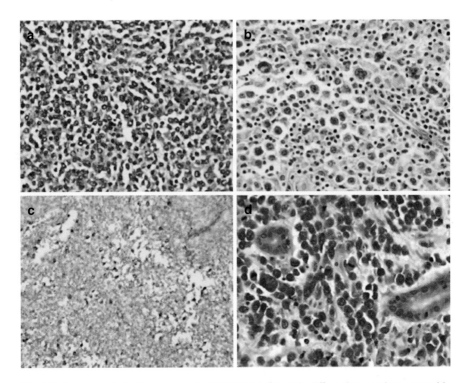

Fig. 8.6 Large neoplastic lymphoma cells in DLBCL infiltrate in diffuse sheets and may resemble centroblasts or immunoblasts (**a**). EBV-positive DLBCL shows Hodgkin/Reed-Sternberg-like cells, large lymphocyts, and reactive small lymphocytes (**b**) positive nuclear staining pattern demonstrated by in situ hybridization for Epstein-Barr virus encoded RNA (EBER) (**c**). Discohesive large neoplastic cells, which resemble immunoblasts or plasmablasts, are found in gastric plasmablastic lymphoma (**d**)

BCL6 immunoreactivity is variable. Typically, the transformed gastric DLBCLs from MALT lymphoma are CD10-negative but often BCL-6 positive. In contrast, gastric de novo DLBCL is often CD10-positive, and some are BCL2-positive.

For plasmablastic lymphoma, neoplastic large plasmacytoid cells are positive for CD38 (Fig. 8.8a), CD138, and MUM1 (Fig. 8.8b), but negative for B-cell markers, such as PAX5, CD20 (Fig. 8.8c), CD79a (Fig. 8.8d), and T-cell markers. Ki67 proliferative index is often very high (not shown). In situ hybridization for EBV-encoded RNA (EBER) may be positive in 70% of cases, especially in HIV-positive patients [10]. The rearrangement involving *MYC* gene can be found with interphase fluorescence in situ hybridization in 67% of cases [10, 25].

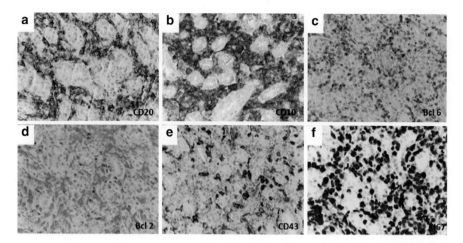

Fig. 8.7 Immunophenotypic characteristics of the lymphoma case shown in Fig. 8.5. Neoplastic large lymphoid cells are strongly immunoreactive to CD20 (**a**), CD10 (**b**), variably positive to BCL6 (**c**), but negative for BCL2 (**d**). These cells show aberrant expression of CD43 (**e**) and strong positivity to Ki67 in over 90% of cells (**f**)

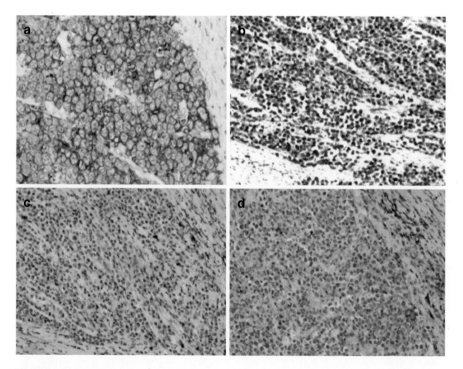

Fig. 8.8 Neoplastic large plasmacytoid cells are positive for CD38 (**a**) and MUM1 (**b**) but negative for CD20 (**c**) and CD79a (**d**), supporting the diagnosis of plasmablastic lymphoma

Cytogenetic Abnormalities

Gastric DLBCL may have complex cytogenetic abnormalities with clonal rearrangements of immunoglobulin (IG) heavy- and light-chain genes. Translocations involving *BCL6* and *MYC* genes may play a key role not only in the progression of gastric MALT lymphoma to DLBCL but also in the tumorigenesis of de novo DLBCL as well. *BCL2* gene rearrangement, however, is rare. Thus, "double-hit" lymphoma is very rare among primary gastric lymphoma, while patients with multiple gene amplifications and/or copy number gains in *BCL6*, and "MYC, BCL2 double-expresser" gastric DLBCL, have a poor clinical outcome [26]. Mutations with loss of heterozygosity in regions 5q21 (*APC* gene locus), 9p21 (*INK4A/ARF*), 13q14 (*RB*), and 17p13 (*P53*), and allelic imbalances in 2p16, 6p23, and 12p12-13 have been reported in gastric DLBCL [27]. Cytogenetic abnormalities such as t(11;18) and trisomy 3 (most often involving chromosomes 12 and 18) can be detected in some cases of gastric MALT lymphoma but rare in both de novo and transformed DLBCLs. Some gastric DLBCL tumors may be positive for EBV markers [28] and granular cytoplasmic anaplastic lymphoma kinase (ALK) expression [29, 30]. Very rarely, *MYC* gene rearrangement can be found in plasmablastic lymphoma without EBV infection in an immunocompetent young adult [25].

The case illustrated in Fig. 8.5 showed clonal *IGH* gene rearrangement. Further fluorescence in situ hybridization analysis for high-grade B-cell lymphoma demonstrated the majority of neoplastic cells with one copy of *MYC* and two copies of *BCL6*. Rearrangements of *MYC* and *BCL6* genes were observed in about 70% of cells analyzed, and unusual *IGH-BCL2* single fusion pattern was identified in about 20% of cells. The overall changes were consistent with high-grade B-cell lymphoma with the features intermediate between DLBCL and Burkitt's lymphoma, which was renamed as high-grade B-cell lymphoma, NOS (not otherwise specified) in the 2016 revision of World Health Organization (WHO)Classification of Hematopoietic and Lymphoid Neoplasms [31].

Prognosis

Primary gastric DLBCL is a highly heterogeneous malignant tumor. The 5-year survival of patients with gastric DLBCL is significantly worse than that of patients with MALT lymphoma. There is no significant difference in clinical behaviors between transformed MALT lymphoma and primary DLBCL [32, 33]. DLBCLs are further divided into germinal center B- (GCB) and non-GCB subtypes by Hans, Choi, and Tally immunohitochemical algorithms. Primary gastric DLBCL tends to show a higher prevalence of GCB subtype with a better 5-year overall survival rate than that of other DLBCL types [32]. *IGH*-involved translocation in DLBCL has been found to be an independent prognostic factor, in addition to younger age and early stage, for better overall survival and event-free survival [9]. *H.*

pylori-positive gastric "pure" DLBCL, as a distinct subtype, may be less aggressive and respond to *H. pylori* eradication and conventional chemotherapy [34]. Expression of BCL6 by tumor cells is also regarded as a favorable factor [8]. In contrast, poor outcomes in patients with gastric DLBCL are associated with advanced clinical stages, expression of BCL2 [8, 33] and BLIMP-1 [33], elevated serum levels of lactate dehydrogenase [8], and EBV infection, likely due to resistance to standard chemoradiotherapy [35]. Plasmablastic lymphoma is rapidly progressive and almost invariably fatal.

Summary

Non-Hodgkin lymphoma in the gastric cardia shows a predominance of lowgrade marginalzone B-cell lymphoma, also known as MALToma, which is primarily related to *H. pylori* infection. Highgrade non-Hodgkin lymphoma in the gastric cardia is rare and occurs mainly in the elderly population. It is heterogeneous in cell type, pathogenesis, and prognosis. Accurate morphologic pathologicdiagnosis and molecular characterization is essential for patient management.

References

1. Koch P, del Valle F, Berdel WE, et al. Primary gastrointestinal non-Hodgkin's lymphoma: I. Anatomic and histologic distribution, clinical features, and survival data of 371 patients registered in the German Multicenter Study GIT NHL 01/92. J Clin Oncol. 2001;19:3861–73.
2. Papaxoinis G, Papageorgiou S, Rontogianni D, et al. Primary gastrointestinal non-Hodgkin's lymphoma: a clinicopathologic study of 128 cases in Greece. A Hellenic Cooperative Oncology Group study (HeCOG). Leuk Lymphoma. 2006;47:2140–6.
3. Freeman C, Berg JW, Cutler SJ. Occurrence and prognosis of extranodal lymphomas. Cancer. 1972;29:252–60.
4. Cogliatti SB, Schmid U, Schumacher U, et al. Primary B-cell gastric lymphoma: a clinicopathological study of 145 patients. Gastroenterology. 1991;101:1159–70.
5. Radaszkiewicz T, Dragosics B, Bauer P. Gastrointestinal malignant lymphomas of the mucosa-associated lymphoid tissue: factors relevant to prognosis. Gastroenterology. 1992;102:1628–38.
6. Muller AF, Maloney A, Jenkins D, et al. Primary gastric lymphoma in clinical practice 1973-1992. Gut. 1995;36:679–83.
7. Wang T, Gui W, Shen Q. Primary gastrointestinal non-Hodgkin's lymphoma: clinicopathological and prognostic analysis. Med Oncol. 2010;27:661–6.
8. Chung KM, Chang ST, Huang WT, et al. Bcl-6 expression and lactate dehydrogenase level predict prognosis of primary gastric diffuse large B-cell lymphoma. J Formos Med Assoc. 2013;112:382–9.
9. Nakamura S, Ye H, Bacon CM, et al. Translocations involving the immunoglobulin heavy chain gene locus predict better survival in gastric diffuse large B-cell lymphoma. Clin Cancer Res. 2008;14:3002–10.
10. Loghavi S, Alayed K, Aladily TN, et al. Stage, age, and EBV status impact outcomes of plasmablastic lymphoma patients: a clinicopathologic analysis of 61 patients. J Hematol Oncol. 2015;8:65.

11. Tio TL, den Hartog Jager FC, Tijtgat GN. Endoscopic ultrasonography of non-Hodgkin lymphoma of the stomach. Gastroenterology. 1986;91:401–8.
12. Caletti G, Ferrari A, Brocchi E, Barbara L. Accuracy of endoscopic ultrasonography in the diagnosis and staging of gastric cancer and lymphoma. Surgery. 1993;113:14–27.
13. Fujishima H, Misawa T, Maruoka A, Chijiiwa Y, Sakai K, Nawata H. Staging and follow-up of primary gastric lymphoma by endoscopic ultrasonography. Am J Gastroenterol. 1991;86:719–24.
14. Suekane H, Iida M, Yao T, Matsumoto T, Masuda Y, Fujishima M. Endoscopic ultrasonography in primary gastric lymphoma: correlation with endoscopic and histologic findings. Gastrointest Endosc. 1993;39:139–45.
15. Fischbach W, Goebeler-Kolve ME, Greiner A. Diagnostic accuracy of EUS in the local staging of primary gastric lymphoma: results of a prospective, multicenter study comparing EUS with histopathologic stage. Gastrointest Endosc. 2002;56:696–700.
16. Wiersema MJ, Gatzimos K, Nisi R, Wiersema LM. Staging of non-Hodgkin's gastric lymphoma with endosonography-guided fine-needle aspiration biopsy and flow cytometry. Gastrointest Endosc. 1996;44:734–6.
17. Wotherspoon AC, Doglioni C, Isaacson PG. Low-grade gastric B-cell lymphoma of mucosa-associated lymphoid tissue (MALT): a multifocal disease. Histopathology. 1992;20:29–34.
18. Chang KJ, Katz KD, Durbin TE, et al. Endoscopic ultrasound-guided fine-needle aspiration. Gastrointest Endosc. 1994;40:694–9.
19. Wiersema MJ, Kochman ML, Cramer HM, Tao LC, Wiersema LM. Endosonography-guided real-time fine-needle aspiration biopsy. Gastrointest Endosc. 1994;40:700–7.
20. Vilmann P, Hancke S, Henriksen FW, Jacobsen GK. Endoscopic ultrasonography-guided fine-needle aspiration biopsy of lesions in the upper gastrointestinal tract. Gastrointest Endosc. 1995;41:230–5.
21. Suekane H, Iida M, Kuwano Y, et al. Diagnosis of primary early gastric lymphoma. Usefulness of endoscopic mucosal resection for histologic evaluation. Cancer. 1993;71:1207–13.
22. Papageorgiou SG, Sachanas S, Pangalis GA, et al. Gastric involvement in patients with primary mediastinal large B-cell lymphoma. Anticancer Res. 2014;34:6717–23.
23. Erbersdobler A, Petri S, Lock G. Russell body gastritis: an unusual, tumor-like lesion of the gastric mucosa. Arch Pathol Lab Med. 2004;128:915–7.
24. Di Bernardo A, Mussetti A, Aiello A, De Paoli E, Cabras AD. Alternate clonal dominance in richter transformation presenting as extranodal diffuse large B-cell lymphoma and synchronous classic Hodgkin lymphoma. Am J Clin Pathol. 2014;142:227–32.
25. Huang X, Zhang Y, Gao Z. Plasmablastic lymphoma of the stomach with C-MYC rearrangement in an immunocompetent young adult: a case report. Medicine (Baltimore). 2015;94:e470.
26. He M, Chen K, Li S, et al. Clinical Significance of "Double-hit" and "Double-protein" expression in Primary Gastric B-cell Lymphomas. J Cancer. 2016;7:1215–25.
27. Starostik P, Patzner J, Greiner A, et al. Gastric marginal zone B-cell lymphomas of MALT type develop along 2 distinct pathogenetic pathways. Blood. 2002;99:3–9.
28. Sumida T, Kitadai Y, Masuda H, et al. Rapid progression of Epstein-Barr-virus-positive gastric diffuse large B-cell lymphoma during chemoradiotherapy: a case report. Clin J Gastroenterol. 2008;1:105–9.
29. McManus DT, Catherwood MA, Carey PD, Cuthbert RJ, Alexander HD. ALK-positive diffuse large B-cell lymphoma of the stomach associated with a clathrin-ALK rearrangement. Hum Pathol. 2004;35:1285–8.
30. Rudzki Z, Rucinska M, Jurczak W, et al. ALK-positive diffuse large B-cell lymphoma: two more cases and a brief literature review. Pol J Pathol. 2005;56:37–45.
31. Swerdlow SH, Campo E, Pileri SA, et al. The 2016 revision of the World Health Organization classification of lymphoid neoplasms. Blood. 2016;127:2375–90.
32. Chen Y, Xiao L, Zhu X, et al. [Immunohistochemical classification and prognosis of diffuse large B-cell lymphoma in China]. Zhonghua Bing Li Xue Za Zhi. 2014;43:383–8.

33. Martin-Arruti M, Vaquero M, Diaz de Otazu R, et al. Bcl-2 and BLIMP-1 expression predict worse prognosis in gastric diffuse large B cell lymphoma (DLCBL) while other markers for nodal DLBCL are not useful. Histopathology. 2012;60:785–92.
34. Kuo SH, Yeh KH, Chen LT, et al. Helicobacter pylori-related diffuse large B-cell lymphoma of the stomach: a distinct entity with lower aggressiveness and higher chemosensitivity. Blood Cancer J. 2014;4:e220.
35. Yoshino T, Nakamura S, Matsuno Y, et al. Epstein-Barr virus involvement is a predictive factor for the resistance to chemoradiotherapy of gastric diffuse large B-cell lymphoma. Cancer Sci. 2006;97:163–6.

Chapter 9
Diagnosis

Chenggong Yu, Guifang Xu, Qin Huang, Tingshan Lin, and Edward Lew

Introduction

There is considerable geographic variability in the incidence of gastric cardiac cancer (GCC). Even among East Asian countries with high rates of gastric cancer, the proportion of GCC radical resection cases is tenfold higher in China (>25%) than in Japan and Korea (2.5–3%) [1, 2]. The reasons for such variations in GCC incidence remain unclear. Early diagnosis of GCC is essential for improving survival and outcomes but challenging, because of the lack of specific clinical symptoms. As a result, many patients with GCC are diagnosed at advanced stages and have a poor prognosis because of extensive locoregional nodal and distant metastases. Despite recent advances in gastric cancer treatment, the best chance to cure this

C. Yu (✉)
Department of Gastroenterology, Nanjing Drum Tower Hospital, The Affiliated Hospital of Nanjing University Medical School, Nanjing, Jiangsu, People's Republic of China
e-mail: chenggong_yu@nju.edu.cn

G. Xu
Department of Gastroenterology, Affiliated Nanjing Drum Tower Hospital of Nanjing University Medical School, Nanjing, People's Republic of China

Q. Huang
Pathology and Laboratory Medicine, Veterans Affairs Boston Healthcare System, West Roxbury, MA, USA

Harvard Medical School and Brigham and Women's Hospital, Boston, MA, USA

T. Lin
Nanjing Drum Tower Hospital, Nanjing, People's Republic of China

E. Lew
Harvard Medical School, VA Boston Healthcare System and Brigham and Women's Hospital, Boston, MA, USA
e-mail: Edward.Lew@va.gov

© Springer International Publishing AG, part of Springer Nature 2018   161
Q. Huang (ed.), *Gastric Cardiac Cancer*, https://doi.org/10.1007/978-3-319-79114-2_9

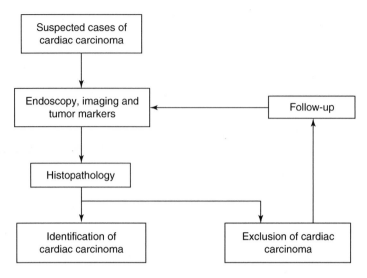

Fig. 9.1 Algorithm for diagnosis of gastric cardiac carcinoma

fatal cancer depends on early diagnosis. This can then lead to subsequent curative resection with an excellent prognosis and 5-year survival rates of over 90%, as reported in Japan, Korea, and China [1, 3]. To date, upper endoscopy and imaging studies such as barium swallow are the main methods used for diagnosing GCC. Pathologic diagnosis based on the findings in biopsy tissue samples, immu-nohistochemistry, flow cytometry, and molecular markers remains the gold standard. An algorithm to diagnose GCC is outlined in Fig. 9.1.

Clinical Manifestations

At early stages, most patients who develop GCC are asymptomatic, but some may present with nonspecific, mild epigastric discomfort, dyspepsia, nausea, anorexia, or a change in eating habits [4]. Patients with ulcerated GCC may also have gastro-intestinal bleeding and anemia. Dysphagia with difficulty in swallowing solids is the most common symptom and may progress to difficulty in swallowing liquids [5]. Regurgitation, odynophagia, weight loss, coughing, and pain more often occur in advanced cases [6]. In a retrospective clinical study on risk factors of 115 con-secutive Chinese patients with radically resected early GCCs, several independent risk factors were significantly associated with early GCC [7]. These included advanced age over 50 years, personal cancer history, obesity, and exposure to envi-ronmental toxins. In contrast, GCC was not significantly associated with male gen-der (although male patients outnumbers female patients), unusual dietary habits, *H. pylori* infection, tobacco or alcohol abuse, hiatal hernia, gastroesophageal reflux disease, or columnar-lined esophagus [7]. As a result, these differences in characteristics may help distinguish early GCC from distal gastric non-cardiac carcinoma and distal esophageal adenocarcinoma. It is interesting that GCC rarely occurs in patients younger than 40 years of age [1]. Because most early GCC tumors (61.9%) are grossly protruding or elevated with only 16.8% cases having an excavated morphology, the ulcerated gastric cancer-associated symptoms are typically very rare. Due to the fact that clinical signs and symptoms arising from early GCC are often minimal and nonspecific, most early GCC tumors are unexpectedly found during upper endoscopy performed for other purposes or during screening programs for gastric carcinoma. In contrast, alarming symptoms and signs, such as anemia, weight loss, and gastrointestinal tract bleeding, are primarily seen in patients with advanced GCC. Therefore, it is crucial to routinely scrutinize the entire gastric cardiac region in elderly patients at upper endoscopy for other reasons.

Screening for Early Carcinoma

The nonspecific symptoms in GCC patients and the absence of reliable clinical or laboratory tests to detect GCC unfortunately lead to delays in diagnosis and complicate optimal management. At present, there is no specific screening program for GCC. No reliable serology biomarkers have been proven to be sensitive enough for detection of GCC. In a recent meta-analysis of 16 studies in 1193 patients [8], the use of circulating tumor DNA (ctDNA) had a sensitivity of 62% and a specificity of 95% in diagnosing gastric cancer. There was a correlation of detecting ctDNA with larger tumors at advanced stages with an overall worse prognosis. The use of ctDNA for early detection of GCC is thus limited. The only proven reliable and accurate screening method for diagnosis of GCC is upper endoscopy with biopsies, especially in the high-risk regions and for the most vulnerable populations, which include (1) the person at or older than 50-year-old from a high-risk region on esophageal and/or gastric cancer, (2) the individual with a family history of esophageal and/or gastric cancer, and (3) the patient with biopsy-proven chronic atrophic gastritis or intestinal metaplasia.

Upper Endoscopy

Upper endoscopy is an important tool in the diagnosis, staging, treatment, and surveillance of patients with GCC. The most widely used endoscopy modality is the conventional white-light endoscopy. Among several high-volume centers, however, advanced endoscopic techniques have been used to increase the detection rate for early GCC, such as chromoendoscopy, magnification endoscopy with indigo carmine and acetic acid spray, narrow-band imaging with or without magnification, and autofluorescence imaging. Overall, these methods increase the accuracy of detecting early GCC tumors with high sensitivity and specificity.

Endoscopic Gastric Carcinoma Gross Classification

During endoscopy, there are two main tumor gross classification systems for gastric carcinoma:

1. The Bormann system is used for advanced carcinomas and consists of four categories: Type I for polypoid tumors, Type II for fungating tumors, Type III for ulcerated tumors, and Type IV for diffusely infiltrating tumors. Representative images are illustrated in Chap. 7.
2. The Paris classification, which is similar to the Japanese classification, includes three categories for early gastric carcinoma as shown in Table 9.1 and Fig. 9.2.

Endoscopically, a Type 0-I lesion is greater than 2.5 mm above the mucosal surface, estimated as the width of the closed cups of a biopsy forceps, and similar to Type 0-IIa, which is, however, less than 2.5 mm in height (Fig. 9.2a, b). By histology, the height of Type 0-I lesion is greater than twice as the thickness of the adjacent mucosa. Types 0-IIc and 0-III lesions are similar and covered with the fibrinopurulent exudate, but the former is slightly depressed (Fig. 9.2c), and the latter is ulcerated to the muscularis mucosae and probably to submucosa (Fig. 9.2d). Endoscopic diagnosis of Type 0-III tumors is frequently overdiagnosed by inclusion of Type 0-IIC lesions. Several endoscopic studies of early GCC have confirmed that most early GCC tumors are Types 0-I and 0-IIa; Type 0-III tumors are significantly less common in the gastric cardia than those in distal non-cardiac carcinomas [7–9].

Upper Endoscopy Examination

Flexible upper endoscopy with histopathologic examination of biopsies is the primary method for diagnosing GCC [6] and has been proven to be more sensitive and specific for the detection of early GCC than any other diagnostic modality. During upper endoscopy, the entire cardiac region must be carefully examined using the retroflex view. Because of the challenging anatomy in the cardiac region and a high

Table 9.1 The Paris classification of endoscopic gross types of early gastric carcinoma

Type	Subtype	Description
0-I	Polypoid are subcategorized as	
	0-Ip	Protruded, pedunculated
	0-Is	Protruded, sessile
0-II	Nonpolypoid, subcategorized as	
	0-IIa	Slightly elevated
	0-IIb	Flat
	0-IIc	Slightly depressed
0-III		Excavated

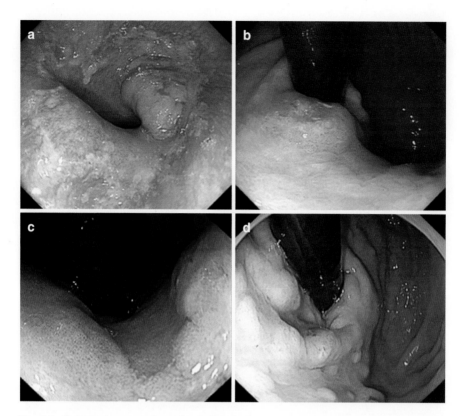

Fig. 9.2 Endoscopic types of gastric cardiac carcinoma, according to the Paris classification (**a**: 0-Is, **b**: 0-IIa; **c**: 0-IIc, and **d**: 0-III)

missing rate of greater than 42% for GCC at endoscopy [10], the endoscopist should carefully inspect the entire cardiac mucosa by rotating the scope for 360° to ensure a complete visualization and close examination of the cardiac mucosa. During this meticulous inspection, several high-quality digital images should be taken for future inspection and comparison [11].

Using conventional white-light endoscopy, early GCC may have characteristic endoscopic appearances that include an irregular, uneven, asymmetric surface and discoloration in a demarcated lesion (Fig. 9.3a), which can be highlighted by indigo carmine chromoendoscopy (Fig. 9.3b).

Acetic acid spray may help delineating the border of slightly elevated early tumors. Further investigation with magnifying narrow-band imaging may be useful for differentiating neoplasia from non-neoplasia, determining the tumor border, and demonstrating irregular microvascular and abnormal micromucosal surface patterns of an EGC tumor (Fig. 9.3c). At upper endoscopy, a clear demonstration of a tumor demarcation line and irregular vascular network along with abnormal mucosal surface of a lesion are highly predictive of EGC.

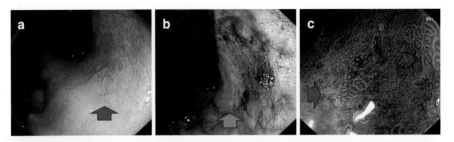

Fig. 9.3 Endoscopic appearances of an early gastric cardiac carcinoma (arrows) with poorly defined erythematous discoloration and irregular mucosal and vascular patterns, as shown by conventional white-light endoscopy as a 0-IIb flat lesion (**a**). The borders of this cardiac lesion are accentuated by indigo carmine chromoendoscopy (**b**) or by narrow-band imaging (**c**)

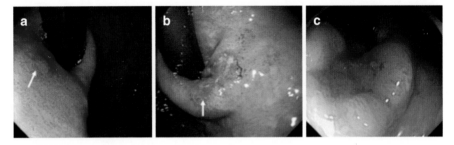

Fig. 9.4 Endoscopic appearances of gastric cardiac carcinoma with erythema (**a**, arrow), erosion (**b**, arrow), and ulceration (**c**)

Among patients suspected of harboring GCC, it is critically important to perform systematic and targeted endoscopic biopsies for diagnosis because histopathology remains the gold standard for EGC diagnosis. If there are no suspicious abnormalities found in the entire cardiac region after careful inspection with white-light endoscopy, the endoscopist should obtain systematic biopsies. In this scenario, at least three to four biopsies should be obtained from the distal esophagus, cardia at the lesser curvature, antrum-angular at the lesser curvature, and duodenum for comparison of pathologic changes among the different locations and surveillance of the most cancer-prone mucosa along the lesser curvature [9]. However, if the cardiac mucosa shows any protruding polypoid changes (Fig. 9.4a), erythema, erosion (Fig. 9.4b), superficial plaque, discoloration, or depressed, ulcerated lesions (Fig. 9.4c), the endoscopist must also obtain targeted biopsies. The diagnostic endoscopy can also provide important information about the likely stage of the tumor. Large and circumferential tumors (Fig. 9.5) are almost always transmural, and approximately 80% of cases also have lymph node metastasis [12].

During endoscopy, a complete visual assessment of gross tumor characteristics should be made not only for the lesion length but also the distance to and relationship with the esophagogastric junction (EGJ) line that is defined as the most proximal end of the gastric longitudinal mucosal folds. In addition, the distal esophageal

Fig. 9.5 A large gastric cardiac carcinoma circumscribes the esophagogastric junction

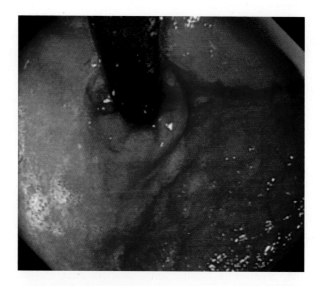

Fig. 9.6 Endoscopic appearance of distal esophageal salmon-red columnar-lined metaplastic lesion with a tongue-like pattern (blue arrow). Note the smooth surface and a short distance from the squamocolumnar junction (black arrow)

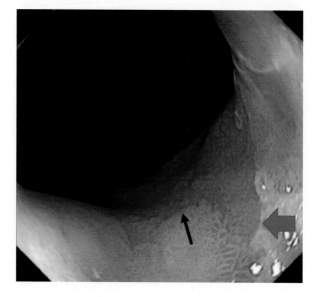

mucosa should be carefully examined for the presence of salmon-red discoloration that may suggest columnar metaplasia (Fig. 9.6). The identified lesion needs to be accurately assessed and characterized with regard to the size, number, shape, surface, consistency, and relationship to the EGJ. Biopsies must be obtained at the time of endoscopy for histopathologic evaluation.

Obtaining multiple biopsies increases the diagnostic accuracy. The diagnostic yield is close to 100% when greater than five samples are obtained using a standard endoscopic biopsy protocol [13]. Therefore, the 2015 practice guidelines of the

American Society of Gastrointestinal Endoscopy recommend taking at least seven biopsy samples from gastric masses or heaped-up edges of ulcers suspicious for carcinoma [14]. Biopsy of the mucosa adjacent to the tumor lesion is crucial for assessment of underlying diseases, such as atrophic gastritis, intestinal metaplasia, and dysplasia, and also for investigation of baseline risk of gastric malignancy. Brush cytology may be helpful in cases of tight malignant strictures where performing conventional biopsies may prove to be difficult [15]. In such cases, brushings can maximize the diagnostic yield and should be obtained before biopsies [16]. Advanced high-resolution endoscopy and narrow-band imaging may enhance visualization of early GCC with improved detection [17].

Advanced Endoscopic Techniques

Mucosal image-enhanced endoscopy such as magnifying chromoendoscopy can help improve the localization, characterization, and diagnosis of suspicious lesions by instilling dyes to enhance the detail of the mucosa [18, 19]. Other techniques such as magnifying narrow-band imaging can also show a sharply demarcated early carcinoma with abnormal mucosal microarchitectures and microvascular features. These techniques often require additional preparation of the gastric mucosa. In practice, systematic examination of the entire gastric mucosa by conventional white-light endoscopy is first used to screen for any suspicious lesions that can be subsequently further investigated with these advanced chromoendoscopy and magnifying narrow-band imaging techniques. Such strategies are routine in large high-volume centers. Because many early gastric cancers are small or flat or have focal subtle mucosal discoloration and depression (Fig. 9.7), which cannot be visualized

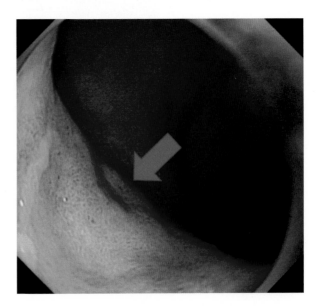

Fig. 9.7 Focal subtle mucosal depression and discoloration (arrow)

well by the conventional white-light endoscopy, magnifying narrow-band imaging together with a comprehensive "vessel plus surface classification" system has been shown very useful for detecting primarily intestinal-type early gastric carcinoma, but not for poorly differentiated or signet-ring cell carcinoma [18]. As such, the intestinal-type gastric carcinoma can be diagnosed endoscopically with high accuracy to determine the tumor size, border, presence or absence of associated ulceration, and possible invasion depth. In the gastric cardia, the majority of early GCC are polypoid protruding; the flat pattern is uncommon, and the excavated lesion is only about 16%, which is significantly less than that in the distal non-cardiac stomach [1]. For poorly differentiated and signet-ring cell carcinomas, the diagnosis relies upon histopathologic determination. Recent studies suggest that the detection of poorly differentiated carcinoma and signet-ring cell carcinoma can be significantly improved through magnifying narrow-band imaging [20]. In an endoscopic study of 78 consecutive early gastric undifferentiated carcinomas, Okada et al. reported the diagnostic accuracy of early carcinoma and the lateral extent of undifferentiated carcinomas by magnifying narrow-band imaging to be similar to that of histopathology. For depressed early gastric carcinoma, a combination of use of conventional white-light endoscopy along with magnifying narrow-band imaging, enhanced by 1.5% acetic acid spread, was able to improve endoscopic predication of both differentiated and undifferentiated early gastric carcinomas that are grossly depressed and difficult to be identified and diagnosed [21].

Moreover, using a novel flexible mini-contact microscope that can be inserted into a conventional endoscopy channel, the endocytoscopy system takes advantage of the magnifying power to ×900 with a digital lens (×1.8) to facilitate endoscopic observations at the cellular level of the gastric mucosal surface, which makes the true "target" biopsy possible [22]. This is a step further than the narrow-band imaging system. However, the diagnostic value of both endocytoscopy and narrow-band imaging on the tumor invasion depth remains problematic. In contrast, optical coherence tomography (OCT) with spatial resolution up to 7 μm is able to penetrate the mucosa up to 2 mm and generate histopathology-like digital images (Fig. 9.8). A pilot study was able to visualize the mucosal vascular structure up to the muscularis mucosae [23, 24]. However, the clinical application of this technology on gastric cancer diagnosis has not yet been thoroughly investigated.

Endoscopic Ultrasound

Endoscopic ultrasonography (EUS) has an important role in the diagnosis and staging workup of gastric carcinoma, including GCC. This exam should be especially useful in cases where standard biopsy or brushings do not yield a diagnosis among patients with high suspicion [25]. In addition, EUS can be used to determine whether or not a tumor invades the submucosal layer (Fig. 9.9), as required by the 2015 practice guideline of the American Society of Gastrointestinal Endoscopy [14]. However, EUS probes are typically larger in size, and care should be taken when biopsies are attempted in lesions with strictures, which may need to be dilated first

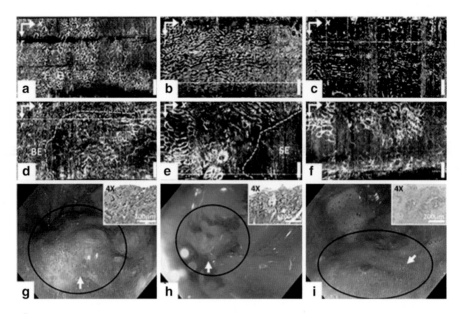

Fig. 9.8 En face OCT angiography (**a–f**) imaging from about 180 μm beneath the mucosal surface allows rapid evaluation of the mucosal vascular network in the esophagogastric junction region with the resolution similar to narrow-band imaging (**g–i**). Compared to non-dysplastic columnar-lined esophagus in (**a–c**), dysplastic lesions shown in (**d–f**) demonstrated abnormal vessel branching (arrows in **d**), heterogeneous size of vessels (arrows in **e**), or both patterns (**f**), as high-grade (**d, e**) and low-grade (**f**) dysplasia in the corresponding histopathologic diagnoses depicted in the right upper corners of images (**g–i**) in three different patients (**d, g; e, h;** and **f, i**). Note the sharp demarcation of abnormal vessels in dysplastic mucosal lesions outlined by yellow lines in (**d**) and (**e**). Arrows in (**a–c**) show the regular honeycomb microvascular pattern in non-dysplastic mucosa. Yellow arrows in (**b** and **c**) refer to respiration-related motion artifact. BE in (**d**): Barrett's esophagus. SE in (**e**): squamous epithelium. Modified from [23]

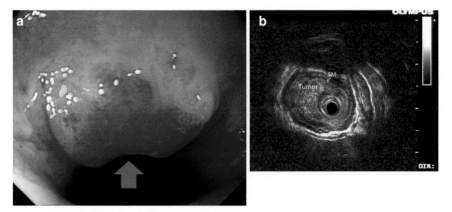

Fig. 9.9 By conventional white-light endoscopy, a broad-based protruding lesion (arrow) is visualized primarily in the gastric cardia with the possible involvement of the gastroesophageal junction (**a**). By endoscopic ultrasonography, the tumor (arrow) appears to invade the muscular mucosae into the submucosal (SM) layer (**b**)

before the use of EUS [6]. To investigate the predictive value of EUS on tumor depth, Okada et al. studied 542 early gastric carcinomas and reported a diagnostic accuracy of EUS in tumor invasion depth to be 87.8% (259/295) for differentiated carcinoma which is 30 mm or smaller and 75% (42/56) for undifferentiated carcinoma which is 20 mm or smaller. However, the EUS diagnostic accuracy decreases significantly for ulcerous lesions and tumors larger than 30 mm in size [20]. Using a combination of conventional white-light endoscopy for mass-like lesions with irregular mucosal surface and a submucosal tumor-like marginal elevation along with optimal use of EUS, the diagnostic accuracy for tumor depth can exceed 85%, as reported by Tsujii et al. [26].

The use of EUS with or without fine-needle aspiration (FNA) of suspicious locoregional lymph nodes or thoracoscopic and laparoscopic lymph node sampling is recommended to stage the nodal disease before endoscopic submucosal dissection (ESD) [14], despite concerns about tumor cell seeding along the needle track [27]. The 2015 practice guidelines of the American Society of Gastrointestinal Endoscopy suggest that EUS should focus on identification of metastatic diseases, especially in the liver and other solid organs. Whenever possible, suspicious lesions identified by EUS should be biopsied with FNA to determine both T and N stages. A most recent Cochran review on diagnostic accuracy of EUS for the preoperative locoregional staging of primary gastric cancer identified 66 qualified papers published between 1988 and 2012 in a total of 7747 patients with gastric cancer staged with EUS [28]. The authors performed meta-analysis of 50 studies with 4397 patients and showed that EUS is clinically useful to guide clinicians in the locoregional staging of patients with gastric cancer (Table 9.1). Because of the data heterogeneity and other issues, they caution that EUS diagnostic accuracy is lower for separating superficial pT1a tumors from submucosal pT1b ones and also the specificity for nodal metastasis is only 67% (Table 9.2) [28]. However, when combined with FNA, the EUS-FNA test results changed the patient management plan in up to 15% (34/234) of cases [29]. The EUS test is especially important for advanced GCC because detection of peritoneal metastatic cancer in patients with low-volume ascites by EUS and cytology examinations is an independent indicator for inoperability [30]. Therefore, the additional diagnostic value of EUS in GCC is significant, especially when conventional white-light endoscopy, narrow-band imaging, and FNA in patients with GCC are combined (Table 9.3).

There are other novel endoscopic techniques being developed, including flexible spectral imaging color enhancement (FICE) endoscopy, i-Scan technology, endocytoscopy, confocal laser endomicroscopy (CLE), and autofluorescence endoscopy.

Table 9.2 Cochran meta-analysis of diagnostic values of endoscopic ultrasound on gastric cancer [27]

Diagnostic test	Number of paper	Number of patients	Sensitivity (%)	Specificity (%)
T1/T2 vs. T3/T4	50	4397	86	90
T1 vs. T2	46	2742	85	90
T1a vs. T1b	20	3321	87	75
Nodal metastasis	44	3573	83	67

Table 9.3 Comparison of major advanced endoscopic techniques on gastric cancer diagnosis [23]

Feature	Narrow-band imaging	Optical coherence tomography	Endoscopic ultrasound
Technology	Light of specific blue and green wavelengths	Laser	High-frequency sound waves
Spatial resolution	500 μm	7 μm (in water)	110 μm at 25 MHz
Penetration depth	500 μm	2 mm	5 micro
Coupling medium	Air	Air or water	Water
Image analogue	Histopathology	Histopathology	Ultrasound
Application	Mucosal surface changes only	Mucosal surface changes in the entire thickness	Mucosal surface changes only

Endoscopic Surveillance After Successful ESD Resection

In patients with a history of malignancy, especially esophageal and gastric carcinoma, the risk of developing synchronous or metachronous multiple gastric carcinoma including GCC is substantial [7]. After endoscopic or surgical resection, periodic systematical endoscopic surveillance is essential to monitor and control any secondary cancers. In a 12-center study of 1258 Japanese patients [31], 175 (13.9%) patients developed secondary gastric cancer within a mean of 26.8 months after resection. Synchronous and metachronous tumors accounted for 110 (62.9%) and 65 (36.3%) cases, respectively. Surprisingly, 21 of 110 (19.1%) synchronous cancers were missed primarily in the upper stomach including the cardia, a finding that parallels the results of another study [10]. The cumulative incidence of metachronous cancers increased at the rate of 3.5% and was correlated with time, but not with the status of *H. pylori* eradication. In that study, all recurrent cancers were successfully resected again endoscopically.

The American Society of Gastrointestinal Endoscopy has published practice guidelines in 2015 on the role of endoscopy in management of pre- and cancerous diseases [14]. Their recommendations include that patients undergoing resection of lesions with a pathologic diagnosis of low-grade dysplasia/adenoma should also undergo a surveillance exam 1 year after resection.

Correlation Between Endoscopic and Pathologic Diagnoses

In the hands of experienced endoscopists using advanced endoscopic techniques, the correlation in pathologic diagnosis between endoscopic biopsies and resections, such as ESD, is high, especially for intestinal-type early gastric carcinoma including GCC. Sometimes, there are discrepancies among cases with missed synchronous early gastric carcinoma. In a retrospective study [32], Yoo et al. investigated predictive factors with missed synchronous early gastric carcinoma detected within 1 year after ESD in 250 patients. Missed tumors were smaller but located in the same third of the stomach as the primary tumor. The incidence was 11.6% (29/250) and significantly correlated with the number of tumors at the time of ESD resection and advanced age of patients. Therefore, careful endoscopic surveillance after ESD should be carried out, especially for multiple lesions and in elderly patients who are the main GCC patient population. On the other hand, pathologic evaluation of the ESD-resected specimen sometimes fails to demonstrate invasive carcinoma that was diagnosed in the mucosal biopsies. Jeong et al. recently retrospectively reviewed 1379 cases and identified negative pathology in 2% (28/1379) ESD-resected lesions. They reported that the tumors present only in the biopsy specimens were significantly smaller in size and in the surface area. Therefore, most tumors were completely removed by biopsies (71.4%, 20/28); overdiagnosis occurred only in 17.9% (5/28), and tumors in a different ESD site were 10.7% (3/28) [33].

Diagnostic Discrepancy Between Endoscopic Biopsy and Resection

Gastric carcinoma diagnosis is defined as histologic identification of invasion of neoplastic cells or glands through the basement membrane into the lamina propriety, according to the WHO criteria [34]. Unfortunately, there is considerable disagreement among pathologists especially on the diagnosis of intramucosal carcinoma, or high-grade dysplasia, which is similar to the difficulties in distinguishing Barrett's intramucosal adenocarcinoma from high-grade dysplasia arising in Barrett's esophagus. The debate for the pathologic diagnosis of high-grade adenoma (dysplasia) and intramucosal carcinoma between the West and East pathologists has become meaningless in recent years because the same management strategies are employed for both lesions [18]. Lesions that are labeled as either intramucosal carcinoma or as high-grade adenoma/dysplasia are removed using endoscopic or open surgical resection. Surprisingly, underdiagnosis of invasive carcinoma in resection specimens is quite common in cases with biopsies having being read as low- or high-grade dysplasia [35, 36]. In a recent retrospectively study [36], Xu et al. analyzed diagnostic discrepancy between biopsy and resection specimens in 57 early gastric carcinomas diagnosed with the WHO criteria. Although concordant diagnosis was found in most (74.9%) cases, the diagnosis of intramucosal carcinoma was upgraded in over 25% resection cases, in which 60.5% were initially diagnosed as high-grade dysplasia and 29.5% as low-grade dysplasia, especially in lesions larger than 2 cm in size and a depressed endoscopic gross pattern. Since both high-grade dysplasia and intramucosal carcinoma carry a minimal risk of lymph node metastasis, both lesions are resected, most commonly by ESD [18, 19].

Helicobacter pylori Testing

Multiple studies have shown that *H. pylori* infection is a significant risk factor and likely carcinogen for the development of gastric carcinoma, although its role in the tumorigenesis of GCC remains unclear. Nevertheless, all patients suspected of having GCC should be tested for *H. pylori* infection. There are several validated clinical tests for detecting *H. pylori*. For example, the ^{13}C urea breath test as well as the stool antigen test are noninvasive and have high sensitivities and specificities. They are recommended for both the screening and confirming successful eradication of *H. pylori* after treatment. A serology test for the specific antibody to this bacterium is also available. Other tests include the rapid urease test, histology, and culture.

Clinical Staging

Once a carcinoma is diagnosed in the gastric cardia, the tumor needs to be staged, according to the tumor node metastasis (TNM) classification system of the American Joint Committee on Cancer. The detailed procedure is described in Chap. 10. In the 2015 practice guidelines of the American Society of Gastrointestinal Endoscopy [14], EUS is required for evaluation of gastric submucosal lesions and local staging of gastric cancer, with or without FNA.

Barium Swallow

Traditionally, barium swallow is used as a diagnostic tool in GCC and provides a so-called road map before the era of endoscopy. Polypoid tumors, strictures with mucosal irregularity, and "apple core" constrictions (Fig. 9.10) are typical findings on barium studies to suggest malignancy.

The barium swallow examination may also provide information to help with surgical planning, including tumor location and the presence of other pathological conditions, such as a hiatal hernia or diverticulum. However, features of GCC tumors, such as size and location, can be more accurately assessed using upper endoscopy than a barium study [37]. The value of the barium study as an initial diagnostic test remains controversial [38]. The main advantages of a barium study are convenient, inexpensive, and noninvasive. It may also provide the valuable evidence to support the differentiation of GCC from distal gastric tumors, especially in situations where large tumors are seen on retroflexion that obscures the anatomy (Fig. 9.11) [39]. Early manifestations of GCC are usually subtle with minimal mucosal changes. In advanced GCC, tumors may be large, ulcerated, invading into the gastric wall, surrounding tissues, organs, and sometimes the distal esophagus, which can be clearly visualized by barium swallow. Therefore, despite the

Fig. 9.10 Typical radiologic appearances of gastric cardiac carcinoma revealed by barrow swallow feature marked strictures with mucosal irregularity (arrow)

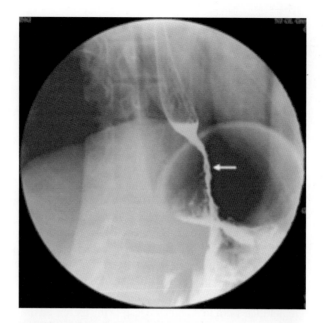

Fig. 9.11 An ulcerated gastric cardiac carcinoma (arrow) is visualized by retroflex view of conventional white-light endoscopy

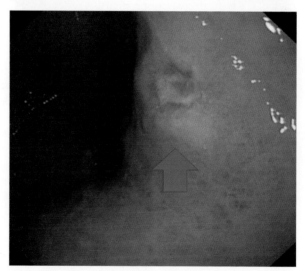

widespread use of upper endoscopy, barium swallow can be a useful and valuable diagnostic tool in selected cases. The shortcomings of this diagnostic test lie in the inability to take biopsies and limited utility to detect early carcinoma. Among studies that examined pathologically proven early gastric carcinomas, one report suggested that the barium study had a sensitivity of only 28.6% (4/14) [40], and another found that the barium test missed all 15 early gastric carcinoma cases [41].

In Japan, the X-ray photofluorography along with barium swallow is recommended for screening gastric cancer [42]. For this test, the patient swallows effervescent granules and then drinks 200–300 mL of barium for several plain radiographs. This test is costly and has a low sensitivity and specificity for detection of early gastric cancer.

Computed Tomography (CT) and Magnetic Resonance Imaging (MRI)

Recent advances in technology have made CT and MRI more effective in staging, assessing tumor resectability, radiotherapy planning, and evaluating treatment responses. For early GCC, CT (especially contrast-enhanced CT with both oral and intravenous contrast) of the chest and abdomen is used as one of initial evaluation tests [6]. Axial CT images of a GCC tumor (Fig. 9.12) may visualize an abnormal area of gastric wall thickening, usually defined as being greater than 5 mm [43].The accuracy of CT in assessing the depth of tumor penetration is 80–85%. Strong enhancement and heterogeneous enhancement patterns have been used as the criteria for gastric carcinoma. In fact, CT can detect all of hepatic metastatic lesions greater than 1 cm in diameter. Despite the increased diagnostic sensitivity, the drawback of CT is the decreased specificity. A series of the CT data on the esophagus and the stomach can be obtained by modern multi-slice CT (MSCT) scanners with a resolution of 1 mm. MSCT is able to easily detect enlarged lymph nodes but difficult to define the nature of an enlarged lymph node.

The inherent multi-planar feature of MRI is no longer advantageous over CT. In fact, CT and MRI are largely comparable in terms of staging accuracy, but CT is significantly less expensive. Two interesting enhancements are under development: miniaturized MR receiver coils can be mounted within an endoscope, giving a much higher resolution at the expense of a smaller field of view. Novel contrast agents are also being studied for use in MRI.

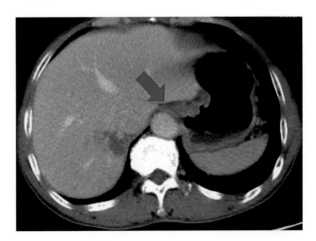

Fig. 9.12 An advanced gastric cardiac carcinoma is demonstrated by axial CT scan (arrow)

Fig. 9.13 A metastatic lesion from a patient with advanced gastric cardiac carcinoma is demonstrated in the spinal vertebral body as a high signal (arrow)

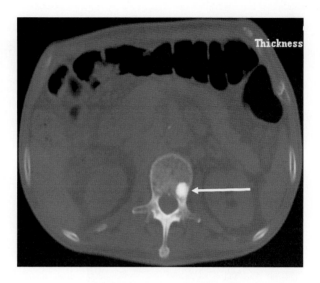

Currently, preoperative staging in GCC includes the use of CT and MRI examinations to determine locoregional and distant organ metastases in peri-gastric lymph nodes, the liver, pancreas, peritoneum, mediastinum, chest, head-neck, and other organs (such as bone metastasis) (Fig. 9.13), which is superior over EUS in this respect. In addition, MSCT scanning and three-dimensional reconstruction of simulated endoscopic techniques are also being used for the diagnosis and staging of GCC [44, 45].

Positron Emission Tomography

Whole-body 18Fdeoxyglucose (FDG)-positron emission tomography (PET) scanning has been shown to be a useful tool primarily in preoperative staging. For early GCC, the PET scan is an optional test for staging [6]. For detection of distant lymph node metastasis, the PET scan has a higher sensitivity than CT or EUS. Because most malignancies are FDG-avid (Fig. 9.14), the PET scan is able to effectively illustrate a tumor with the high-signal location to provide the necessary information for radiation therapy and surgery decisions [46]. However, false-positive results are common. Mucosal ulcerations, inflammations, and previous interventions (biopsy or stent placement) may appear as linear or focal FDG-avid lesions and become common causes of false-positive FDG uptake. For these reasons, evaluation of the apparent metabolic activity in GCC should be combined with the results of upper endoscopy and biopsy pathology. PET scans can be complementary to endoscopy and reveal occult submucosal diseases [6].

As a new diagnostic combination, PET/CT systems can provide both anatomic and functional information, thus contributing significantly to improving the clinical

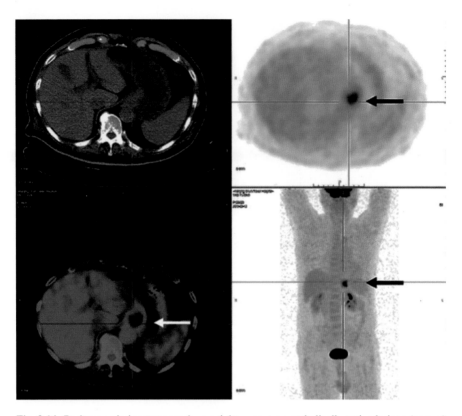

Fig. 9.14 Positron emission tomography on right uncovers metabolically active lesions (arrows) in the whole body, as in the case of advanced gastric cardiac carcinoma

Table 9.4 Diagnostic and staging investigations in gastric cardiac cancer [47]

Procedure	Purpose
Endoscopy and biopsy	Obtain tissue for diagnosis, histological classification, and molecular biomarkers
CT	Staging of tumor—to detect local/distant lymphadenopathy and metastatic disease
EUS	Accurate assessment of T and N stage in potentially operable tumors Determine the proximal and distal extent of tumor
PET (if available)	Improve detection of occult metastatic disease

decision-making process (Table 9.4) [27]. Studies involving patients with biopsy-proven GCC showed that the addition of PET/CT to standard staging may change the choice of follow-up management modalities [47, 48].

Differential Diagnosis

Because of the surgical anatomical location between the lower thorax and upper abdomen, the differential diagnosis of GCC is broad, ranging from distal esophageal-cardiac achalasia; stricture; stenosis, as a result of chronic inflammation and erosion of the lower esophagus; and ulcerative lesions in the gastric cardia and EGJ, due to severe bile reflux diseases. In some cases, the radiologic imaging studies of the gastric cardia or the EGJ show alarming changes in the gastric cardiac region. However, a simple conventional white-light upper endoscopy with biopsies for histopathologic confirmation is usually diagnostic and uncovers a nonneoplastic disease process.

During endoscopy, lesions that may mimic GCC include hyperplastic polyps, gastritis cystica profunda, and mesenchymal tumors such as leiomyoma and gastrointestinal stromal tumors.

Summary

GCC is usually asymptomatic at the early stage and occurs primarily in elderly patients with a male predominance. Early diagnosis relies upon a thorough and systematic endoscopic investigation with biopsies in the gastric cardia. Once GCC is diagnosed pathologically, the patient needs to be completely worked up for nodal metastasis and clinical staging to guide further management.

References

1. Huang Q, Fang C, Shi J, et al. Differences in clinicopathology of early gastric carcinoma between proximal and distal location in 438 Chinese patients. Sci Rep. 2015;5:13439.
2. Sano T, Coit DG, Kim HH, et al. Proposal of a new stage grouping of gastric cancer for TNM classification: International Gastric Cancer Association staging project. Gastric Cancer. 2017;20(2):217–25.
3. Nashimoto A, Akazawa K, Isobe Y, et al. Gastric cancer treated in 2002 in Japan: 2009 annual report of the JGCA nationwide registry. Gastric Cancer. 2013;16(1):1–27.
4. Schmitz KJ, König C, Riesener KP. Intramural carcinoma of the oesophagogastric junction. BMJ Case Rep. 2011;2012(2dHalf):169–80.
5. Daly JM, Fry WA, Little AG, et al. Esophageal cancer: results of an American College of Surgeons Patient Care Evaluation Study. J Am Coll Surg. 2000;190(5):562–72.
6. Varghese TK Jr, Hofstetter WL, Rizk NP, Low DE, et al. The Society of Thoracic Surgeons guidelines on the diagnosis and staging of patients with esophageal cancer. Ann Thorac Surg. 2013;96(1):346.

7. Fang C, Huang Q, Lu L, et al. Risk factors of early proximal gastric carcinoma in Chinese diagnosed using WHO criteria. J Dig Dis. 2015;16(6):327–36.
8. Gao Y, Zhang K, Xi H, et al. Diagnostic and prognostic value of circulating tumor DNA in gastric cancer: a meta-analysis. Oncotarget. 2017;8(4):6330–40.
9. Huang Q, Shi J, Sun Q, et al. Clinicopathological characterisation of small (2 cm or less) proximal and distal gastric carcinomas in a Chinese population. Pathology. 2015;47(6):526–32.
10. Ren W, Yu J, Zhang ZM, Song YK, Li YH, Wang L. Missed diagnosis of early gastric cancer or high-grade intraepithelial neoplasia. World J Gastroenterol. 2013;19(13):2092–6.
11. Emura F, Gralnek I, Baron TH. Improving early detection of gastric cancer: a novel systematic alphanumeric-coded endoscopic approach. Rev Gastroenterol Peru. 2013;33(1):52–8.
12. Nigro JJ, Demeester SR, Hagen JA, et al. Node status in transmural esophageal adenocarcinoma and outcome after en bloc esophagectomy. J Thorac Cardiovasc Surg. 1999;117(5):960–8.
13. Lal N, Bhasin DK, Malik AK, Gupta NM, Singh K, Mehta SK. Optimal number of biopsy specimens in the diagnosis of carcinoma of the oesophagus. Gut. 1992;33(6):724.
14. Committee AS, Evans JA, Chandrasekhara V, et al. The role of endoscopy in the management of premalignant and malignant conditions of the stomach. Gastrointest Endosc. 2015;82(1):1–8.
15. Evans JA, Early DS, Chandraskhara V, et al. The role of endoscopy in the assessment and treatment of esophageal cancer. Gastrointest Endosc. 2003;57(7):817–22.
16. Zargar SA, Khuroo MS, Jan GM, Mahajan R, Shah P. Prospective comparison of the value of brushings before and after biopsy in the endoscopic diagnosis of gastroesophageal malignancy. Acta Cytol. 1991;35(5):549–52.
17. Ajani JA, D'Amico TA, Almhanna K, et al. Esophageal and esophagogastric junction cancers, version 1.2015. J Natl Compr Canc Netw. 2011;9(8):830–87.
18. Yao K, Nagahama T, Matsui T, Iwashita A. Detection and characterization of early gastric cancer for curative endoscopic submucosal dissection. Dig Endosc. 2013;25(Suppl 1):44–54.
19. Uedo N, Yao K. Endoluminal diagnosis of early gastric cancer and its precursors: bridging the gap between endoscopy and pathology. Adv Exp Med Biol. 2016;908:293–316.
20. Okada K, Fujisaki J, Kasuga A, et al. Endoscopic ultrasonography is valuable for identifying early gastric cancers meeting expanded-indication criteria for endoscopic submucosal dissection. Surg Endosc. 2011;25(3):841–8.
21. Matsuo K, Takedatsu H, Mukasa M, et al. Diagnosis of early gastric cancer using narrow band imaging and acetic acid. World J Gastroenterol. 2015;21(4):1268–74.
22. Kumagai Y, Takubo K, Kawada K, et al. A newly developed continuous zoom-focus endocytoscope. Endoscopy. 2017;49(2):176–80.
23. Lee HC, Ahsen OO, Liang K, et al. Endoscopic optical coherence tomography angiography microvascular features associated with dysplasia in Barrett's esophagus (with video). Gastrointest Endosc. 2017;86(3):476–84, e473.
24. Nishioka NS. Optical biopsy using tissue spectroscopy and optical coherence tomography. Can J Gastroenterol. 2003;17(6):376–80.
25. Faigel DO, Deveney C, Phillips D, Fennerty MB. Biopsy-negative malignant esophageal stricture: diagnosis by endoscopic ultrasound. Am J Gastroenterol. 1998;93(11):2257–60.
26. Tsujii Y, Kato M, Inoue T, et al. Integrated diagnostic strategy for the invasion depth of early gastric cancer by conventional endoscopy and EUS. Gastrointest Endosc. 2015;82(3):452–9.
27. Wallace MB, Nietert PJ, Earle C, et al. An analysis of multiple staging management strategies for carcinoma of the esophagus: computed tomography, endoscopic ultrasound, positron emission tomography, and thoracoscopy/laparoscopy. Ann Thorac Surg. 2002;74(4):1026–32.
28. Mocellin S, Pasquali S. Diagnostic accuracy of endoscopic ultrasonography (EUS) for the preoperative locoregional staging of primary gastric cancer. Cochrane Database Syst Rev. 2015;(2):CD009944.
29. Hassan H, Vilmann P, Sharma V. Impact of EUS-guided FNA on management of gastric carcinoma. Gastrointest Endosc. 2010;71(3):500–4.
30. Sultan J, Robinson S, Hayes N, Griffin SM, Richardson DL, Preston SR. Endoscopic ultrasonography-detected low-volume ascites as a predictor of inoperability for oesophagogastric cancer. Br J Surg. 2008;95(9):1127–30.

31. Kato M, Nishida T, Yamamoto K, et al. Scheduled endoscopic surveillance controls secondary cancer after curative endoscopic resection for early gastric cancer: a multicentre retrospective cohort study by Osaka University ESD study group. Gut. 2013;62(10):1425–32.
32. Yoo JH, Shin SJ, Lee KM, et al. How can we predict the presence of missed synchronous lesions after endoscopic submucosal dissection for early gastric cancers or gastric adenomas? J Clin Gastroenterol. 2013;47(2):e17–22.
33. Jeong DI, Kim HW, Choi CW, et al. Clinical features of negative pathologic results after gastric endoscopic submucosal dissection. Surg Endosc. 2017;31(3):1163–71.
34. Lauwers GY, Carneiro F, Graham DY, et al. Gastric carcinoma. In: Bosman FT, Carneiro F, Hruban RH, Theise ND, editors. WHO classification of tumours of the digestive system. Lyon: IARC Press; 2010. p. 48–58.
35. Choi CW, Kim HW, Shin DH, et al. The risk factors for discrepancy after endoscopic submucosal dissection of gastric category 3 lesion (low grade dysplasia). Dig Dis Sci. 2014;59(2):421–7.
36. Xu G, Zhang W, Lv Y, et al. Risk factors for under-diagnosis of gastric intraepithelial neoplasia and early gastric carcinoma in endoscopic forceps biopsy in comparison with endoscopic submucosal dissection in Chinese patients. Surg Endosc. 2016;30(7):2716–22.
37. Dooley CP, Larson AW, Stace NH, et al. Double-contrast barium meal and upper gastrointestinal endoscopy. A comparative study. Ann Intern Med. 1984;101(4):538–45.
38. Esfandyari T, Potter JW, Vaezi MF. Dysphagia: a cost analysis of the diagnostic approach. Am J Gastroenterol. 2002;97(11):2733–7.
39. Maric R, Cheng KK. Classification of adenocarcinoma of the oesophagogastric junction. Br J Surg. 1998;85(11):1457–9.
40. Longo WE, Zucker KA, Zdon MJ, Modlin IM. Detection of early gastric cancer in an aggressive endoscopy unit. Am Surg. 1989;55(2):100–4.
41. Ballantyne KC, Morris DL, Jones JA, Gregson RH, Hardcastle JD. Accuracy of identification of early gastric cancer. Br J Surg. 1987;74(7):618–9.
42. Sugano K. Screening of gastric cancer in Asia. Best Pract Res Clin Gastroenterol. 2015;29(6):895–905.
43. Yoon YC, Lee KS, Shim YM, Kim BT, Kim K, Kim TS. Metastasis to regional lymph nodes in patients with esophageal squamous cell carcinoma: CT versus FDG PET for presurgical detection prospective study. Radiology. 2003;227(3):764–70.
44. Zhao Q, Li Y, Hu Z, Tan B, Yang P, Tian Y. [Value of the preoperative TNM staging and the longest tumor diameter measurement of gastric cancer evaluated by MSCT]. Zhonghua Wei Chang Wai Ke Za Zhi. 2015;18(3):227–31.
45. Feng XY, Wang W, Luo GY, et al. Comparison of endoscopic ultrasonography and multislice spiral computed tomography for the preoperative staging of gastric cancer—results of a single institution study of 610 Chinese patients. PLoS One. 2013;8(11):e78846.
46. Walker AJ, Spier BJ, Perlman SB. Integrated PET/CT fusion imaging and endoscopic ultrasound in the pre-operative staging and evaluation of esophageal cancer. Mol Imaging Biol. 2011;13(1):166.
47. Blencowe NS, Whistance RN, Strong S, et al. Evaluating the role of fluorodeoxyglucose positron emission tomography-computed tomography in multi-disciplinary team recommendations for oesophago-gastric cancer. Br J Cancer. 2011;109(6):1445–50.
48. Waddell T, Verheij M, Allum W, et al. Gastric cancer: ESMO–ESSO–ESTRO Clinical Practice Guidelines for diagnosis, treatment and follow-up. Ann Oncol. 2013;23(Suppl 6):40–8.

Chapter 10
Prognosis and Staging

Qin Huang and Jason S. Gold

Introduction

The tumor-node-metastasis (TNM) staging system has been proven to be the best predictor of outcomes in patients with solid malignant tumors. Based on the TNM system, the Union for International Cancer Control (UICC) and the American Joint Committee on Cancer (AJCC) have developed the cancer staging manual to guide the worldwide clinical practice on cancer classification and staging. Historically, gastric cardiac cancer (GCC) had always been part of gastric cancer and staged as such until January 2010, when the UICC/AJCC published the seventh edition of the cancer staging manual (AJCC 7) [1]. In this most important cancer staging guideline, GCC was classified as part of esophageal adenocarcinoma and required to be staged as such. This dramatic paradigm shift was based on the research results accumulated primarily in the Caucasian population in the West, in which adenocarcinoma arising in the esophagogastric junction (EGJ) region often results from Barrett's esophagus, predominantly in the elderly Caucasian men. Some authorities believe that carcinomas arising in the distal esophagus, across the EGJ line, or in the gastric cardia share similar epidemiologic, clinicopathologic, and molecular characteristics and should be grouped as adenocarcinomas of the distal esophagus [2–4].

Q. Huang (✉)
Pathology and Laboratory Medicine, Veterans Affairs Boston Healthcare System, West Roxbury, MA, USA

Harvard Medical School and Brigham and Women's Hospital, Boston, MA, USA

J. S. Gold
Department of Surgery, Harvard Medical School/Brigham and Women's Hospital, Boston, MA, USA

Veterans Affairs Boston Healthcare System, West Roxbury, MA, USA
e-mail: jgold@bwh.harvard.edu

© Springer International Publishing AG, part of Springer Nature 2018
Q. Huang (ed.), *Gastric Cardiac Cancer*, https://doi.org/10.1007/978-3-319-79114-2_10

Fig. 10.1 The Siewert classification of adenocarcinomas in the esophagogastric junction (EGJ) region. Tumors with epicenters located between 1 and 5 cm above the EGJ are classified as Siewert I, tumors with epicenters located within 2 cm below the EGJ are grouped as Siewert II, and tumors with epicenters located 3–5 cm below the EGJ are grouped as Siewert III [2]

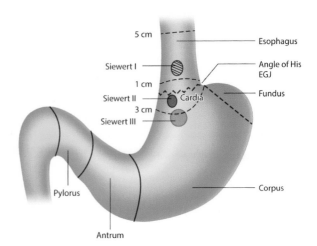

For adenocarcinomas arising from the 10-cm region in the EGJ region (5 cm above and 5 cm below the EGJ line), the German thoracic surgeon, Dr. Siewert, along with his colleagues, divided EGJ adenocarcinomas into three types [2]. As shown in Fig. 10.1, Siewert I adenocarcinomas arise between 1 cm and 5 cm above the EGJ line, Siewert II tumors refer to adenocarcinomas with epicenters from 1 cm above to 2 cm below the EGJ, and Siewert III tumors show epicenters 2–5 cm below the EGJ. In the Siewert system, GCC corresponds mainly to Siewert type II and some type III tumors. The AJCC 7 adopted the Siewert classification and required all adenocarcinomas in this 10-cm-long region to be classified, staged, and treated as esophageal adenocarcinoma [1]. Since the publication of the AJCC 7 in 2010, a number of studies have been published with the following key findings [5–9]:

1. The Siewert classification may be useful for surgical resection of EGJ adenocarcinomas.
2. The value of this classification is minimal for post-resection prognosis stratification.
3. Siewert I adenocarcinoma is Barrett esophageal adenocarcinoma and occurs primarily in the elderly Caucasian male population in the West but very infrequently in East Asian countries.
4. Clinicopathology and prognosis of Siewert III adenocarcinomas are similar to those of gastric adenocarcinomas, but not those of Siewert I esophageal adenocarcinomas.
5. By definition, the Siewert classification of the EGJ cancer was intended for adenocarcinomas only. In fact, a substantial proportion of carcinomas in the 10-cm-long EGJ region are not adenocarcinomas, especially in Chinese patients [10, 11]. Therefore, the applicability of the Siewert classification for non-adenocarcinoma tumors is in question, especially in the Chinese population
6. As required by AJCC 7, staging GCC as esophageal adenocarcinoma cannot effectively stratify patient prognosis. Instead, the most recent data published by the International Gastric Cancer Association (IGCA) indicate that GCC should be

staged as gastric cancer for a much better stratification of patient outcomes after radical resection [12]. As such, the updated AJCC 8 published in 2017 changed the rules set previously by AJCC 7 on classification and staging of GCC [13].

In this chapter, we will provide readers with the most important high-quality evidence on this critical issue in clinical practice on staging and prognosis of GCC.

New Stage Groupings of the International Gastric Cancer Association and Eighth Edition of the American Joint Committee on Cancer (AJCC 8)

Since 2009, the IGCA leadership has established an international expert group specifically charged with the task on classification and prognostic stage stratification of GCC, i.e., Siewert type II and III tumors [12]. As a result, the task force collected and analyzed 25,411 cases of radical resection of GCC tumors from 15 countries in patients without neoadjuvant therapy but with at least 5-year follow-up survival information [12]. The IGCA panel proposed in 2017 expanding the pIIIC subgroup in the TNM staging system for gastric cancer by including GCC cases primarily staged at pN3a, pN3b, and pT4b as well as some at pN2 and pT4a. Their analysis showed substantial improvement in prognostic stratification of the previously problematic pIII subgroup defined by AJCC 7. Table 10.1 exhibits the new 2017 IGCA pathologic TNM stage groupings for GCC [12].

This new 2017 pTNM grouping system by IGCA has successfully resolved the defect in AJCC 7 for pIII staging in GCC, which is a unique feature of GCC [7, 14]. By grouping pN3 disease into the pIIIC category, the prognosis stratification becomes meaningful for patients with pIII GCC. Similarly, using the same IGCA database with 25,411 radical resection cases, AJCC 8, published in 2017, has modified the classification of adenocarcinoma in the EGJ region and requires staging tumors involving the EGJ with epicenters 2 cm below the EGJ, i.e., some Siewert II GCCs, with the rules for esophageal squamous cell carcinoma, not gastric cancer [13], as did AJCC 7 (Fig. 10.2).

However, for Siewert II tumors with epicenters 2 cm below the EGJ without extension through the EGJ into the distal esophagus, as well as Siewert III tumors with epicenters more than 2 cm below the EGJ (Fig. 10.3), AJCC 8 changed AJCC 7 rules and required staging those tumors with the schemes for gastric carcinoma. Apparently at present, accurate determination of the EGJ line and the exact relationship between the EGJ and the tumor epicenter is critically important for classification and staging of tumors in this region.

Adenocarcinoma is defined as neoplastic glands breaking through the basement membrane and infiltrating the gastric wall from the lamina propria to muscularis mucosae and beyond. Because tumor differentiation also affects patient prognosis, all adenocarcinomas should be graded by the criteria of the World Health

Table 10.1 pTNM stage grouping proposed by the International Gastric Cancer Association [12]

pStage	T	N	M
IA	1	0	0
IB	1	1	0
	2	0	0
IIA	1	2	0
	2	1	0
	3	0	0
IIB	1	3a	0
	2	2	0
	3	1	0
	4a	1	0
IIIA	2	3a	0
	3	2	0
	4a	1	0
	4a	2	0
IIIB	1	3b	0
	2	3b	0
	3	3a	0
	4a	3a	0
	4b	2	0
	4b	1	0
IIIC	3	3b	0
	4a	3b	0
	4b	3a	0
	4b	3b	0

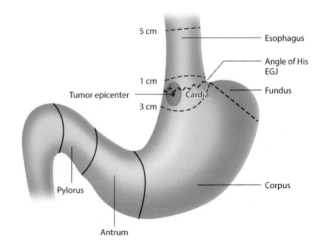

Fig. 10.2 The AJCC 8 requires staging gastric cardiac carcinoma with epicenters 2 cm below but crossing the esophagogastric junction (EGJ) with the rules for esophageal squamous cell carcinoma

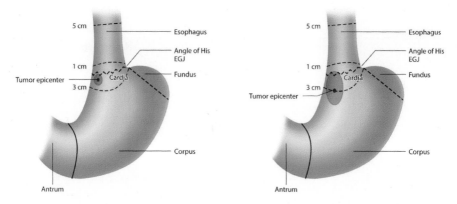

Fig. 10.3 Tumors with epicenters located 2 cm below the esophagogastric junction (EGJ) without the esophageal involvement (left) or epicenters 3 cm below the EGJ but with esophageal invasion (right) are required by AJCC8 to be staged as gastric carcinoma

Table 10.2 Grading of gastric adenocarcinoma by the rules of the WHO [15]

G (grading)	Criteria
1	Well differentiated, >95% of the tumor is composed of well-formed neoplastic glands
2	Moderately differentiated, 50–94% of the tumor shows discernable neoplastic glands
3	Poorly differentiated, <49% of the tumor exhibits neoplastic glandular structure

Table 10.3 Clinical TNM rules (cTNM) for esophageal adenocarcinoma [13]

Grouping	T	N	M
0	Tis	0	0
I	1	0	0
IIA	1	1	0
IIB	2	0	0
III	2	1	0
	3	0–1	0
	4a	0–1	0
IVA	1–4a	2	0
	4b	0–2	0
	Any T	3	0
IVB	Any T	Any N	1

Organization (WHO) on the basis of the estimated proportion of discernable neoplastic glands in a tumor (Table 10.2) [15].

Clinical staging of esophageal adenocarcinoma, including Siewert II GCC invading the esophagus before resection, is important for patient management but may not be as accurate as pathologic staging. Therefore, AJCC 8 also sets the rules for clinical TNM staging (cTNM) [13], as listed in Table 10.3.

Table 10.4 AJCC 8 Pathologic TNM (pTNM) rules for esophageal adenocarcinoma/GCC [13]

Grouping	T	N	M	Differentiation (G)
0	Is (in situ)	0	0	Not available
IA	1a	0	0	1
	1a	0	0	X
IB	1a	0	0	2
	1b	0	0	1–2
	1b	0	0	X
IC	1	0	0	3
	2	0	0	1–2
IIA	2	0	0	3
	2	0	0	X
IIB	1	1	0	Any
	3	0	0	Any
IIIA	1	2	0	Any
	2	1	0	Any
IIIB	2	2	0	Any
	3	1–2	0	Any
	4a	0–1	0	Any
IVA	4a	2	0	Any
	4b	0–2	0	Any
	Any T	3	0	Any
IVB	Any T	Any N	1	Any

After resection, pathologic TNM (pTNM) staging of esophageal adenocarcinoma, including GCC tumors smaller than 2 cm in size but involving the esophagus, is critical for patient triage, management, and follow-up. For pTNM grouping, AJCC 8 sets the following rules listed in Table 10.4.

It must be pointed out that the new 2017 guideline on GCC staging by the IGCA is significant and should have considerable positive impact on survival analysis of patients with GCC, although the data used for the analysis are primarily (>84%) from patients in Japan and Korea where GCC is uncommon with Siewert type II and III adenocarcinomas (GCC), accounting for only 2.5% for the Japanese data and 3% of the Korean data [12]. In contrast, the prevalence of GCC tumors is substantial in the Chinese population and reported in over 25% of gastric cancer resection cases [9, 16]. According to the 2012 epidemiology data accumulated by WHO on gastric cancer [17], over 42% of new gastric cancer cases are from China. Inclusion of Chinese GCC patients with solid clinicopathologic data in the future staging update would make the pTNM system on GCC more universally applicable and reliable.

Pathologic Tumor Staging (PT)

The complexity of pathologic staging of GCC is mainly due to the pathologic T (pT) and N (pN) stage groupings [6, 18]. In advanced GCC, the overall tumor volume is usually larger, and invasion depth is deeper than for that of distal

Table 10.5 AJCC 8 pathologic tumor stage grouping (pT) criteria for primary gastric carcinoma [13]

Group	Criteria
TX	Primary tumor cannot be assessed
T0	No primary tumor identified
Tis	Carcinoma in situ with no evidence of invasion, high-grade dysplasia
T1	Invasion into the lamina propria, muscularis mucosae, and submucosa
T1a	Invasion into the lamina propria, muscularis mucosae
T1b	Invasion into the submucosa
T2	Invasion into the muscularis propria
T3	Invasion into the subserosal fat, omentum, but not visceral peritoneum[a]
T4	Invasion through the visceral peritoneum (T4a) or into adjacent structures (T4b)
T4a	Invasion through the visceral peritoneum
T4b	Invasion into the adjacent structures such as diaphragm, esophagus, colon, pancreas, spleen, abdominal wall, adrenal gland, kidney, small intestine, and retroperitoneum

[a]Gastric cardiac carcinoma invading intramurally into the esophagus is NOT classified as pT4b for invasion of adjacent structure, but staged with the depth of the greatest invasion in the esophagus

esophageal adenocarcinoma and gastric non-cardiac carcinoma [16, 19], which are well-known to be correlated with a high frequency of nodal metastasis [7, 20–22]. In a single-center German study with 224 radical resections of GCC involving the distal esophagus, the nodal metastasis rate was reported to be zero (0/71) for pT1a and 18% (27/153) for pT1b, in which 19 (70.4%, 19/27) were pN1, 5 (18.5%, 5/27) were pN2, and 2 (7.4%, 2/27) were pN3 [23]. In a retrospective study of 291 radical resections performed at a single center in China, over 95% of carcinomas were diagnosed at advanced stages with a mean size of 5.9 cm [24]. As a result, by the AJCC 7 rules for gastric cancer, the pT staging for GCC in Chinese patients is monotonous in subgroups [24], except for indiscriminate separation between pT2 and pT3 and pT4a and pT4b [24]. In contrast, by the rules for esophageal adenocarcinoma, the pT stage becomes neither monotonous nor distinct. The 5-year survival rate is incorrectly worse for patients staged pT4a than those staged pT4b [24] or between pIIIA and pIA [7]. The data suggest inadequate stratification of prognosis by applying the staging rules of esophageal cancer to GCC in Chinese patients. In AJCC 8 [13], gastric carcinomas, including some GCC tumors, are stage-grouped into four categories as shown in Table 10.5. The effectiveness of this prognostic grouping remains to be validated independently.

In East Asian countries where Siewert type I adenocarcinoma is rare [5, 8, 24, 25], GCC most commonly arises in the gastric cardia and may invade the distal esophagus. The prognosis of patients with GCC invading into the esophagus has been shown to be significantly ($p < 0.001$) worse with a 5-year survival rate of 48.7% ($N = 222$) than those without esophageal invasion (80.8%, $N = 108$) after stratification by the pathologic stage and nodal status in a Japanese study [26]. In fact, esophageal invasion was shown by multivariate analysis to be an independent risk factor for poor prognosis [26]. The results have been confirmed in a Korean study [8]. The outcomes of patients with Siewert type II and III tumors (i.e., GCC) are similar [8], supporting the classification of those tumors as gastric carcinoma.

Pathologic Nodal Staging (pN)

Overall, nodal metastasis in GCC is similar to that in other gastric cancers, but not to that in esophageal cancer [6, 26–28]. In a case series study from China with 142 GCC cases, nodal metastasis occurs most commonly, in the decreasing order of frequency, in the paracardial, the lesser and greater curvatures, and the celiac axis regions [29]. Celiac axis nodal metastasis accounts for 25% of cases [29], a rate similar to that reported in the literature [30–32]. There was no metastasis discovered in lymph nodes in the retropancreatic, para-aortic, and paraesophageal regions in that study [29]. However, mediastinal nodal metastasis was reported to be substantial for EGJ adenocarcinomas including some GCC tumors [30–34]. In a small sample of 50 D1 or D2 resection cases, Monig et al. reported nodal metastases in the lower mediastinum in 24%, 11%, and 13% for Siewert type I, II, and III carcinomas, respectively, and no nodal metastasis discovered in the upper mediastinum in all 13 patients with transthoracic en bloc resection and D2 lymphadenectomy [33]. In a multicenter study of 315 R0 or R1 EGJ adenocarcinoma resection cases including GCC, Japanese investigators reported nodal metastasis rates in the upper, middle, and lower mediastinum in 4%, 7%, and 11%, respectively [35]. They also described that the only independent risk factor for mediastinal nodal metastasis was the distance from the tumor proximal edge to the EGJ: >3 cm for the upper and middle mediastinal nodal metastasis and >2 cm for the lower mediastinal metastasis [35]. In that report, the median tumor size was 5.5 cm (range 0.8–10.0), and most (63.5%, 200/315) tumors likely belonged to Siewert I esophageal adenocarcinoma, which explains the high frequency of mediastinal nodal metastasis described in that study. In a systematic review of nodal metastasis in patients with GCC, the highest incidence of lymph node metastasis, according to the Japan Gastric Cancer Association, was, in fact, in the upper abdomen, in the descending order, stations 1–3 (range 13.7–72.7%), station 4 (range 0–31.8%), and stations 7, 9, and 11 (range 0–45.5%), on the basis of D1 or D2 dissection findings [22]. These results have been confirmed by the most recent comprehensive Japanese multicenter study of 400 Siewert II GCC radical resections, in which nodal metastasis most frequently occurs in the abdomen in station 1 (40.8%), station 2 (31.7%), station 3 (43.2%), station 7 (27.6%), station 9 (13%), station 10 (9.7%), the para-aortic area (16.1%), station 16a2 (13.6%), and station 16b1 (20%) [36]. Surprisingly, upper, middle, and lower mediastinal nodal metastases were also considerable and found in 17.3% (4/23), 25% (12/48), and 17.7% (37/208) of cases, respectively [36]. Importantly, the initial carcinoma recurrence rate was 37.7%, and the nodal recurrence in more than one region occurred in 15.8% of cases with 9.8% in abdominal para-aortic lymph nodes. In that study, the most common organ recurrences included the liver (11%), lung (7.3%), peritoneum (6.8%), and esophagus (1%) [36]. Because of the unique location of GCC at the boundary between the thoracic azygos venous return and the abdomen portal venous system, the high frequency of thoracic mediastinal and abdominal nodal metastases is not surprising and should be thoroughly investigated and validated by investigators from other countries for better pathologic N staging. Although in a single-center retrospective study in China, the investigators did not find a statistically significant difference in the number of mediastinal nodal

Fig. 10.4 The extent of lymphadenectomy after total gastrectomy in gastric cardiac carcinoma. The numbers correspond to the lymph node station as defined in the Japanese classification of gastric carcinoma. The numbers in blue denote D1 dissection for nodal stations from 1 to 7; those in orange D1+ dissection with additional nodal stations 8a, 9, 11p; and those in red for D2 dissection with additional nodal stations 10, 11d, 12a [37]

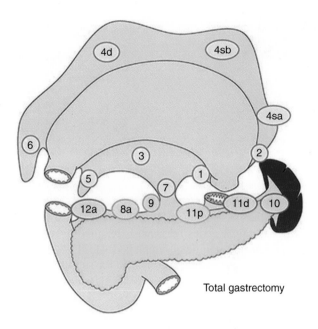

Total gastrectomy

Fig. 10.5 The extent of lymphadenectomy after proximal gastrectomy. The numbers correspond to the lymph node station as defined in the Japanese classification of gastric carcinoma. The numbers in blue denote D1 dissection for nodal stations 1, 2, 3a, 4sa, and 7 and those in orange for D1+ nodal dissection in stations 8a, 9, 11p. For the tumor with esophageal invasion, nodal dissection may include nodal station 110 in the lower thoracic paraesophageal region [37]

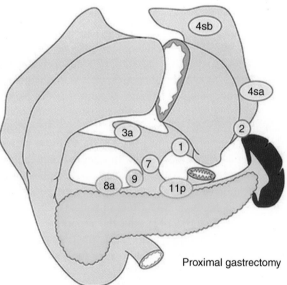

Proximal gastrectomy

metastasis between adenocarcinomas of EGJ/GCC ($N = 291$) and carcinomas from the upper stomach ($N = 176$) [24].

The most recently published 2014 gastric cancer treatment guidelines by the Japanese Gastric Cancer Association requires extensive dissection of lymph nodes for total gastrectomy [37] (Fig. 10.4), which is frequently used for radical resection of GCC. For GCC cases with proximal gastrectomy, the extent of nodal dissection is not widespread (Fig. 10.5).

Table 10.6 The AJCC 8 pN
stage grouping criteria for
gastric carcinoma [13]

Subgroup	Criteria
pNx	Regional lymph nodes cannot be assessed
pN0	No regional lymph node metastasis
pN1	Metastasis in 1–2 regional lymph nodes
pN2	Metastasis in 3–6 regional lymph nodes
pN3	Metastasis in >7 regional lymph nodes
pN3a	Metastasis in 7–15 regional lymph nodes
pN3b	Metastasis in more than 16 regional lymph nodes

For the pN staging in gastric carcinoma, a minimum of 16 (preferably >30) regional lymph nodes retrieved is required by AJCC 8 for appropriate pathologic evaluation and staging of lymph nodes [13].

Metastatic carcinoma deposits in the subserosal fat of GCC without evidence of residual lymph node morphology are classified as regional nodal metastasis, regardless of the shape, contour, or size of the deposits [13].

For GCC, the difference in pN staging by AJCC 8 between the rules for esophageal and gastric carcinomas is the pN3 stage that is further divided into pN3a (7–15 lymph nodes with metastasis) and pN3b (16 or more nodes with metastasis) subgroups for gastric, but not for esophageal carcinoma (Table 10.6). By the staging rules of AJCC 7 for gastric or esophageal cancer [1], the pN stage of GCC is monotonous and distinct because patient survival becomes worse as the number of metastatic lymph nodes increases, except for the pN3 group [6, 7, 24]. The AJCC 7 gastric cancer staging scheme separates pN3a from pN3b subgroups, while the AJCC 7 esophageal rule combines both pN3a and pN3b subgroups into one pN3. In fact, the GCC patients staged at pN3b have a 5-year survival rate significantly worse than those at pN3a or at pM1 [7]. In Chinese patients with GCC, the pN stage grouping with the rules for gastric cancer is better able to stratify patient outcomes, compared to that with the rules for esophageal cancer, which supports the classification of GCC as part of gastric cancer [12]. In a case series of GCC involving the esophagus in 142 Chinese patients [29], the nodal metastasis rate was as high as 74.6% (106/142), and the proportions of the pN stage subgroups were 20.8%, 33%, and 46.2% for pN1, pN2, and pN3, respectively, by the rules for esophageal carcinoma of AJCC 7. In the pN3 group, 35 (33%, 35/106) cases were staged as pN3a and the remaining 14 cases (13.2%, 14/106) as pN3b, by the rules for gastric cancer set by AJCC 7. The cases staged at pN3 were universally associated with advanced tumor stages in most pIIIB and pIV cases. Further analysis of patient survival revealed that the patients staged as pN3B had prognosis worse than those staged as pN3A or pM1; they had 3- and 5-year survival rates worse than those staged at pT4, pM1, and pIV [29]. As a result, the summary pTNM becomes unpredictable for prognosis stratification in GCC tumors staged as esophageal carcinoma as shown in Fig. 10.6. Apparently, it is the pN3 subgroup that becomes a major problem in the pN grouping of GCC patients for prognostic stratification [7, 12, 24, 29].

Fig. 10.6 Prognostic stratification of patients with gastric cardiac carcinoma involving the esophagus staged as esophageal cancer becomes unpredictable with apparent erroneously better survival for the subgroups staged as pIIA and pIIIA than those staged as pIA and equivalent survival for groups staged as pIIB and pIIIB. The data indicate the limitations of using esophageal cancer staging rules to stratify post-resection outcomes of Chinese patients with gastric cardiac carcinoma involving the esophagus [7]

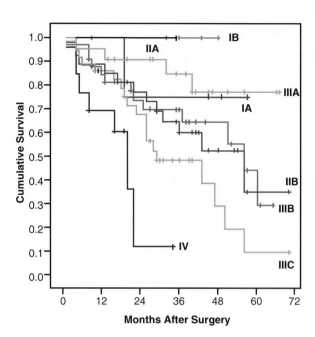

Pathologic Metastatic Tumor Staging (PM)

By definition, carcinoma metastasis involving distant organs and lymph nodes constitutes pM1 disease. The most common organs with metastatic GCC include the liver, peritoneum, lung, and rarely the esophagus and brain. Therefore, tumor cells identified in the peritoneal washings or biopsies of peritoneal nodules/implants are classified as pM1 disease by AJCC 8 [13]. In contrast, bulky tumors with direct local extension into the adjacent organs such as the diaphragm, esophagus, transverse colon, tail of the pancreas, etc. should be classified as pT4b stage, not pM1 disease, as defined by AJCC8 [13].

Metastasis to distant lymph nodes in patients with GCC is staged as pM1. Those distant lymph nodes are located in the retropancreatic, pancreaticoduodenal, peripancreatic, superior mesenteric, middle colic, para-aortic, and retroperitoneal regions. However, lymph nodes along the common hepatic artery, such as celiac, hepatoduodenal, and left gastric arterial nodes, are classified as regional nodes for gastric carcinoma, although GCC patients with nodal metastasis in this region have been shown to have a worse prognosis [29]. It has been reported that the patients with advanced pIII GCC with esophageal invasion and metastasis in the celiac lymph nodes have 3- and 5-year survival rates worse than those without celiac nodal metastasis (Fig. 10.7) [5, 7, 38].

If confirmed by large samples in multicenter studies, nodal metastasis in the common hepatic arterial region may be justified as being classified as pM1. Because of the dismal prognosis in patients with GCC involving the esophagus and metastasis to lymph nodes in the celiac axis region [7], total gastrectomy with en bloc resection of carcinoma and dissection of lymph nodes in the celiac axis region has been advocated to improve patient survival [39].

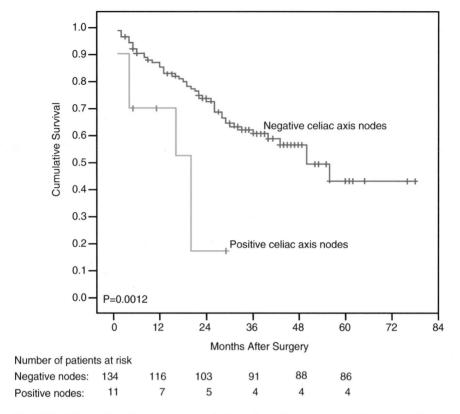

Number of patients at risk

Negative nodes:	134	116	103	91	88	86
Positive nodes:	11	7	5	4	4	4

Fig. 10.7 Patients with celiac nodal metastasis of gastric cardiac carcinoma with esophageal invasion have worse outcomes than those without celiac nodal metastasis [7]

In the same context, much work is needed for prognostic stratification of nodal metastasis in the upper, middle, and lower mediastinum in patients with GCC involving the esophagus in order to determine whether or not mediastinal nodal metastasis should be classified as regional or distant metastasis in GCC patients.

Pathologic Evaluation of Neoadjuvant Therapy (ypTNM)

As neoadjuvant therapy becomes popular in clinical practice for patients with GCC, adequate pathologic assessment of radical resection specimens after neoadjuvant therapy is crucial for objective and accurate evaluation of tumor responses. In AJCC 8, pathologists are required to use the post-neoadjuvant therapy classification staging system in this setting [13]. In this new AJCC 8 system, both macro- and microscopic features of the tumor should be clearly described and documented [13]. By histopathologic evaluation, the effectiveness of neoadjuvant therapy is semiquantitatively estimated and reported as the percentage of residual viable neoplastic cells identified in the tumor section in relation to areas of necrosis, granulation tissue, fibrosis, and inflammation. Oftentimes, immunohistochemistry is used to highlight residual neoplastic cells embedded in the deep tissues by key biomarkers of GCC (Figs. 10.8 and 10.9).

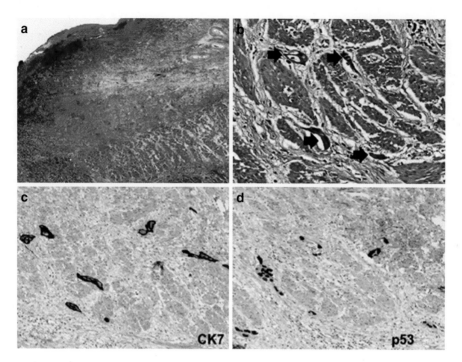

Fig. 10.8 Residual gastric cardiac adenocarcinoma after neoadjuvant therapy exhibited complete ablation of the surface tumor mass with a necrotic surface ulcer and granulation tissues in (**a**). Careful examination of the deep muscularis propria demonstrates scattered large bazar atypical cells (blue arrows in **b**). By immunohistochemistry, those cells were highlighted by CK7 (**c**) and p53 (**d**), supporting the diagnosis of viable residual deeply infiltrating neoplastic cells

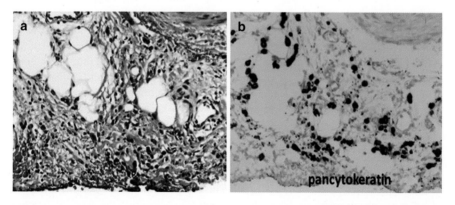

Fig. 10.9 Residual GCC neoplastic cells after neoadjuvant therapy are difficult to discern in the subserosal area on routine hematoxylin and eosin stain (**a**) but can be easily highlighted by positive brown immunostaining for pan-cytokeratin (**b**)

The therapy response varies widely from 100% (i.e., no residual viable neoplastic cells identified in the entire gross lesion) to 0% (i.e., no effect on the tumor as evidenced by the absence of necrosis, fibrosis, and inflammation). The presence of residual neoplastic cells indicates an incomplete response to the neoadjuvant therapy and needs to be reported as a percentage of residual viable neoplastic cells estimated by a pathologist from the overall tumor volume on a tumor histology section. Sometimes, acellular mucin pools are noted in the area of the lesion indicating a therapy effect, but not as evidence of residual carcinoma.

For the yT stage, AJCC 8 requires using the distance of the deepest focus of neoplastic cells in the gastric wall [13], frequently highlighted by a routine pancytokeratin immunostain (Fig. 10.9). For the ypN stage, at least one focus of metastatic neoplastic cells should be identified in a lymph node. If no additional diagnostic tests are carried out after the neoadjuvant therapy, the pM stage will be the same as cM; otherwise, a ypM stage will be assigned, based on the new findings [13].

Other Prognostic Factors

In addition to the well-known pTNM system for prognostic stratification in esophageal and gastric carcinomas [40, 41], other prognostic factors have also been found to be significantly correlated with outcomes for GCC patients. Because of unique clinicopathologic characteristics, GCC does not perfectly fit the prognostic profile of either genuine esophageal or gastric carcinoma [7, 21], by the rules of the AJCC7 pTNM stage groupings. Gertler et al. analyzed pTNM stage groupings of 1141 GCC (Siewert types II–III) patients and reported that the staging rules for either esophageal or gastric carcinomas cannot optimally stratify GCC patient prognosis [21]. For American patients with Siewert II GCC tumors staged as pIII, the prognosis is considerably better than those of genuine esophageal Siewert I adenocarcinomas at the same pIII stage [14, 19]. These findings are parallel to those shown in Korean and Chinese patients [7, 28]. One reason explaining the heterogeneity of the pTNM stage groupings with respect to prognosis of GCC is related to lymph node metastasis, which occurs in the majority of patients with advanced GCC. In those patients, metastasis in more than 15 lymph nodes is common, and patient prognosis cannot be adequately stratified by the rule for esophageal cancer that has only a single subgroup of pN3 [1, 6, 7]. In contrast, a subclassification of pN3 into pN3a and pN3b diseases may effectively separate patient groups with respect to prognosis by the rules for gastric cancer, but not by the rules for esophageal cancer, as shown convincingly by the 2017 IGCA data [12].

In a case series study of 142 eligible Chinese patients with GCC involving the esophagus, investigators analyzed the relationship of prognosis to 13 clinicopathologic features including age, gender, *H. pylori* infection, surgical modality, Siewert type, Bormann's type, tumor size, differentiation, histologic type, surgical margin, lymphovascular and perineural invasion, and pathologic TNM stage after radical resection with curative intent [29]. They reported that by univariate analysis, age > 70 years, poor tumor differentiation, >15 total lymph nodes retrieved, lymph node metastasis, and distant metastases predicted poor postoperative overall survival, while male gender, *H. pylori* infection, Bormann's type, size, histologic type, surgical modality, positive surgical margin, lymphovascular and perineural invasion, and pT stage were not predictive of overall survival. By multivariate analysis, age > 70 years, ≥16 positive lymph nodes, lymph node ratio (the ratio of the number of positive nodes to the number of total nodes retrieved) >0.2, and summary pTNM stage were independent predictors of poor overall survival after resection [29].

Other prognostic factors used to predict post-resection outcomes in patients with GCC include elevated serum levels of CA19-9, alpha-fetal protein (AFP), and CA 125, but not carcinoembryonic antigen (CEA) [42]. According to a recent serological study of 1477 Chinese patients with gastric cancer, including 507 (34%) GCC cases, high serum levels of CA19-9, AFP, and CA125 were significantly associated with poor post-resection prognosis with CA19-9 and AFP being independent prognostic predictors [42]. In contrast, serum levels of CEA did not have prognostic values in this group of Chinese patients [42].

Essential Information on Cancer Reporting

For cancer registry data collection and also for clinical management and research, the following structured tumor data may need to be reported in every case of GCC radical resection:

1. Clinical study results (endoscopy with biopsy, endoscopic ultrasound, endoscopic ultrasound-guide fine needle aspiration, computed tomography (CT), PET/CT)
2. Serum levels of AFP, CA125, and CA 19-9
3. Type of surgical resection
4. Tumor location and macro- and microscopic histologic types
5. WHO tumor differentiation grade
6. pT stage with tumor size in length, width, and invasion depth
7. pN stage with the number of lymph nodes retrieved and the number of lymph nodes with metastasis, extranodal invasion, as well as the location of nodal metastasis
8. pM stage with metastatic site
9. Summary pTNM grouping
10. Number of primary tumors and distance between tumors
11. Lymphovascular invasion
12. Perineural invasion
13. Status of resection margins (macro- and microscopically negative or positive) and the distance of the tumor edge to the nearest margin of resection
14. Neoadjuvant (ypTNM) and adjuvant chemotherapy and/or radiation therapy
15. HER2 status (positive or negative)

16. Other pathologic diseases, especially the presence or absence of Barrett's esophagus in the tissues adjacent to the tumor
17. Status of *H. pylori* infection
18. Special molecular study results
19. Family and personal history of cancer and hereditary diseases

Summary

The most recently published pathologic staging rules by the 2017 IGCA and 2017 AJCC 8 greatly improve post-resection outcome stratification in patient with GCC. The most controversial staging issue is related to how to appropriately stage pN3 tumors with celiac nodal metastasis, which requires further investigation with large samples from multicenter studies. Because of the widespread use of neoadjuvant therapy, pathologic staging needs to be standardized as required by 2017 AJCC 8. After radical resection, all GCC tumors should be thoroughly investigated by pathologists, using a complete synoptic report for patient triage, cancer registry data collection, and clinicopathologic research.

References

1. American Joint Committee on Cancer. Chapter 10. Esophagus and esophagogastric junction. In: AJCC cancer staging manual. 7th ed. New York, NY: Springer; 2009. p. 129–44.
2. Siewert JR, Stein HJ. Classification of adenocarcinoma of the oesophagogastric junction. Br J Surg. 1998;85:1457–9.
3. Wijnhoven BP, Siersema PD, Hop WC, et al. Adenocarcinomas of the distal oesophagus and gastric cardia are one clinical entity. Rotterdam Oesophageal Tumour Study Group. Br J Surg. 1999;86:529–35.
4. Chandrasoma P, Wickramasinghe K, Ma Y, et al. Adenocarcinomas of the distal oesophagus and "gastric cardia" are predominantly esophageal carcinomas. Am J Surg Pathol. 2007;31:569–75.
5. Fang WL, Wu CW, Chen JH, et al. Esophagogastric junction adenocarcinoma according to Siewert classification in Taiwan. Ann Surg Oncol. 2009;16(12):3237–44.
6. Kwon SJ. Evaluation of the 7th UICC TNM Staging System of Gastric Cancer. J Gastric Cancer. 2011;11(2):78–85.
7. Huang Q, Shi J, Feng AN, et al. Gastric cardiac carcinomas involving the esophagus are more adequately staged as gastric cancers by the 7th edition of the American Joint Commission on Cancer staging system. Mod Pathol. 2011;24:138–46.
8. Suh YS, Han DS, Kong SH, et al. Should adenocarcinoma of the esophagogastric junction be classified as esophageal cancer? A comparative analysis according to the seventh AJCC classification. Ann Surg. 2012;255:908–15.
9. Huang Q. Unique clinicopathology of proximal gastric carcinoma: a critical review. Gastroint Tumors. 2014;1:115–22.
10. Huang Q, Zhang LH. The histopathologic spectrum of carcinomas involving the gastroesophageal junction in the Chinese. Int J Surg Pathol. 2007;15:38–42.

11. Huang Q. Carcinoma of the gastroesophageal junction in Chinese patients. World J Gastro. 2012;18(48):7134–40.
12. Sano T, Coit DG, Kim HH, et al. Proposal of a new stage grouping of gastric cancer for TNM classification: International Gastric Cancer Association staging project. Gastric Cancer. 2017;20:217–25.
13. American Joint Committee on Cancer. Chapter 17. Stomach. In: AJCC cancer staging manual. 8th ed. New York, NY: Springer; 2017. p. 203–20.
14. Whitson BA, Groth SS, Li Z, Kratzke RA, Maddaus MA. Survival of patients with distal esophageal and gastric cardia tumors: a population-based analysis of gastroesophageal junction carcinomas. Thorac Cardiovasc Surg. 2010;139(1):43–8.
15. Lauwers GY, Carneiro F, Graham DY, et al. Gastric carcinoma. In: Bosman FT, Carneiro F, Hruban RH, Theise ND, editors. WHO classification of tumours of the digestive system. Lyon: IARC Press; 2010. p. 48–58.
16. Huang Q, Sun Q, Fan XS, Zhou D, Zou XP. Recent advances in proximal gastric carcinoma. J Dig Dis. 2016;17(7):421–32.
17. Ferlay J, et al. Estimates of worldwide burden of cancer in 2008: GLOBOCAN 2008. Int J Cancer. 2010;127:2893–917.
18. Patel MI, Rhoads KF, Ma Y, et al. Seventh edition (2010) of the AJCC/UICC staging system for gastric adenocarcinoma: is there room for improvement? Ann Surg Oncol. 2013;20(5):1631–8.
19. Huang Q, Fan XS, Agoston AT, et al. Comparison of gastroesophageal junction carcinomas in Chinese versus American patients. Histopathology. 2011;59(2):188–97.
20. Li R, Chen TW, Hu J, et al. Tumor volume of resectable adenocarcinoma of the esophagogastric junction at multidetector CT: association with regional lymph node metastasis and N stage. Radiology. 2013;269(1):130–8.
21. Gertler R, Stein HJ, Loos M, Langer R, Friess H, Feith M. How to classify adenocarcinomas of the esophagogastric junction: as esophageal or gastric cancer? Am J Surg Pathol. 2011;35:1512–22.
22. Okholm C, Svendsen LB, Achiam MP. Status and prognosis of lymph node metastasis in patients with cardia cancer—a systematic review. Surg Oncol. 2014;23(3):140–6.
23. Gertler R, Stein HJ, Schuster T, Rondak IC, Höfler H, Feith M. Prevalence and topography of lymph node metastases in early esophageal and gastric cancer. Ann Surg. 2014;259(1):96–101.
24. Zhao E, Ling T, Xu J, et al. Turning left or right? A comparative analysis in adenocarcinomas of the esophagogastric junction according to the seventh AJCC TNM classification for cancers of the esophagus and stomach: experience in a Chinese single institution. Int J Clin Exp Med. 2015;8(7):10668–77.
25. Huang Q, Shi J, Sun Q, et al. Distal esophageal carcinomas in Chinese patients vary widely in histopathology, but adenocarcinomas remain rare. Hum Pathol. 2012;43(12):2138–48.
26. Tokunaga M, Tanizawa Y, Bando E, Kawamura T, Tsubosa Y, Terashima M. Impact of esophageal invasion on clinicopathological characteristics and long-term outcome of adenocarcinoma of the subcardia. J Surg Oncol. 2012;106(7):856–61.
27. Ielpo B, Pernaute AS, Elia S, et al. Impact of number and site of lymph node invasion on survival of adenocarcinoma of esophagogastric junction. Interact Cardiovasc Thorac Surg. 2010;10(5):704–8.
28. Kim HI, Cheong JH, Song KJ, et al. Staging of adenocarcinoma of the esophagogastric junction: comparison of AJCC 6th and 7th gastric and 7th esophageal staging systems. Ann Surg Oncol. 2013;20(8):2713–20.
29. Zhang YF, Shi J, Yu HP, et al. Factors predicting survival in patients with proximal gastric carcinoma involving the esophagus. World J Gastro. 2012;18(27):3602–9.
30. Zhang HD, Ma Z, Tang P, et al. Prognostic value of metastatic lymph node ratio in adenocarcinoma of the gastroesophageal junction. Zhonghua Wei Chang Wai Ke Za Zhi. 2013;16(9):822–6. (in Chinese).
31. Roviello F, Marrelli D, Morgagni P, et al. Survival benefit of extended D2 lymphadenectomy in gastric cancer with involvement of second level lymph nodes: a longitudinal multicenter study. Ann Surg Oncol. 2002;9(9):894–900.

32. de Manzoni G, Verlato G, Guglielmi A, et al. Classification of lymph node metastases from carcinoma of the stomach: comparison of the old (1987) and new (1997) TNM systems. World J Surg. 1999;23(7):664–9.
33. Mönig SP, Baldus SE, Zirbes TK, et al. Topographical distribution of lymph node metastasis in adenocarcinoma of the gastroesophageal junction. Hepato-Gastroenterology. 2002;49(44):419–22.
34. Matsuda T, Takeuchi H, Tsuwano S, Nakahara T, Mukai M, Kitagawa Y. Sentinel node mapping in adenocarcinoma of the esophagogastric junction. World J Surg. 2014;38(9):2337–44.
35. Kurokawa Y, Hiki N, Yoshikawa T, et al. Mediastinal lymph node metastasis and recurrence in adenocarcinoma of the esophagogastric junction. Surgery. 2015;157(3):551–5.
36. Matsuda T, Kurokawa Y, Yoshikawa T, et al. Clinicopathological characteristics and prognostic factors of patients with Siewert Type II esophagogastric junction carcinoma: a retrospective multicenter study. World J Surg. 2016;40(7):1672–9.
37. Japanese Gastric Cancer Association. Japanese gastric cancer treatment guidelines 2014 (ver. 4). Gastric Cancer. 2017;20:1–19.
38. Nunobe S, Ohyama S, Sonoo H, et al. Benefit of mediastinal and para-aortic lymph-node dissection for advanced gastric cancer with esophageal invasion. J Surg Oncol. 2008;97(5):392–5.
39. Schomas DA, Quevedo JF, Donahue JM, Nichols Iii FC, Romero Y, Miller RC. The prognostic importance of pathologically involved celiac node metastases in node-positive patients with carcinoma of the distal esophagus or gastroesophageal junction: a surgical series from the Mayo Clinic. Dis Esophagus. 2010;23(3):232–9.
40. Mariette C, Castel B, Toursel H, Balon JM, Triboulet JP. Surgical management of and long-term survival after adenocarcinoma of the cardia. Br J Surg. 2002;89:1156–3.
41. Lagarde SM, ten Kate FJ, Reitsma JB, Busch OR, van Lanschot JJ. Prognostic factors in adenocarcinoma of the esophagus or gastroesophageal junction. J Clin Oncol. 2006;24(26):4347–55.
42. Feng F, Sun L, Liu Z, et al. Prognostic values of normal preoperative serum cancer markers for gastric cancer. Oncotarget. 2016;7(36):58459–69.

Chapter 11
Endoscopic Resection of Early Gastric Cardiac Cancer

Guifang Xu, Rui Li, Dongtao Shi, Qin Huang, and Hiroshi Mashimo

Introduction

At present, endoscopic resection, such as endoscopic mucosal resection (EMR) or endoscopic submucosal dissection (ESD), for early gastric carcinoma (EGC), including early gastric cardiac carcinoma, has become the treatment of choice in East Asian countries because of long-term excellent outcomes comparable to open surgical resection. In this chapter, we discuss the most relevant information and results of key clinical studies regarding a multidiscipline team approach for decision on endoscopic therapy, techniques and procedures for ESD resection, post-resection management, and follow-ups.

G. Xu (✉)
Department of Gastroenterology, Affiliated Nanjing Drum Tower Hospital of Nanjing University Medical School, Nanjing, People's Republic of China
e-mail: 13852293376@163.com

R. Li
Soochow University First Hospital, Soochow University, Soochow, People's Republic of China

D. Shi
Department of Gastroenterology, Soochow University First Hospital, Soochow University, Soochow, People's Republic of China

Q. Huang
Pathology and Laboratory Medicine, Veterans Affairs Boston Healthcare System, West Roxbury, MA, USA

Harvard Medical School and Brigham and Women's Hospital, Boston, MA, USA

H. Mashimo
VA Boston Healthcare System and Brigham and Women's Hospital, Harvard Medical School, Boston, MA, USA
e-mail: hmashimo@hms.harvard.edu

© Springer International Publishing AG, part of Springer Nature 2018
Q. Huang (ed.), *Gastric Cardiac Cancer*, https://doi.org/10.1007/978-3-319-79114-2_11

Risk Factors of Lymph Node Metastasis

Once a diagnosis of early gastric cardiac carcinoma is rendered, based on character-istic tumor endoscopic imaging and histopathologic evidence of invasive carcinoma in a biopsy specimen, the decision for endoscopic versus open surgical resection of the tumor should be made with the multidiscipline team. The decision relies heavily upon clinical risk assessment for lymph node metastasis because nodal metastasis is an absolute contraindication for endoscopic resection of EGC. Historically, the rationale behind this endoscopic resection strategy is based on the extremely low risk of nodal metastasis in EGC, according to a study of 5265 EGC radical gastrec-tomy cases accumulated before the year 2000 at the Japanese National Cancer Center Hospital [1]. In that study, Gotoda et al. reported the absence of nodal metas-tasis in four groups of EGC patients. As a result, the current ESD practice guidelines in Japan and China suggest three major indications [2, 3]:

1. Intestinal-type intramucosal carcinoma of any size without ulcer
2. Intestinal-type intramucosal carcinoma with ulcer but smaller than 3 cm in size
3. Diffuse-type EGC smaller than 3 cm in size with superficial (<0.5 mm in depth) submucosal invasion but without lymphovascular invasion

While lymphovascular invasion has been confirmed worldwide as the most impor-tant risk factor for nodal metastasis in EGC (Fig. 11.1) [4–6], the reported extremely low frequency of nodal metastasis in EGC for intramucosal carcinoma smaller than 2 cm in size and superficial submucosal invasion without lymphovascular invasion [1] has not been universally confirmed (Table 11.1).

Several recent Chinese and Korean studies have revealed other risk factors for nodal metastasis in EGC, such as the female gender [6–10], intestinal type [5, 9], and distal gastric location [9–11], but not ulceration [9, 11–13]. A recent systematic review of the worldwide literature in 42 qualified studies showed low, but substan-tial, nodal metastasis rates of 6% for intramucosal carcinoma, 9% for EGC without lymphovascular invasion, 13% for the intestinal-type EGC, 13% for EGC with an

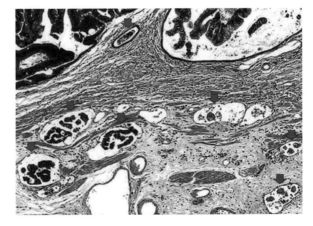

Fig. 11.1 Lymphovascular invasion (blue arrows) in the submucosa is associated with an overlying papillary adenocarcinoma in the gastric cardia

Table 11.1 Comparison in endoscopic resection criteria of lymph node metastasis incidence in early gastric carcinoma among Japanese, Korean, and Chinese patients

Risk factor of nodal metastasis	Gotoda et al. 2000 (%) [1]	Kang et al. 2010 (%) [7]	Huang et al. 2015 (%) [8, 9]
Intramucosal cancer, intestinal type, no LVI, ≤3 cm, irrespective of ulceration (%)	0/1230 (0)	2/126 (1.6)	1/76 (1.3)
Intramucosal cancer, intestinal type, no LVI, any size, without ulceration (%)	0/929 (0)	2/146 (1.4)	0/64 (0)
Intramucosal cancer, diffuse type, no LVI, ≤3 cm, without ulceration (%)	0/141 (0)	6/108 (5.6)	3/30 (10)
Submucosal cancer, sm1 (≤500 μm), intestinal type, no LVI, ≤3 cm (%)	0/145 (0)	3/20 (15.0)	3/27 (11.1)

Note: *LVI* lymphovascular invasion

elevated growth pattern, and 8% for EGC smaller than 2 cm in size [5]. The data are similar to those of Chinese studies, which reported nodal metastasis rates of 6.3% for intramucosal and 19.6% for submucosal carcinomas [8, 9]. In Korea, Kang et al. [7] reported an overall 12.6% nodal metastasis rate in 478 EGC radical resection cases, and no relationship was found between clinicopathologic features and nodal metastasis in 270 pT1a tumors (Table 11.1), in concert with the findings in Chinese patients [8, 9].

Even for undifferentiated EGC, such as poorly differentiated adenocarcinoma, poorly cohesive carcinoma, and signet ring cell carcinoma, a recent meta-analysis of 23 qualified studies on risk factors of nodal metastasis identified eight significant risk factors, including female gender, age >60 years, tumor size >2 cm, non-corpus location, the presence of an ulcer, submucosal invasion, the presence of lymphovascular invasion, and non-signet ring cell type [14].

Apparently, the current criteria concerning relative indications for ESD on EGC have been found to be problematic for accurately predicting nodal metastasis. A growing body of evidence acquired in recent years raises a serious legitimate concern over the low but considerable risk of nodal metastasis of EGC in patients with presumed risk factors that were considered minimal or none in the earlier study [1]. The discrepancy in nodal metastasis of EGC between Japanese and Chinese patients is at least partially related to a much higher prevalence of gastric cardiac carcinoma in the Chinese patient population. Early gastric cardiac carcinoma accounted for over 25% of radical gastrectomies for EGC in a Chinese report [8], which is about tenfold higher in frequency than that (2.5% of all gastric cancer resections) in Japan [15]. Surprisingly, the nodal metastasis rate was significantly lower in early gastric cardiac carcinoma (2.9%, 3/104) than in early non-cardiac carcinoma (16.7%, 46/275) ($p < 0.001$) [8]. Interestingly, the vast majority (97.1%) of early gastric cardiac carcinoma tumors were staged as pIA, while pIB was rare (2.9%) [3].

EGCs with papillary adenocarcinoma have been shown to have frequent lymph node and liver metastases and worse overall 5-year survival outcomes [16, 17]. This cancer is frequently associated with the recently established micropapillary adenocarcinoma of the stomach for a propensity (50%, $N = 4$) of nodal metastasis [8].

Compared to tubular EGC, papillary EGC was associated with a higher frequency of lymphovascular invasion, nodal and distant metastases, and with worse 5-year survival [16]. Importantly, the nodal metastasis rate for papillary EGC was alarmingly high and found in 13.6% of cases in a Chinese cohort [16], over 18% in a Korean study [18], and 18.2–29.2% in two Japanese reports [19, 20].

The prevalent view is that gastric signet ring cell carcinoma is associated with widespread nodal and distant metastases and has fatal outcomes. Thus, this carcinoma is classified as undifferentiated carcinoma, unsuitable for endoscopic resection in EGC. However, a growing body of evidence acquired in recent years suggests otherwise. Early signet ring cell carcinoma not only has been shown to have a better prognosis than early non-signet ring cell carcinoma with a better 5-year overall survival rate but is also more suitable for endoscopic resection [21–25]. Recent clinicopathologic studies show that intramucosal signet ring cell carcinoma generally arises in the isthmus/neck region of a gastric unit, is found in the distal stomach as flat and depressed growth patterns, and is more common in young women. Compared to well-differentiated intestinal-type EGC, intramucosal signet ring cell carcinoma has been shown to have a similar incidence of submucosal spread, lymphovascular invasion, and nodal metastasis [23, 25]. Since the report by Hyung et al. of a very low (1.6%, 3/185) rate of nodal metastasis for signet ring cell carcinoma at the pT1a stage [24], a number of other studies have confirmed this finding [19–23]. The independent risk factors of nodal metastasis in 1544 mucosa-confined signet ring cell carcinomas, reported by a Korean multicenter study, include tumor size >1.7 cm, elevated growth pattern, and lymphovascular invasion [26]. Kim et al. most recently discovered that none of 189 surgical resections of early signet ring cell carcinoma smaller than 2 cm in size without ulceration demonstrated nodal metastasis [27], suggesting endoscopic resection as an effective and safe alternative to surgical gastrectomy for intramucosal signet ring cell carcinoma under certain circumstances. The features are summarized in Table 11.2.

However, not all patients with early signet ring cell carcinoma should undergo endoscopic resection, especially for those with associated hereditary CDH1 gene mutation for which total gastrectomy may be a better and safer option because of

Table 11.2 Risk of lymph node metastasis (LNM) in pT1 early signet ring cell carcinoma (SRC)

pT1 (N)	SRC (%)	M/F (%)	Location (%)		Endoscopic feature (%)		pT1a (%)	pT1b (%)	Overall LNM (%)	Reference
			Cardia	Non-cardia	Flat/depressed	Ulcer Mixed				
933	28.2	1.1	6.5	93.5	90.9	0	1.6	15.4	5.7	[24]
1520	25.5	0.96	7.7	92.3	60.3	38	1.6	25.3	9.5	[29]
1362	32.9	1	0	100	87.9	12.1	6.3	26.3	12	[21]
422	24.2	2	3	97	95.1	0	4	28.9	15	[30]
1462	28.7	1.2	5.5	94.5	NA	NA	2.9	12.3	5.7	[31]
1067	172	1.1	1	99	87.2	0	11	26.7	15.1	[25]

Note: N number, M/F male/female, pT1a intramucosal, pT1b submucosal

the multifocal tumor growth pattern of this carcinoma [28]. Therefore, an individualized approach may maximize the benefits of modern endoscopic resection technology and minimize the risk of nodal metastasis [29–31].

In general, early gastric cardiac carcinoma may metastasize primarily to the abdominal lymph nodes and may also spread to the lower mediastinum. However, using both radial-active colloid and blue dye to label sentinel lymph nodes in 15 cT1 gastric cardiac/esophagogastric junctional adenocarcinoma tumors, Matsuda et al. recently demonstrated the absence of nodal metastasis in the lower mediastinum and no cancer recurrence at 38-month follow-up of these patients [32]. Although the number of patients in this study was small, the results are encouraging for less invasive endoscopic resection of early gastric cardiac carcinoma.

In summary, the risk of nodal metastasis for early gastric cardiac carcinoma at the pT1a stage is very low for intramucosal tubular adenocarcinoma, signet ring cell carcinoma, carcinoma with lymphoid stroma, neuroendocrine carcinoma, and adenosquamous carcinoma [8, 9]. The most important risk factor for nodal metastasis is lymphovascular invasion, which is not appropriate for endoscopic therapy.

Principles of Endoscopic Resection

Traditionally, gastric cardiac carcinoma is resected surgically. With the widespread use of upper endoscopy, gastric cardiac carcinoma has been detected much earlier and more frequently.

Endoscopic resection of early gastric cardiac carcinoma includes endoscopic mucosal resection (EMR) and endoscopic submucosal dissection (ESD). EMR was first reported by Japanese investigators in 1984 to resect EGC for pathologic diagnosis and tumor invasion depth [36]. Subsequently in 1994, Takekoshi et al. used a novel IT (insulated tip) endoscopic knife for en bloc resection [37]. This technique was further modified in 1999 and eventually became a standard ESD endotherapy technique in 2013 [38]. Unlike EMR that is used primarily for small intramucosal lesions, ESD is used for lesions of any size, even for superficial submucosal (SM1) lesions, with the advantage of much higher en bloc complete resection rates, lower local recurrence rates, and better tissue reservation for histopathologic evaluation and tumor staging, albeit with a higher frequency of perforation [39, 40].

Endoscopic Mucosal Resection

In general, EMR can be carried out by two methods: (1) non-suction techniques, such as submucosal injection resection (polypectomy), submucosal injection-elevation resection, or submucosal injection-pre-resection resection, and (2) suction techniques, such as EMR with small-caliber-tip transparent cap (EMRC) (Fig. 11.2) or EMR with band ligation.

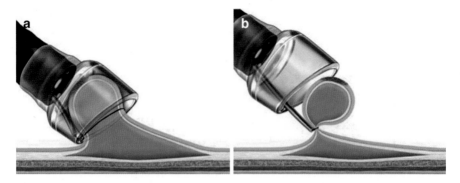

Fig. 11.2 The most commonly used endoscopic mucosal resection (EMR) technique is usually carried out with a transparent cap (EMRC). After injection of saline solution with an injection needle into the submucosal layer beneath the lesion, a small-diameter snare (SD-7P; Olympus Co.) loop passed through the biopsy channel is opened inside the cap, the lesion is drawn inside the cap by endoscopic suction, and the snare loop is closed in (**a**). After confirming the snared mucosal lesion size and consistency for safety under endoscopic direct view, a high-frequency electric current is applied to resect the lesion in (**b**) (Modified from the Olympus website, http://medical.olympuysamerica.com, accessed on 6/13/2017)

For the EMRC method, a transparent cap is placed at the tip of the scope for suction and resection so that the EMR resection procedure becomes simpler and easier to perform in a narrow space to resect larger lesions with minimal complications. However, EMRC is used mainly for removal of small lesions because of the limited size of the transparent cap. In 1994, Chaves et al. were the first to report the application of the tissue banding ligation method for EMR [41]. This method is adopted from that used for banding esophageal venous varices, subsequently resected using an electrocautery snare. The resected field is generally well visualized for controlling bleeding, and the depth of resection is controllable with minimal local tissue injury and bleeding. Thus, it is safe and the success is not affected by the location of a lesion. The general experience with this method for removal of EGC is limited, due to scarcity ($N = 8$) of reported cases with this method. In those eight cases reported, the lesion size is small (<2 cm), and all tumors are not EGC. EMR can also be performed piecemeal, particularly for flat and large (>2 cm) lesions that cannot be successfully removed by a traditional EMR procedure. Because the resected specimen is fragmented, accurate evaluation of the lateral and vertical margins is not possible. Therefore, it is difficult to assess the completeness of resection, and in fact, local recurrence after resection is quite high. As such, after piecemeal EMR for EGC, it is crucial to monitor lateral and deep margins and subsequently resect further lesions as en bloc as possible. In addition, all patients should be closely followed up for at least 5 years after the procedure [42]. Overall, with the EMR methods used for resection of EGC, the en bloc resection rate is 56–75.8%, and the complete resection rate is 66.1–77.6% [43–45]. In China, EMR for early gastric cardiac carcinoma shows the en bloc resection rate of 23.1–45.1% and the curative complete resection rate of 23.1–43.1% [46, 47]. Compared to open surgical resection of gastric cardiac carcinoma, EMR therapy demonstrates similar post-resection survival and morbidity rates but much lower post-resection bleeding rate and mortality rate, shorter hospital stay, and lower overall cost [34].

Endoscopic Submucosal Dissection (ESD)

ESD is the technique used for lesions that are too large for EMR. Based on differences in tumor location, size, and depth of invasion, the operator may use different endoscopic resection knives (Fig. 11.3) to dissect the submucosal space and separate the muscularis mucosa from the muscularis propria with the goal of completely resecting a mucosal lesion.

The gastric cardia is a narrow region underneath the gastroesophageal junction (GEJ) containing hyperplastic fibromuscular tissues, extending from the muscularis mucosae to the entire submucosal space with frequent individual smooth muscle fibers admixed with loose fibrovascular tissues. When a tumor invades the GEJ into the distal esophagus, successful dissection of this submucosal space can be challenging. In addition to control the scope stability, the endoscopist needs operative skills to carry out successful ESD of gastric cardiac carcinoma.

The ESD procedure starts with defining the tumor margin, marking mucosal borders at 5 mm away from the tumor margin and mucosal incision at 5 mm farther

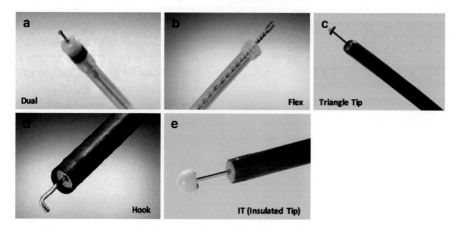

Fig. 11.3 Various common single-use electrosurgical knives for endoscopic submucosal dissection from the vender Olympus. In general, the dual knife in (**a**) is used for marking, incision, and dissection at all directions. The flex knife in (**b**) is able to deliver a flexible cutting and dissection. The triangle-tip knife in (**c**) is frequently used for controlling minor bleeding and cutting without rotating (**d**) The hook knife is used for cutting and dissecting. The direction of the hook can be controlled via handle rotation. The IT (insulated tip) knife in (**e**) helps in minimizing injury to deep tissues in organs with a thin submucosal layer, such as the esophagus and colon (Modified from the Olympus website http://medical.olympuysamerica.com, accessed on 6/13/2017). The detailed techniques on how to use various endoscopic resection knives have been published [48]

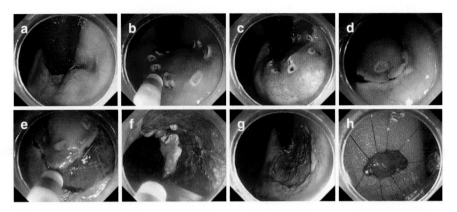

Fig. 11.4 Key steps of endoscopic submucosal dissection procedures. (**a**) A lesion was found at the lesser curvature side of the gastric cardia. (**b**) Marking the lesion borders. (**c**) Submucosal injection. (**d**) Incision was made around the lesion. (**e**) Submucosal dissection was started at the anal side of the lesion. (**f**) Submucosal dissection was carried out at the oral side of the lesion. (**g**) The lesion was completely removed to expose the operative field. (**h**) The removed lesion was slightly stretched and pinned down on a plate with fine needles with appropriate orientation for oral and anal directions, measurement of the size of the entire tissue removed and the size of the tumor, photography, and then immediate placement of the entire plate into the 10% neutral buffered formalin solution for histopathologic tissue processing

away from the mucosal borders to ensure a safe horizontal margin of a total of 10 mm away from the tumor margin. Submucosal dissection begins preferably at the anal end for submucosal injection, pre-resection, and submucosal dissection. Then, the procedure is repeated from the proximal aspect of the lesion for submucosal injection, pre-resection, and dissection. The two dissection procedures meet at the middle of the lesion in order to remove the entire lesion. For stump gastric carcinoma after distal gastrectomy, the procedure is usually started from the oral end. As shown in Fig. 11.4a–c, the tumor border is clearly illustrated with indigo carmine and well defined under narrowband imaging (Fig. 11.4c). In cases where the border of the mucosal lesion is obscured by marked inflammation, the patient first needs to be treated with proton-pump inhibitors (PPI) and, if applicable, antibiotics for *H. pylori* eradication to minimize mucosal tissue edema and inflammation. Once the border is clearly defined and the lesion is well demonstrated on retroflex view, the border is then marked at the sites 3–5 mm away from the lesion border (Fig. 11.4b). Subsequently, the scope is positioned appropriately to start submucosal injection at the distal border of the lesion. The injection solution may be a mixture of 0.9% saline and methylene blue with 0.0005% epinephrine and glycerol fructose or sodium hyaluronate. Other agents with better sustained lifting (less diffusion) are also available. In general, the injection begins at multiple lateral sites of the border marked at the 45 or lower degree of injection angles. The injection should be quick to elevate the lesion sufficiently. To minimize bleeding after injection, the needle tip is pulled back and reinserted at a different position (Fig. 11.4c). In the same way, the lesion can be precut with a dual knife (KD-650L) up to the proximal border of the lesion (Fig. 11.4d). Once the precut is completed, the scope needs to be rotated so that dissection can proceed in the submucosal space along the base of the lesion with a dual knife (KD-650L) or IT knife (KD-610L) toward the lesion proximal border. During the dissection procedure, repeated injections may help elevate the lesion sufficiently to facilitate dissection. Often, when the tumor is poorly exposed, owing to fibrosis obscuring the operative field, a transparent cap is used to push back the submucosal fibroconnective tissue. In addition, the patient may be repositioned so that the lesion can gradually fall off by gravity, thereby making the operative field more visible and facilitating the ESD dissection procedure (Fig. 11.4e). While submucosal injection is carried out at the proximal border of the lesion and the incision is made at the lateral border of the lesion separately, submucosal dissection at the proximal border of the lesion is progressed distally in order to meet the distal dissection front at the middle of the lesion (Fig. 11.4f). Submucosal dissection from the proximal border to the distal is facilitated with the dual knife (KD-650L) or IT knife (KD-610L) (Fig. 11.4g).

Once the dissection is finished and the lesion is removed, the operating field should be carefully inspected for any bleeding and potential bleeding sites. Any visible bleeding needs to be stopped immediately with hemostatic clips or argon plasma coagulation. All deep tissue injury or damage to the muscularis propria should be repaired with metal clips. Early gastric cardiac carcinoma sometimes involves the posterior greater curvature. In this case, the primary incision is made at the lateral border of the lesion, and submucosal dissection starts from the posterior greater curvature, proceeding from the oral to the anal side by gradually dissecting the submucosa up to the greater curvature so that, after appropriate repositioning of the patient, gravity allows the dissected portion of the lesion to fall off the gastric wall and to expose the entire operative field clearly (Fig. 11.4g). Because of the rich blood supply in the gastric cardia, the ESD endoscopist needs to be cautious for submucosal dissection and completely control all visible bleeding sites to prevent delayed bleeding.

Efficacy

In general, curative resection of EGC with ESD en bloc resection is lower for early gastric cardiac carcinoma (range 68–84%), compared to early gastric non-cardiac carcinoma (range 98–100%) [48–55]. In Japan, ESD has been considered as an effective and widely used therapeutic modality for EGC. Based on the data from the Japanese government, a total of 2111 ESD procedures were carried out in June 2007 in Japan, and the annual estimated ESD procedure is about 25,000 cases [56]. In China, the ESD procedure has been successfully utilized to remove early gastric cardiac carcinoma. The en bloc resection and curative resection rates are 92.9–98.7% and 75.6–78.6%, respectively [46, 47].

A recent study indicates that overall efficacy and prognosis are similar between ESD and surgical resection of gastric carcinoma, but the recurrence rate is relatively higher in the ESD treatment group [33–35]. Jang et al. [57] reported the en bloc resection rate, complete resection rate, and curative resection rate were 87%, 79%, and 66%, respectively, similar to those reported by Japanese investigators.

Compared to EMR for early gastric cardiac carcinoma, ESD is preferred because of the higher en bloc resection rate and more complete histopathologic resection, which is especially important because of considerable fibromuscular hyperplasia in the gastric cardia and deeper invasion of early gastric cardiac carcinoma in this region [8].

Other Endotherapeutic Modalities

In recent years, several endoscopic therapies have been reported, such as radiofrequency ablation, laser therapy, and argon plasma coagulation. Although the lesion can be effectively ablated by these thermoablative methods, an intact and undamaged tissue specimen is not available for pathologic evaluation to confirm a diagnosis or assess the status of resection margins, tumor stage, and factors related to risk of lymph node metastasis, such as the tumor invasion front and perineural and lymphovascular invasion. These ablative methods may be useful for endoscopic therapy of premalignant lesions with close clinical and endoscopic follow-ups after ablation. These modalities have not been well studied for EGC.

Indications for EMR/ESD

Intramucosal Early Gastric Cardiac Carcinoma

Early gastric cardiac carcinoma demonstrates a slow progression. Based on the most recent multicenter study of 1620 EGC radical gastrectomies, none of 162 intramucosal gastric cardiac carcinomas had lymph node metastasis, regardless of tumor size, gross growth pattern, histology type, and differentiation [58].

EGC with Lymphoid Stroma and Adenosquamous and Neuroendocrine Carcinomas in the Gastric Cardia

These uncommon types of early gastric cardiac carcinomas demonstrate slow growth features with a pushing invasion front and the absence of lymph node metastasis [8, 58].

Contraindications for EMR/ESD

There are several advisable contraindications for EMR/ESD. These include:

1. Confirmed lymph node metastasis
2. Lymphovascular invasion

The risk of lymphovascular invasion for submucosal invasive gastric cardiac carcinoma is high, with over fivefold increased risk for lymph node metastasis [8, 9, 58].

1. *Tumor size >3 cm*

 According to the results of clinicopathologic study of 1620 EGC tumors, tumor size >3 cm is an independent risk factor for lymph node metastasis with an odds ratio of 1.932 (95% confidence interval 1.052–3.948) [58].

2. *Poor differentiation*

 Poorly differentiated early gastric cardiac carcinoma has been found to be an independent risk factor for lymph node metastasis with an odds ratio of 2.546 (95% confidence interval: 1.521–4.242), on the basis of the data on 1620 EGC radical resections [58].

3. *Tumor invasion into the muscularis propria*

4. *Coagulopathy*

5. *High risk for endoscopic and surgical resection procedures*

 This includes poor functionality, severe coronary artery disease/severe congestive heart failure, etc.

6. *Patient or family refusal*

Relative Contraindications

The inability to elevate a lesion after submucosal injection is considered as a relative contraindication because of adhesion between the submucosa and muscularis propria, which has been shown to be associated with high frequency of perforation during the ESD procedure. However, even in this scenario, ESD may be successfully carried out by an experienced endoscopist.

Other Guidelines

The National Comprehensive Cancer Network guideline published in 2015 in the United States [59] recommended that an EGC tumor ≤2 cm in size, with well-moderate differentiation, at pT1 stage, and without lymphovascular invasion may be removed endoscopically. In cases with poor differentiation, lymphovascular invasion, deep submucosal invasion, positive lateral or deep margins, or lymph node metastasis, or endotherapy considered as incomplete, the guideline recommended that additional surgical resection such as gastrectomy with nodal dissection should be considered [59].

Clinical practice and follow-up guidelines of the 2013 ESMO-ESSO-ESTRO (European Society of Medical Oncology, European Society of Surgical Oncology, European Society for Radiotherapy and Oncology) groups suggested the following indications for endoscopic resection on EGC [60]: lesions with better differentiation, ≤2 cm in size, confined to the mucosa, and non-ulcerated tumors. They referenced the 2014 Japanese guidelines on EGC [61].

The 2011 British practice guidelines on gastric cancer also considered EMR and ESD for potential cure of early gastric mucosal carcinoma as supported by level B evidence [62]. Such endoscopic resection procedures were recommended to be carried out in major surgical centers with well-trained endoscopists in collaboration with a multidiscipline team. As for intraepithelial neoplasms, the guidelines recommended that the Vienna classification be used [63]: low-grade intraepithelial neoplasm needs to be clinically and endoscopically followed up or endoscopically resected; high-grade intraepithelial neoplasm should be removed either endoscopically or surgically [63]. Because of the under-sampling limitations of biopsies, pathologic diagnosis may not be accurate [64]. In one report, about 10–18% of ESD resection cases with a pre-ESD biopsy diagnosis of low-grade intraepithelial neoplasm were upgraded to high-grade intraepithelial neoplasms or EGC [65]. This frequency was even higher in 25% in a Chinese study [66]. The independent risk factors for underdiagnosis of biopsies based on ESD-resected specimens included tumor size >2 cm (odds ratio of 5.778 with 95% confidence interval of 2.893–11.542) and depressed/excavated gross patterns (odds ratio 2.535, 95% confidence interval 1.257–5.111) [66]. Because of the diagnostic uncertainty of biopsies, a thorough investigation before ESD is required to determine the tumor size and invasion depth. Several advanced endoscopic imaging techniques may be useful, such as narrowband imaging, Fuji intelligent chromoendoscopy, confocal endomicroscopy, and optical coherence tomography, to determine the best therapy modality for early gastric cardiac carcinoma.

Pre-ESD Preparation

A preoperative multidiscipline conference including radiologists, pathologists, surgeons, and oncologists should be routinely conducted for a complete assessment of the indications, contraindications, relative indications, and patient safety concerns before ESD is performed. All patients should be routinely assessed for tumor invasion depth and clinical staging with endoscopic ultrasound and CT for perigastric cardiac lymphadenopathy. All contraindications for anesthesia and endoscopic resection should be ruled out. A preoperative conference with the patient and the family should be carried out in a relaxed environment with detailed information on clinical findings, diagnosis, therapeutic options, operative procedures, expected results, possible complications, risk of tumor recurrence and metastasis, as well as the possible need for additional surgical resection with lymph nodal dissection. Patient consent forms for endoscopic resection and possible clinical research are obtained from the patient before the endotherapy procedure is started. The endoscopist and the treatment team should provide adequate time to educate and address concerns of the patient and family, using clear and understandable language to assure optimal understanding among the endoscopist, patient, and family.

Approximately 5–7 days before an ESD procedure, medications that affect coagulation functions need to be discontinued, including aspirin and other nonsteroidal anti-inflammatory drugs [67]. Complete blood count and INR (international normalized ratio) should be assessed to ensure a normal coagulation function. Shortly before the ESD procedure, all patients need to be monitored for cardiovascular function with routine electrocardiography and blood pressure; an intravenous line is established.

For patients on chronic dialysis, because of chronic renal dysfunction, blood transfusion may be considered to minimize the risk of potential post-ESD bleeding. Goto et al. reported ESD procedures in 12 patients with blood dialysis [68]: one patient had delayed bleeding after ESD and required transfusion; another had delayed perforation that required emergency surgical repair. For patients with chronic renal failure, a multidiscipline team conference including specialists from nephrology and general surgery, the patient, and family should be organized to evaluate the overall function of the patient and consider the best options of management. At present, the administration of PPI before ESD remains controversial. The report by Myung et al. suggested that the use of PPI before ESD could facilitate healing of the ulcerative differentiated EGC and reduce the ESD operative time [69], which remains to be validated.

Post-ESD Management

Most delayed ESD complications occur within the first day after ESD. The patient needs to remain fasting and be closely monitored for vital signs, symptoms, vomitus, and stool. During this critical period, delayed bleeding and perforation may occur in about 5% or less after endoscopic colorectal tumor resections [70, 71], although the reports on post-ESD resection complications of early gastric cardiac carcinoma remain limited. If clinical signs and symptoms for delayed bleeding or perforation are discovered, immediate measures should be carried out with the chest and abdominal X-rays for possible perforation. On the other hand, if there is no evidence on post-ESD complications, the patient may be allowed to have semiliquid and soft food. The necessity of a repeat of upper endoscopy 1 week after ESD remains controversial.

The ESD-resected fresh specimen needs to be immediately slightly stretched and pinned down on a dental wax plate, oriented, photographed, measured, promptly submerged in 10% buffered formalin solution, and shipped to the pathology laboratory for investigation, as detailed in Chap. 12.

PPI or H2 receptor antagonists (H2RA) are routinely administered to facilitate healing after ESD, but the choice of medications remains controversial. According to a meta-analysis [72], PPIs are better than H2RA for preventing post-ESD delayed bleeding. However, a recent study from Japan did not find a statistically significant difference between these two types of medications [73]. PPIs were suggested for 8 weeks [74], but Korean investigators preferred a 2-week protocol [75].

Kajiura et al. compared post-ESD mucosal healing with PPI and reported no significant difference between one group that took PPI for 1 week and another group that took PPI for 8 weeks [76]. The results of this small ($N = 45$) single-center retrospective study require validation in future larger prospective studies. Another study confirms that PPI may be used for 1 week after EMR resection [77]. A recent study also suggests that a combination therapy with PPI plus mucosal protective agents may accelerate the mucosal defect healing process [78]. Nakamura et al. reported that a combination therapy with PPI for the first 4 weeks plus rebamipide for 8 weeks is better for post-ESD mucosal defect healing than the use of PPI alone for 8 weeks [79].

In China, PPIs are the first choice for preventing post-ESD delayed bleeding and promoting ESD-related mucosal defect healing. A widely used protocol is to administer PPI intravenously at post-ESD day 1 and orally thereafter for 4–8 weeks. For cases with resection of large lesions or a long resection procedure, PPI may be used for 8 weeks with appropriately increased dosage or combination therapy with mucosal protective agents.

In general, prophylactic use of antibiotics has not been proven useful or effective. Itaba et al. reported a temporary, very low level of bacteremia during the EMR/ESD procedure but the absence of significant difference in bacteremia before and after the EMR/ESD procedure [80]. Another study also concludes that it is not necessary to use antibiotics in this situation [81]. However, for large lesions, longer EMR/ESD resection time, or cases with a high probability of perforation, prophylactic use of antibiotics may be prudent. For EMR/ESD resection of early gastric cardiac carcinoma, use of first- and second-generation cephalosporins, with or without nitroimidazole medication, is recommended and used for a period shorter than 72 h.

The *H. pylori* infection-related gastritis is considered to be a risk factor for ulcer recurrence after EMR/ESD, and *H. pylori* eradication should be carried out after the EMR/ESD procedure [82]. It was reported that eradication of *H. pylori* after EMR/ESD resection of early gastric cardiac carcinoma might reduce the recurrence of gastric cardiac carcinoma [83]. Therefore, patients with early gastric cardiac carcinoma should be tested for *H. pylori* infection. The chemotherapy for eradication of *H. pylori* infection, once confirmed, should be administered, according the fifth edition of the Maastricht consensus report [84].

Management of Post-EMR/ESD Complications

Despite minimal injury to the patient, EMR/ESD procedures may be associated with some complications, such as delayed bleeding, perforation, stenosis, abdominal pain, and infection, which may be related to the operator's experience, techniques, skills, and instruments and the patient's underlying conditions. Close monitoring of the patient's vital signs and clinical signs/symptoms is mandatory to allow immediate management.

Bleeding

Studies on ESD/EMR-related bleeding after resection of early gastric cardiac carcinoma are scarce. The prevalence of EMR/ESD-related bleeding was reported to be between 1.8 and 15.6% [85–90]. Generally, bleeding may occur during the resection procedure or afterward. Acute mild bleeding is defined as tiny bleeding sites on the operative field or bleeding from small arteries for 1 min or longer (Fig. 11.5), which can be successfully controlled endoscopically. Acute massive bleeding refers to active bleeding from the operative field or arterial bleeding that cannot be controlled endoscopically and requires transfusion. In contrast, delayed bleeding refers to post-EMR/ESD bleeding occurring within or beyond 48 h after EMR/ESD procedures, which is defined as a reduction of blood hemoglobin levels over 2 g/dL, compared to that before EMR/ESD procedures [91]. The incidence of acute bleeding during the ESD procedure is about 22.6–90.6%, and delayed bleeding is 0–6.0% [92, 93]. Overall, the risk of bleeding is much higher for the ESD procedure in the upper 2/3 of the stomach including the cardia, compared to that in the lower 1/3 of the stomach [94]. Yosuke et al. analyzed the risk factors of ESD procedure-related bleeding and reported the lesion size >4 cm as the only independent risk factor of delayed bleeding [95]. In China, the prevalence of bleeding was reported between 7.1 and 7.7% [46, 47]. Jang et al. reported a prevalence of 6% (5/82 cases) in five cases: two occurred 2 weeks after ESD procedures as delayed bleeding, and all five bleeding incidences were successfully controlled endoscopically [57].

The most commonly used method for bleeding control during the endoscopic procedure is direct electrocautery, using heated biopsy forceps or other direct electrocautery ESD instruments. For arterial bleeding, heated biopsy forceps are recommended [96]. It is very important to prevent bleeding during the procedure. Whenever a naked blood vessel is exposed, endoscopic clipping and electrocautery are performed to prevent bleeding [97]. For delayed bleeding at the early stage, the operative field is soft and edematous. The bleeding can be easily controlled with

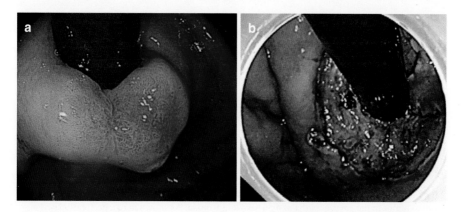

Fig. 11.5 A 0–IIa early gastric cardiac carcinoma (**a**). The post-ESD operative field shows a fresh mucosal defect (**b**) with small bleeding sites that need to be controlled as completely as possible

hemostatic clips or endoscopically heated biopsy forceps. In contrast, for delayed bleeding at a late stage, the operative field has been undergoing extensive fibrosis. In this scenario, submucosal sclerosant injection may be better for achieving hemostasis [96]. It is a common practice to use coagulation promoting medications and PPI in sufficient dosage to prevent post-EMR/ESD bleeding.

Perforation

Perforation during or after an EMR/ESD procedure is one of rare but potentially serious complications. In general, perforation occurs most commonly during the ESD procedure, especially for endoscopic resection of gastrointestinal stromal tumor, but very rarely for endoscopic resection of early gastric cardiac carcinoma. This complication can be readily diagnosed during the procedure and closed successfully by endoscopic clips in most cases. If perforation is discovered after the procedure, the patient may have typical abdominal peritoneal irritation signs and demonstrate free air under the diaphragm on abdominal X-ray or CT. Perforations should be diagnosed and treated immediately. The risk factors for gastric perforation during endotherapy include lesions in the markedly thinned proximal gastric wall, deep ulcerations, serious gastric atrophy, and other diseases [98]. Kojima et al. reported a perforation incidence of about 0.5% for EMR- and 1.2–4.1% for ESD-related procedures [92, 93]. The most important risk factors for perforation included a lesion size >2 cm and lesion location in the upper stomach [99].

If perforation occurs during the EMR/ESD procedure, the site may be closed with metallic clips (Fig. 11.6) [100]. If the perforation site is large, a large amount of air may enter the abdomen, leading to serious complications affecting vital signs such as blood pressure, pulse, and respiration. In this urgent situation, inserting a

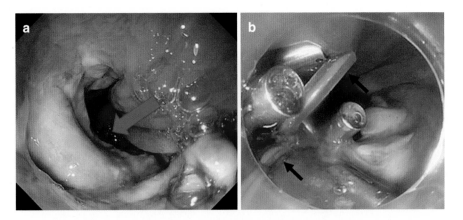

Fig. 11.6 Perforation of 1 day after an endoscopic submucosal dissection for a gastrointestinal stromal tumor in the gastric cardia of a 56-year-old woman. As shown in (**a**), perforation was associated with mucosal necrosis (arrow). After discovery, the perforated gastric wall was successfully closed with metallic clips along with a purse-string suture (arrows in **b**)

transcutaneous needle into the abdomen may be effective to reduce intra-abdominal pressure. During the ESD procedure, use of CO_2 instead of air may reduce pneumo-peritoneum and ESD-related gastric perforation [101] and pneumoabdomen-related instability in circulation and respiration, alleviate post-EMR/ESD-related vomiting and abdominal discomfort, and prevent air emboli [102]. In contrast, EMR/ESD-related small perforations during the procedure may have minimal adverse effects and be generally managed with continued abstaining of food intake, nasogastric tubing for decompression with intermittent suction, and antibiotic use. Therefore, small perforation may be self-contained, requiring only conservative management and observation. However, large and serious delayed perforations involving a large defect in the muscularis propria may not be easily repaired endoscopically. In that scenario, the perforated wall may be repaired by larger over-the-scope clips, endo-scopic full-thickness suturing devices, and cardiac septal defect occluders [103], although urgent surgical intervention may be necessary.

Stenosis

Post-ESD-related gastric cardiac stenosis occurs in 1.7–8% of cases [50–55]. As shown in Fig. 11.7, the post-ESD stenosis may narrow the opening of the GEJ with scar. The most important risk factors include mucosal resection involving over 3/4 of the circumference or longitudinal resection length >5 cm [51]. However, in a small case series report, Jang et al. described post-ESD-related circumferential mucosal defect >3/4 in two cases and the longitudinal resection length >5 cm in five cases, of which none had gastric cardiac stenosis [57]. It is believed that endoscopic balloon dilation is an effective therapy for gastric cardiac stenosis but is associated with a high risk for perforation [104].

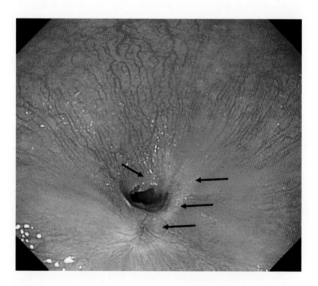

Fig. 11.7 Post-ESD stenosis at the esophagogastric junction with scar (arrows)

Bacteremia and Pneumothorax

Mild temporary bacteremia after EMR/ESD therapy may occur and is generally asymptomatic [105]. No specific therapy is needed, as discussed previously [105]. In the elderly population, ESD is still considered as a safe and effective therapeutic endoscopic procedure for resection of early gastric cardiac carcinoma [106]. However, in patients older than 75 years, post-therapy pneumothorax may occur with an incidence of up to 1.6% [107].

Assessment of Efficacy

There are several methods to evaluate the efficacy of EMR/ESD procedures. The most commonly used parameters include the following:

1. The percentage of en bloc resection, which refers to the frequency of a complete endoscopic resection of lesions with intact single resection specimens during a specific period of the study.
2. The positive horizontal and vertical resection margins, which are documented by histopathologic examination of the EMR/ESD resection specimen revealing tumor involvement of the horizontal and vertical margins of resection after the formalin fixation and complete evaluation of the entire resection specimen sectioned at 2 mm intervals. The horizontal margin refers to the inked lateral margin of resection, while the vertical margin indicates the inked deep margin of resection. In general, patients with a positive lateral margin require close follow-ups; but those with malignant cancerous cells/glands in the vertical margin need additional resection of the lesion [59].
3. Complete resection, which refers to both horizontal and vertical margins of resection being disease-free. This is not the same as the R0 resection because of the absence of lymph node dissection.
4. Curative resection, which is defined as complete resection of early carcinoma without the risk of lymph node metastasis. This can be achieved by endotherapy of early pT1a gastric cardiac carcinoma.
5. Local recurrence, which designates tumor recurrence at the previous EMR/ESD resection site within 6 months after the procedure.
6. Residual carcinoma, which refers to pathologic identification of carcinoma at or within 1 cm of the site of previous resection [59, 108].
7. Synchronous recurrence of carcinoma, which is defined as the discovery of de novo gastric cardiac carcinoma within 12 months after the previous EMR/ESD resection. This may be related to the development of a new carcinoma focus or progression from residual carcinoma that was left over the previous resection [109].
8. Metachronous recurrence, which is defined as a new carcinoma tumor discovered at the time over 12 months after previous complete resection [110]. Most metachronous tumors occur at the previous site of cancer resection and demonstrate similar pathologic features.

Post-EMR/ESD Surveillance

Unfortunately, tumor recurrence after EMR/ESD resection is not uncommon. For EMR procedures, the recurrence rate varies from 1.9 to 18%, and most cases are related to incomplete resection [43, 111]. The recurrence rate after the ESD procedure is about 0–7.7% with the 5-year survival rate of 91.2–100% and 5-year disease-specific survival rate of 100% [50–55]. In China, the recurrence rate after the ESD procedure varies from 2.1 to 5.4% [46, 47]. If the post-EMR/ESD pathologic examination demonstrates a high risk for lymph node metastasis and recurrence, an open surgical resection is recommended with nodal dissection [59].

A repeat endoscopic resection or close endoscopic surveillance is recommended for the following patients who are deemed to have a very low risk of lymph node metastasis: (1) a positive horizontal margin of resection in a well-moderately differentiated gastric cardiac carcinoma smaller than 0.6 cm in size after en bloc resection [98] and (2) well-moderately differentiated adenocarcinoma that is resected piecemeal in the way criteria for a complete resection are satisfied [61]. In general, the positive horizontal margin occurs in about 2% of cases and is associated with a recurrence rate of 0.3%. The main independent risk factor for a positive horizontal margin is a tumor situated in the upper 1/3 stomach (gastric cardia) [112].

All patients must be closely followed endoscopically, in general, at 3, 6, and 12 months after the EMR/ESD procedure. Once normal healing changes are confirmed endoscopically at the resection site, annual upper endoscopy is sufficient for surveillance along with routine monitoring of serological tumor biomarkers and necessary imaging studies. In some patients, colonoscopy may be recommended because many elderly patients with gastric cardiac carcinoma are at higher risk for developing colorectal neoplasms, compared to the general population [113].

Summary

At present, the only hope for improving patient survival is to detect, diagnose, and resect early gastric cardiac carcinoma, for which endoscopic therapy is the method of choice. Pre-resection investigation to rule out the risk of nodal metastasis in early gastric cardiac carcinoma is essential and requires a multidiscipline approach, despite the fact of significantly lower risk, compared to gastric non-cardiac carcinoma. Once decided, endoscopic therapy with ESD is preferred. This is a technically demanding technique, requiring extensive operative experience and also skills on management of post-resection complications.

References

1. Gotoda T, Yanagisawa A, Sasako M, et al. Incidence of lymph node metastasis from early gastric cancer: estimation with a large number of cases at two large centers. Gastric Cancer. 2000;3:219–25.

2. Ono H, Yao K, Fujishiro M, et al. Guidelines for endoscopic submucosal dissection and endoscopic mucosal resection for early gastric cancer. Dig Endosc. 2016;28(1):3–15.
3. Chinese Society of Digestive Endoscopy Consensus for early gastric carcinoma diagnosis and treatment in China. Chin J Dig Endosc. 2014;31:361–377.
4. Ahmad R, Setia N, Schmidt BH, et al. Predictors of lymph node metastasis in Western Early Gastric Cancer. J Gastroint Surg. 2016;20:531–8.
5. Barreto SG, Windsor JA. Redefining early gastric cancer. Surg Endosc. 2016;30:24–37.
6. Jin EH, Lee DH, Jung SA, et al. Clinicopathologic factors and molecular markers related to lymph node metastasis in early gastric cancer. World J Gastroenterol. 2015;21:571–7.
7. Kang HJ, Kim DH, Jeon TY, et al. Lymph node metastasis from intestinal-type early gastric cancer: experience in a single institution and reassessment of the extended criteria for endoscopic submucosal dissection. Gastrointest Endosc. 2010;72:508–55.
8. Huang Q, Fang C, Shi J, et al. Differences in clinicopathology of early gastric carcinoma between proximal and distal location in 438 Chinese patients. Scientific Report. 2015;5:13439.
9. Fang C, Shi J, Sun Q, et al. Risk factors of lymph node metastasis in early gastric carcinomas diagnosed with WHO criteria in 379 Chinese patients. J Dig Dis. 2016;17(8):526–37.
10. Guo TJ, Qin JY, Zhu LL, et al. Feasible endoscopic therapy for early gastric cancer. World J Gastroenterol. 2015;21:13325–31.
11. Yang HJ, Kim SG, Lim JH, et al. Predictors of lymph node metastasis in patients with non-curative endoscopic resection of early gastric cancer. Surg Endosc. 2014. https://doi.org/10.1007/s00464-014-3780-7.
12. Zhao BW, Chen YM, Jiang SS, et al. Lymph node metastasis, a unique independent prognostic factor in early gastric cancer. PLoS One. 2015;10:e0129531.
13. Park JH, Lee SH, Park JM, et al. Prediction of the indication criteria for endoscopic resection of early gastric cancer. World J Gastroenterol. 2015;21:11160–7.
14. Zhao X, Cai A, Xi H, et al. Predictive factors for lymph node metastasis in undifferentiated early gastric cancer: a systematic review and meta-analysis. J Gastrointest Surg. 2017. https://doi.org/10.1007/s11605-017-3364-7. [Epub ahead of print].
15. Sano T, Coit DG, Kim HH, et al. Proposal of a new stage grouping of gastric cancer for TNM classification: International Gastric Cancer Association staging project. Gastric Cancer. 2017;20(2):217–25.
16. Yu HP, Fang C, Chen L, et al. Worse prognosis in papillary, compared to tubular, early gastric carcinoma. J Cancer. 2017;8(1):117–23.
17. Yasuda K, Adachi Y, Shiraishi N, Maeo S, Kitano S. Papillary adenocarcinoma of the stomach. Gastric Cancer. 2000;3:33–8.
18. Lee HJ, Kim GH, Park do Y, et al. Is endoscopic submucosal dissection safe for papillary adenocarcinoma of the stomach? World J Gastroenterol. 2015;21:3944–52.
19. Sekiguchi M, Kushima R, Oda I, et al. Clinical significance of a papillary adenocarcinoma component in early gastric cancer: a single-center retrospective analysis of 628 surgically resected early gastric cancers. J Gastroenterol. 2015;50(4):424–34.
20. Koseki K, Takizawa T, Koike M, et al. Distinction of differentiated type early gastric carcinoma with gastric type mucin expression. Cancer. 2000;89:724–32.
21. Lee SH, Jee SR, Kim JH, Seol SY. Intramucosal gastric cancer: the rate of lymph node metastasis in signet ring cell carcinoma is as low as that in well-differentiated adenocarcinoma. Eur J Gastroenterol Hepatol. 2015;27:170–4.
22. Chiu CT, Kuo CJ, Yeh TS, et al. Early signet ring cell gastric cancer. Dig Dis Sci. 2011;56:1749–56.
23. Gronnier C, Messager M, Robb WB, et al. Is the negative prognostic impact of signet ring cell histology maintained in early gastric adenocarcinoma? Surgery. 2013;154:1093–9.
24. Hyung WJ, Noh SH, Lee JH, et al. Early gastric carcinoma with signet ring cell histology. Cancer. 2002;94:78–83.
25. Guo CG, Zhao DB, Liu Q, et al. Risk factors for lymph node metastasis in early gastric cancer with signet ring cell carcinoma. J Gastroint Surg. 2015;19:1958–65.

26. Pyo JH, Shin CM, Lee H, et al. A risk-prediction model based on lymph-node metastasis for incorporation into a treatment algorithm for signet ring cell-type intramucosal gastric cancer. Ann Surg. 2016;264(6):1038–43.
27. Kim YH, Kim JH, Kim H, et al. Is the recent WHO histological classification for gastric cancer helpful for application to endoscopic resection? Gastric Cancer. 2016;19:869–75.
28. Fujita H, Lennerz JK, Chung DC, et al. Endoscopic surveillance of patients with hereditary diffuse gastric cancer: biopsy recommendations after topographic distribution of cancer foci in a series of 10 CDH1-mutated gastrectomies. Am J Surg Pathol. 2012;36:1709–17.
29. Ha TK, An JY, Youn HK, Noh JH, Sohn TS, Kim S. Indication for endoscopic mucosal resection in early signet ring cell gastric cancer. Ann Surg Oncol. 2008;15:508–13.
30. Tong JH, Sun Z, Wang ZN, et al. Early gastric cancer with signet-ring cell histologic type: risk factors of lymph node metastasis and indications of endoscopic surgery. Surgery. 2011;149:356–63.
31. Kim HM, Pak KH, Chung MJ, et al. Early gastric cancer of signet ring cell carcinoma is more amenable to endoscopic treatment than is early gastric cancer of poorly differentiated tubular adenocarcinoma in select tumor conditions. Surg Endosc. 2011;25:3087–93.
32. Matsuda T, Takeuchi H, Tsuwano S, Nakahara T, Mukai M, Kitagawa Y. Sentinel node mapping in adenocarcinoma of the esophagogastric junction. World J Surg. 2014; 38(9):2337–44.
33. Fukase K, Kawata S. Evaluation of the efficacy of endoscopic treatment for early gastric cancer considered in terms of long-term prognosis more than 10 years: a comparison with surgical treatment. Fertil Steril. 2004;82(3):241–7.
34. Choi KS, Jung HY, Choi KD, et al. EMR versus gastrectomy for intramucosal gastric cancer: comparison of long-term outcomes. Gastrointest Endosc. 2011;73(5):942–8.
35. Chiu PW, Teoh AY, To K F, et al. Endoscopic submucosal dissection (ESD) compared with gastrectomy for treatment of early gastric neoplasia: a retrospective cohort study. Surg Endosc. 2012;26(12):3584–91.
36. Tada M, Shimada M, Murakami F. Development of the strip-off biopsy. Gastroenterol Endosc. 1984;26(6):833–9.
37. Takekoshi T, Baba Y, Ota H, et al. Endoscopic resection of early gastric carcinoma: results of a retrospective analysis of 308 cases. Endoscopy. 1994;26(4):352–8.
38. Gotoda T, Kondo H, Ono H, et al. A new endoscopic mucosal resection procedure using an insulation-tipped electrosurgical knife for rectal flat lesions: report of two cases. Gastrointest Endosc. 1999;50(4):560–3.
39. Lian J, Chen S, Zhang Y, et al. A meta-analysis of endoscopic submucosal dissection and EMR for early gastric cancer. Gastrointest Endosc. 2012;76(4):763–70.
40. Yamamoto H, Kita H. Endoscopic therapy of early gastric cancer. Best Pract Res Clin Gastroenterol. 2006;19(6):909–26.
41. Chaves DM, Sakai P, Mester M, et al. A new endoscopic technique for the resection of flat polypoid lesions. Gastrointest Endosc. 1994;40(2):224–6.
42. Horiki N, Omata F, Uemura M, et al. Risk for local recurrence of early gastric cancer treated with piecemeal endoscopic mucosal resection during a 10-year follow-up period. Surg Endosc. 2012;26(1):72–8.
43. Kojima T, Parra-Blanco A, Takahashi H, et al. Outcome of endoscopic mucosal resection for early gastric cancer: review of the Japanese literature. Gastrointest Endosc. 1998;48(5):550.
44. Kim JJ, Lee JH, Jung HY, et al. EMR for early gastric cancer in Korea: a multicenter retrospective study. Gastrointest Endosc. 2007;66(4):693.
45. Oda I, Saito D, Tada M, et al. A multicenter retrospective study of endoscopic resection for early gastric cancer. Gastric Cancer. 2006;9(4):262.
46. Endoscopic treatment of early cardia cancer, pull the screen for esophageal cancer, head and neck cancer associated with esophageal cancer, Beijing Union Medical College, 刘勇. 内镜治疗早期贲门癌、拉网筛查食管癌、头颈部癌合并食管癌的相关研究[D]. 北京协和医学院, 2016 (in Chinese).

47. Lv Y, Zhang XQ, Zou XP, et al. Comparison of endoscopic submucosal dissection and endoscopic mucosal resection in the treatment of precancerous lesions and early cancer of the gastroesophageal junction. J Dig Endosc. 2012;29(5):243–6. (in Chinese).
48. Shimizu Y, Takahashi M, Yoshida T, et al. Endoscopic resection (endoscopic mucosal resection/endoscopic submucosal dissection) for superficial esophageal squamous cell carcinoma: current status of various techniques. Dig Endosc. 2013;25(Suppl 1):13–9.
49. Choi MK, Kim GH, Park do Y, et al. Long-term outcomes of endoscopic submucosal dissection for early gastric cancer: a single center experience. Surg Endosc. 2013;27:4250–8.
50. Omae M, Fujisaki J, Horiuchi Y, et al. Safety, efficacy, and long-term outcomes for endoscopic submucosal dissection of early esophagogastric junction cancer. Gastric Cancer. 2013;16(2):147–54.
51. Park CH, Kim EH, Kim HY, et al. Clinical outcomes of endoscopic submucosal dissection for early stage esophagogastric junction cancer: a systematic review and meta-analysis. Dig Liver Dis. 2015;47(1):37.
52. Yamada M, Oda I, Nonaka S, et al. Long-term outcome of endoscopic resection of superficial adenocarcinoma of the esophagogastric junction. Endoscopy. 2013;45(12):992–6.
53. Imai K, Kakushima N, Tanaka M, et al. Validation of the application of the Japanese curative criteria for superficial adenocarcinoma at the esophagogastric junction treated by endoscopic submucosal dissection: a long-term analysis. Surg Endosc. 2013;27(7):2436–45.
54. Hirasawa K, Kokawa A, Oka H, et al. Superficial adenocarcinoma of the esophagogastric junction: long-term results of endoscopic submucosal dissection. Gastrointest Endosc. 2010;72(5):960–6.
55. Yoshinaga S, Gotoda T, Kusano C, et al. Clinical impact of endoscopic submucosal dissection for superficial adenocarcinoma located at the esophagogastric junction. Gastrointest Endosc. 2008;67(2):202.
56. Ono, Shunsuke. Ministry of Health, Labour and Welfare (MHLW, Japan). Japanese Scientific Monthly, 2007; p. 60.
57. Jang YS, Lee BE, Kim GH, et al. Factors associated with outcomes in endoscopic submucosal dissection of gastric cardiatumors: a retrospective observational study. Medicine (Baltimore). 2015;94(31):e1201.
58. Huang Q, Shi J, Xu GF, et al. Risk factors of lymph node metastasis in 1620 early gastric carcinoma radical gastrectomies: a multicenter clinicopathologic study in Jiangsu Province in China. The 2017 Annual Meeting of the Chinese Gastroenterology Society in Xian, China.
59. NCCN Guidelines version 2.2015 Gastric Cancer. http://www.cjcpt.org/files/2015/03-06/2015-NCCN/2015%20NCCN-%E8%83%83%E7%99%8C-V2.pdf. Accessed 19 June 2017.
60. Waddell T, Verheij M, Allum W, et al. Gastric cancer: ESMO-ESSO-ESTRO Clinical Practice Guidelines for diagnosis, treatment and follow-up. Ann Oncol. 2013;40(suppl 6):1165–76.
61. Association JGC. Japanese gastric cancer treatment guidelines 2014 (ver. 4). Gastric Cancer. 2017;20(1):1–19.
62. Allum WH, Griffin SM, Watson A, et al. Guidelines for the management of oesophageal and gastric cancer. Gut. 2011;60(11):1449–72.
63. Schlemper RJ, Riddell RH, Kato Y, et al. The Vienna classification of gastrointestinal epithelial neoplasia. Gut. 2000;47(2):251.
64. You Z, Enqiang L, Zhongsheng L, et al. Preoperative biopsy in gastric mucosal lesions endoscopic submucosal dissection in the value of the value. Chin J Dig Endosc. 2012;29(3):151–4. (in Chinese).
65. Kim YJ, Park JC, Kim JH, et al. Histologic diagnosis based on forceps biopsy is not adequate for determining endoscopic treatment of gastric adenomatous lesions. Endoscopy. 2010;42(08):620–6.
66. Xu G, Zhang W, Lv Y, et al. Risk factors for under-diagnosis of gastric intraepithelial neoplasia and early gastric carcinoma in endoscopic forceps biopsy in comparison with endoscopic submucosal dissection in Chinese patients. Surg Endosc. 2016;30(7):2716–22.

67. Veitch AM, Baglin TP, Gershlick AH, et al. Guidelines for the management of antico-agulant and antiplatelet therapy in patients undergoing endoscopic procedures. Gut. 2008;57(9):1322.

68. Goto O, Fujishiro M, Kodashima S, et al. Feasibility of endoscopic submucosal dissection for patients with chronic renal failure on hemodialysis. Dig Endosc. 2010;22(1):45–8.

69. Myung YS, Hong SJ, Han JP, et al. Effects of administration of a proton pump inhibitor before endoscopic submucosal dissection for differentiated early gastric cancer with ulcer. Gastric Cancer. 2017;20(1):200–6.

70. Fujishiro M, Yahagi N, Kakushima N, et al. Outcomes of endoscopic submucosal dissection for colorectal epithelial neoplasms in 200 consecutive cases. Clin Gastroenterol Hepatol. 2007;5:678–83.

71. Saito Y, Uraoka T, Matsuda T, et al. Endoscopic treatment of large superficial colorectal tumors: a case series of 200 endoscopic submucosal dissections (with video). Gastrointest Endosc. 2007;66:966–73.

72. Yang Z, Wu Q, Liu Z, Wu K, Fan D. Proton pump inhibitors versus histamine-2-receptor antagonists for the management of iatrogenic gastric ulcer after endoscopic mucosal resec-tion or endoscopic submucosal dissection: a meta-analysis of randomized trials. Digestion. 2011;84(4):315–20.

73. Imaeda H, Hosoe N, Suzuki H, et al. Effect of lansoprazole versus roxatidine on prevention of bleeding and promotion of ulcer healing after endoscopic submucosal dissection for super-ficial gastric neoplasia. J Gastro. 2011;46(11):1267–72.

74. Goto O, Fujishiro M, Kodashima S, et al. Short-term healing process of artificial ulcers after gastric endoscopic submucosal dissection. Gut Liver. 2011;5(3):293–7.

75. Niimi K, Fujishiro M, Goto O, et al. Prospective single-arm trial of two-week rabepra-zole treatment for healing after gastric endoscopic submucosal dissection. Dig Endosc. 2012;24(2):110–6.

76. Kajiura S, Hosokawa A, Ueda A, et al. Effective healing of endoscopic submucosal dissection-induced ulcers by a single week of proton pump inhibitor treatment: a retrospective study. BMC Res Notes. 2015;8:150.

77. Lee SY, Kim JJ, Lee JH, et al. Healing rate of EMR-induced ulcer in relation to the duration of treatment with omeprazole. Gastrointest Endosc. 2004;60(2):213–7.

78. Shin WG, Kim SJ, Choi MH, et al. Can rebamipide and proton pump inhibitor combination therapy promote the healing of endoscopic submucosal dissection-induced ulcers? A ran-domized, prospective, multicenter study. Gastrointest Endosc. 2012;75(4):739–47.

79. Nakamura M, Tahara T, Shiroeda H, et al. The effect of short-term proton pump inhibitor plus anti-ulcer drug on the healing of endoscopic submucosal dissection-derived artificial ulcer: a randomized controlled trial. Hepato-Gastroenterology. 2015;62(137):219–24.

80. Itaba S, Iboshi Y, Nakamura K, et al. Low-frequency of bacteremia after endoscopic submu-cosal dissection of the stomach. Dig Endosc. 2011;23(1):69–72.

81. Chinese Society of Digestive Endoscopy (CSDE). Expert recommendations for perioperative use of endoscopic submucosal dissection for gastric mucosal lesions (2015, Suzhou). Chin J Dig Endosc. 2015;54(10):905–8.

82. Huang Y, Kakushima N, Takizawa K, et al. Risk factors for recurrence of artificial gastric ulcers after endoscopic submucosal dissection. Endoscopy. 2010;43(3):236–9.

83. Fukase K, Kato M, Kikuchi S, et al. Effect of eradication of Helicobacter pylori, on incidence of metachronous gastric carcinoma after endoscopic resection of early gastric cancer: an open-label, randomised controlled trial. Lancet. 2008;372(9636):392.

84. Malfertheiner P, Megraud F, O'Morain CA, et al. European Helicobacter and Microbiota Study Group and Consensus panel. Management of Helicobacter pylori infection-the Maastricht V/Florence Consensus Report. Gut. 2017;66(1):6–30.

85. Park YM, Cho E, Kang HY, Kim JM. The effectiveness and safety of endoscopic submucosal dissection compared with endoscopic mucosal resection for early gastric cancer: a systematic review and meta-analysis. Surg Endosc. 2011;25:2666–77.

86. Chung IK, Lee JH, Lee SH, et al. Therapeutic outcomes in 1000 cases of endoscopic submucosal dissection for early gastric neoplasms: Korean ESD Study Group multicenter study. Gastrointest Endosc. 2009;69:1228–35.

87. Koh R, Hirasawa K, Yahara S, et al. Antithrombotic drugs are risk factors for delayed postoperative bleeding after endoscopic submucosal dissection for gastric neoplasms. Gastrointest Endosc. 2013;78:476–83.

88. Lim JH, Kim SG, Kim JW, et al. Do antiplatelets increase the risk of bleeding after endoscopic submucosal dissection of gastric neoplasms? Gastrointest Endosc. 2012;75:719–27.

89. Isomoto H, Shikuwa S, Yamaguchi N, et al. Endoscopic submucosal dissection for early gastric cancer: a large-scale feasibility study. Gut. 2009;58:331–6.

90. Goto O, Fujishiro M, Oda I, et al. A multicenter survey of the management after gastric endoscopic submucosal dissection related to postoperative bleeding. Dig Dis Sci. 2012;57:435–9.

91. Lim SM, Park JC, Lee H, et al. Impact of cumulative time on the clinical outcomes of endoscopic submucosal dissection in gastric neoplasm. Surg Endosc. 2013;27(4):1397–403.

92. Jeon SW, Jung MK, Cho CM, et al. Predictors of immediate bleeding during endoscopic submucosal dissection in gastric lesions. Surg Endosc. 2009;67(9):1974–9.

93. Jang JS, Choi SR, Graham DY, et al. Risk factors for immediate and delayed bleeding associated with endoscopic submucosal dissection of gastric neoplastic lesions. Scand J Gastroenterol. 2009;44(11):1370–6.

94. Oda I, Gotoda T, Hamanaka H, et al. Endoscopic submucosal dissection for early gastric cancer: technical feasibility, operation time and complications from a large consecutive series. Dig Endosc. 2004;17(1):54–8.

95. Tsuji Y, Ohata K, Ito T, et al. Risk factors for bleeding after endoscopic submucosal dissection for gastric lesions. Surg Endosc. 2011;16(1):2913–7.

96. Oda I, Suzuki H, Nonaka S, et al. Complications of gastric endoscopic submucosal dissection. Dig Endosc. 2013;25(Suppl S1):71–8.

97. Chan HP, Sang KL. Preventing and controlling bleeding in gastric endoscopic submucosal dissection. Clin Endosc. 2013;46(5):456–62.

98. Toyokawa T, Inaba T, Omote S, et al. Risk factors for perforation and delayed bleeding associated with endoscopic submucosal dissection for early gastric neoplasms: analysis of 1123 lesions. J Gastro Hepatol. 2012;27(5):907–12.

99. Ohta T, Ishihara R, Uedo N, et al. Factors predicting perforation during endoscopic submucosal dissection for gastric cancer. Gastrointest Endosc. 2012;75(4):AB136.

100. Solis-Cohen M. Complete endoscopic closure of gastric perforation induced by endoscopic resection of early gastric cancer using endoclips can prevent surgery (with video). Gastrointest Endosc. 2006;63(4):596–601.

101. Nonaka S, Saito Y, Takisawa H, et al. Safety of carbon dioxide insufflation for upper gastrointestinal tract endoscopic treatment of patients under deep sedation. Surg Endosc. 2010;24(7):1638.

102. Maeda Y, Hirasawa D, Fujita N, et al. A prospective, randomized, double-blind, controlled trial on the efficacy of carbon dioxide insufflation in gastric endoscopic submucosal dissection. Endoscopy. 2013;45(5):335–41.

103. American Society of Gastrointestinal Endoscopy Technology Committee. Endoscopic closure devices. Gastrointest Endosc. 2012;76:244–51.

104. Tsunada S, Ogata S, Mannen K, et al. Case series of endoscopic balloon dilation to treat a stricture caused by circumferential resection of the gastric antrum by endoscopic submucosal dissection. Gastrointest Endosc. 2008;67(6):979.

105. Lee TH, Hsueh PR, Yeh WC, et al. Low frequency of bacteremia after endoscopic mucosal resection. Gastrointest Endosc. 2000;52(2):223–5.

106. Abe N, Gotoda T, Hirasawa T, et al. Multicenter study of the long-term outcomes of endoscopic submucosal dissection for early gastric cancer in patients 80 years of age or older. Gastric Cancer. 2012;15(1):70–5.

107. Akasaka T, Nishida T, Tsutsui S, et al. Short-term outcomes of endoscopic submucosal dissection (ESD) for early gastric neoplasm: multicenter survey by Osaka University ESD Study Group. Dig Endosc. 2011;23(1):73–7.
108. Hong C, Zheng ZY, Shunying L. Endoscopic submucosal dissection for the treatment of early gastric cancer. Chin J Dig Endosc. 2006;23(5):398–400. (in Chinese)
109. Yoo JH, Shin SJ, Lee KM, et al. How can we predict the presence of missed synchronous lesions after endoscopic submucosal dissection for early gastric cancers or gastric adenomas? J Clin Gastroenterol. 2013;47(2):17–22.
110. Nasu J, Doi T, Endo H, et al. Characteristics of metachronous multiple early gastric cancers after endoscopic mucosal resection. Gastrointest Endosc. 2006;63(5):990.
111. Yuan L, Enqiang L, Zhiqiang W, et al. Study on the recurrence rate of gastric intraepithelial neoplasia and early carcinoma after endoscopic mucosal resection (EMR). China Contin Med Educ. 2011;03(12):101–3. (in Chinese).
112. Numata N, Oka S, Tanaka S, et al. Risk factors and management of positive horizontal margin in early gastric cancer resected by en bloc endoscopic submucosal dissection. Gastric Cancer. 2015;18(2):332–8.
113. Lee KJ, Kim JH, Kim SI, et al. Clinical significance of colonoscopic examination in patients with early stage of gastric neoplasm undergoing endoscopic submucosal dissection. Scand J Gastro. 2011;46(11):1349–54.

Chapter 12
Pathologic Evaluation of Endoscopic Resection Specimens

Qi Sun and Qin Huang

Introduction

Endoscopic resection of neoplasms in the stomach is a type of minimally invasive procedures and has a number of advantages over open surgical resection in terms of lower cost, shorter duration of hospital stay, less blood loss, fewer complications, better preservation of gastric function, and more rapid recovery after the procedure [1]. Endoscopic resection, such as endoscopic mucosal resection (EMR) and endoscopic submucosal dissection (ESD), has been widely accepted and used for the treatment of gastric epithelial neoplasms, especially for early gastric carcinoma (EGC) with negligible risk of lymph node metastasis [2]. Since ESD is significantly more effective than EMR with respect to en bloc resection, lower local recurrence, and complete histopathological assessment of the specimen, most gastric superficial neoplasms have been resected with ESD techniques primarily in East Asian countries [3]. In our practice, most early gastric cardiac carcinomas are resected endoscopically with ESD. As such, accurate histopathologic evaluation of the ESD specimen is critically important and provides the critical information not only on the accurate diagnosis, tumor stage, and associated diseases but also on the adequacy of the ESD resection, margin status, and the presence or absence of risk factors for nodal metastasis to guide patient further triage and management. Over the past several years, we have performed a considerable number of pathologic evaluations of

Q. Sun (✉)
Department of Pathology, Nanjing Drum Tower Hospital,
Nanjing, Jiangsu, People's Republic of China

Q. Huang
Pathology and Laboratory Medicine, Veterans Affairs Boston Healthcare System,
West Roxbury, MA, USA

Harvard Medical School and Brigham and Women's Hospital,
Boston, MA, USA

© Springer International Publishing AG, part of Springer Nature 2018   227
Q. Huang (ed.), *Gastric Cardiac Cancer*, https://doi.org/10.1007/978-3-319-79114-2_12

ESD specimens at the Nanjing Drum Tower Hospital, armed with the latest versions of the practice guidelines and protocols issued by the Chinese Society of Digestive Endoscopy [4], the Japan Gastroenterological Endoscopy Society (JGES), and the Japanese Gastric Cancer Association (JGCA) [2, 5] and the World Health Organization *WHO Classification of Tumours of the Digestive System* (4th edition) [6]. In this chapter, we will present our experience on the methods and protocols on histopathologic assessment of the ESD specimen on early gastric cardiac carcinoma.

Processing of ESD Specimens

Once an early gastric carcinoma is resected with the ESD technique, it is the responsibility of the endoscopist, not pathologist, to immediately start appropriate tissue processing within the endoscopic suit, where the fresh specimen is slightly stretched out, pinned down on a dental wax plate with accurate orientation, photographed, and then immediately immersed in the 10% neutral buffered formalin solution. The tissue ischemic time elapsed between complete resection and formalin fixation should be as short as possible (shorter than 30 min) to minimize tissue degradation and better preserve DNA and RNA molecules. As a general rule, the immersion duration in formalin should be 12–48 h at room temperature to ensure adequate fixation for possible molecular studies in the future.

Tips for the endoscopist on initial ESD tissue processing:

1. *Because the muscularis mucosae will contract after endoscopic resection, the most important thing on immediate fresh ESD specimen handling is to preserve the intact normal anatomy by slightly stretching the fresh tissue and pinning it down on the plate. The endoscopist should mark clearly the correct orientation of the specimen with appropriate markings so that the pathologist will evaluate the dissection margins accurately, minimizing the incidence of reporting false-positive or false-negative margins. We use tweezers together with pins to make the stretching process easier* (Figs. 12.1 and 12.2).
2. *Stainless steel thin pins, such as either insect specimen fixation pins (size 1# or 2#) or acupuncture needles, are good choices for pinning down an ESD specimen with minimal tissue distortion or damage.*
3. *The polystyrene board can be easily found and used as an ideal plate for ESD-resected specimen handling* (Fig. 12.3).
4. *Neutral buffered formalin means 10% volume/formalin in water (approx. 4% formaldehyde), pH 7.4. The specimen should be fixed with at least ten times more 10% neutral buffered formalin solution. Therefore, a large container should be used for each ESD specimen.*
5. *During the initial fresh specimen processing procedure in the endoscopic suit, the specimen should be kept wet with normal saline solution to prevent the fresh specimen from drying up and maintain the tissue* in vivo *physiology before immersing into the formalin solution for a better preservation.*

Fig. 12.1 An ESD specimen is slightly stretched with pin (arrow) to preserve the intact normal anatomy

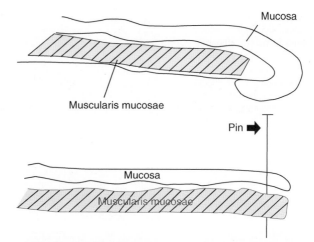

Fig. 12.2 Using tweezers together with pins to stretch and pin down an ESD specimen with accurate orientations

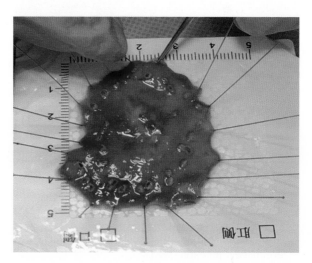

In a well-sealed container, the specimen will be delivered to the pathologist for further processing, such as sectioning of the fully fixed specimen (over 10–24 h), macroscopic photography before and after sectioning, and histology tissue processing.

Once fixed well, the specimen is removed from the plate, and all resection margins are inked, ideally with different colors. Before sectioning, the mucosal surface of an ESD specimen should be washed first to remove mucus, residual food particles, necrotic debris, blood clots, etc. Then, the specimen will be carefully inspected, and the gross characteristics of the tumor and the adjacent uninvolved mucosal tissue should be described, measured, and recorded, including:

1. The specimen size
2. Mucosal surface color (discoloration of the mucosal surface of the lesion, compared to the surrounding normal mucosa)

Fig. 12.3 Once the ESD specimen is pinned down on a polystyrene board with pins, a gross photo is taken, and then the specimen is immediately immersed facedown into the 10% neutral buffered formalin solution in a large container

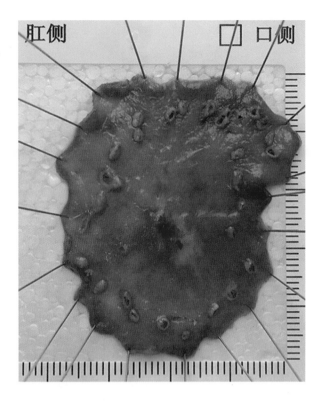

3. The presence or absence of ulceration (UL, lesions with ulcerations or scarring from the previous or current ulcer)
4. The location of the tumor epicenter, size, shape, and color
5. The distance (in millimeter) of the tumor edge to peripheral and deep margins of resection
6. The relationship and distance (in millimeter) of the tumor edge to the gastro-esophageal junction (GEJ)
7. Any mucosal lesions in the adjacent gastric cardia and the distal esophagus, especially columnar-lined esophagus
8. Whether or not the tumor invades into the distal esophagus, if so, the relationship and distance between the tumor in the cardia and the tumor in the distal esophagus, in association with columnar-lined esophagus and other esophageal lesions

Among these observations, the tumor size, margin, and shape (protruding, flat, or ulceration) and the relationship to the GEJ are particularly important. For example, the size of the neoplasm with or without ulcer is critical for the decision of endoscopic therapy and additional surgery [2]. The distance from the tumor edge to the nearest resected margin may help determine the adequacy of the ESD excision and the need for adjuvant or additional resection therapy.

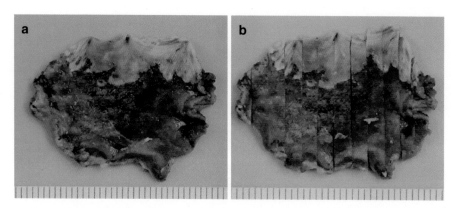

Fig. 12.4 Macroscopic photos before (**a**) and after (**b**) sectioning after formalin fixation

Macroscopic photography should be taken before and after sectioning (Fig. 12.4).

Macroscopic appearances of an early tumor are reclassified, according to the Paris endoscopic classification [7]. Type 0 early tumors are not the same as superficial lesions of the Borrmann classification (proposed for advanced gastric tumors in 1926, which includes Types I–IV) [5]. For Type 0 early tumors, the gross types of the superficial early tumor lesions are divided into polypoid (0-Ip and 0-Is) and non-polypoid subtypes. The non-polypoid subtypes include lesions with a small variation of superficial (0-IIa, slightly elevated; 0-IIb, flat; 0-IIc, depressed) and excavated lesions (0-III). Superficial tumors with O-II or more components should have all components recorded in the order of the surface area occupied, e.g., 0-IIa + IIc (Figs. 12.5 and 12.6). After gross tumor photography, the specimen is cut longitudinally into parallel slices. The first incision is made to allow pathological examination of the lesion with the minimal distance between the margin of the lesion and the lateral edge of a specimen. Then, further sections are made parallel to the first one at interval of 2.0–3.0 mm (Fig. 12.7a–c). As shown in Fig. 12.7a, one can imagine a line tangential to the tumor margin that is the closest to the horizontal margin of the specimen (mucosal dissection margin) and make the first cut perpendicular to this tangential line.

After specimen sectioning is completed, the tissue slices will be sequentially placed in tissue embedding cassettes for paraffin embedding in the correct order of sequence for histology reassembling of the resected tumor. Paraffin tissue blocks will be sliced at 4 μm in thickness and stained with a routine hematoxylin-eosin (H&E) stain.

Tips:

1. *Each tissue slice should be rotated by 90° before being placed into an embedding cassette* (Fig. 12.8a).
2. *To ensure the straightness and correct order, we use a thin sponge to push the tissue slice to the side of an embedding cassette* (Fig. 12.8b).

Fig. 12.5 Schematic representation of the major variants of Type 0 neoplastic lesions of the digestive tract: polypoid (0-Ip and 0-Is), non-polypoid (0-IIa, 0-IIb, and 0-IIc), and excavated (0-III), based on the Paris classification [7]

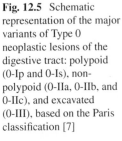

Type 0- I p
Protruded, pedunculated

Type 0- I s
Protruded, sessile

Type 0- I
Protruded

Type 0- II a
Superficial, elevated

Type 0- II b
Superficial, flat

Type 0- II c
Superficial, depressed

Type 0- II
Superficial

Type 0- III
Excavated

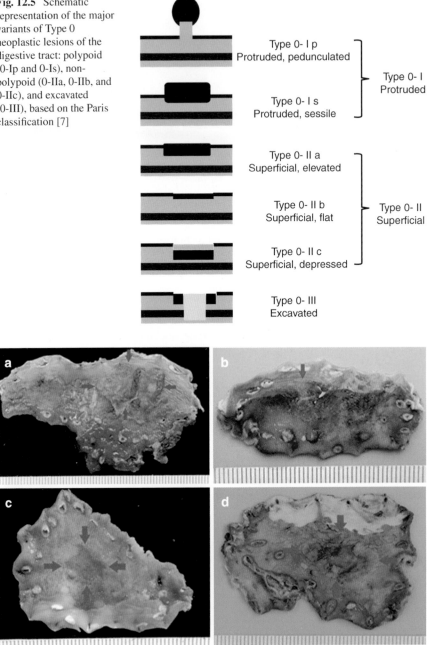

Fig. 12.6 Macroscopic photos of formalin-fixed specimens of early gastric cardiac carcinomas resected by ESD show variations (arrows) in 0-II tumors: (**a**) 0-IIa, slightly elevated; (**b**) 0-IIb, slightly flat; (**c**) 0-IIc, slightly depressed; (**d**) 0-IIa + IIc, depressed area in an elevated lesion

Fig. 12.7 Along an imaginary line tangential to the margin of the blue-colored lesion, closest to the horizontal margin (lateral edge) of the specimen (black dotted line) in (**a**), the first cut is placed perpendicular to this tangential line (red solid line), and additional sequential longitudinal cuts are made parallel to the first cut at interval of 2.0–3.0 mm (red dotted line) (**a**). Actual case (**b**, photographed before sectioning; **c**, photographed after sectioning)

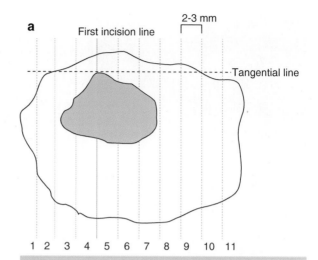

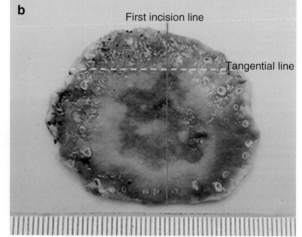

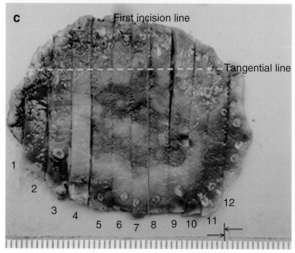

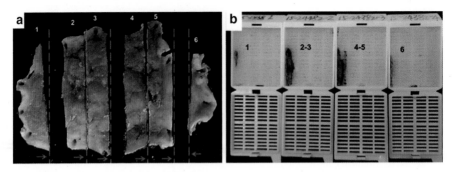

Fig. 12.8 Red dotted lines indicate the sectioning surfaces under a microscope. Tissue slices #1–#5 are turned right, rotated by 90°, and placed in the cassettes facedown. Slice 6# is turned left, the opposite direction, and also rotated by 90° to preserve the far-right lateral edge (**a**). A thin sponge is used to pushing each tissue slice to one side of the cassette to preserve the correct order sequence (**b**)

Fig. 12.9 With a macroscopic photograph of the fixed, sliced specimen, the extent of intramucosal spread and depth of invasion by the tumor can be reconstructed after microscopic evaluation. Green lines indicate the region with low-grade dysplasia, and yellow lines show the area with intramucosal adenocarcinoma in this ESD-resected early gastric cardiac carcinoma specimen

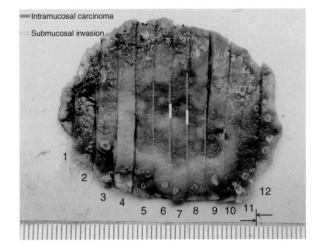

To appropriately reconstruct the extent of intramucosal spread and depth of invasion (Fig. 12.9), it is desirable to take macroscopic photographs of the fixed, sliced specimen before placing tissue slices into cassettes for comparison and tumor mapping purposes.

Histopathological Report

The essential elements in a pathology report on an ESD specimen include:

The size and number of the specimens
The macroscopic type of the tumor (according to the Paris classification)
The size of the tumor (longest and shortest dimensions)

The histological type of the tumor (based on the WHO classification)
Depth of tumor invasion
The presence or absence of lymphovascular invasion
Perineural invasion
The involvement of horizontal and vertical margins (HM and VM) by a dysplastic
    or invasive lesion
Nonneoplastic pathologic lesions in the adjacent uninvolved tissue
Any invasion into the distal esophagus
The presence or absence of columnar-lined esophagus and dysplasia in the distal
    esophagus [4, 5]

According to the WHO diagnostic criteria [6], EGC is defined as an invasive neoplastic epithelial lesion of the stomach confined to the mucosa (M) and/or submucosa (SM), regardless of the lymph node status. Histopathological types of gastric adenocarcinoma include five main categories [tubular, papillary, mucinous, poorly cohesive (including signet ring cell carcinoma and other variants), and mixed carcinomas and rare entities (such as adenosquamous carcinoma, squamous cell carcinoma, hepatoid adenocarcinoma, neuroendocrine carcinoma, carcinoma with lymphoid stroma, etc.)]. For early gastric cardiac carcinoma, most tumors are tubular and/or papillary adenocarcinomas. Because papillary adenocarcinoma is prone to lymph node metastasis and usually with a poor prognosis, the diagnostic criteria should be strictly followed [8]. Unlike distal gastric non-cardiac carcinomas, gastric cardiac carcinoma is more heterogeneous and more likely to be composed of uncommon histological types, such as high-grade neuroendocrine carcinoma, adenosquamous carcinoma, mixed adeno-neuroendocrine carcinoma, hepatoid adenocarcinoma, pancreatic acinar-like adenocarcinoma, carcinoma with lymphoid stroma, choriocarcinoma, squamous cell carcinoma, undifferentiated carcinoma, and carcinosarcoma [8, 9].

Gastric carcinoma categories are similar between WHO and Japanese classifications with only slight differences. According to the Japanese classification of gastric carcinoma, the third English edition [5], all tumors are categorized as either differentiated or undifferentiated (Nakamura's classification). Well- or moderately differentiated tubular and papillary adenocarcinomas of the WHO classification are classified as differentiated cancers, whereas signet ring cell and poorly differentiated adenocarcinomas and others are classified as undifferentiated. Furthermore, when multiple histopathological types coexist, each histopathological type should be recorded, in descending order of relative proportions of each type within the same lesion (e.g., tubular > papillary > poorly differentiated, etc.) (Fig. 12.10).

The depth of tumor invasion needs to be measured and reported in micrometer, including the deepest point at which the cancer has infiltrated. When submucosal invasion is present, the tumor submucosal invasion depth should be measured as the distance from the lowest edge of the muscularis mucosae to the deepest point of an invading cancer. The depth of submucosal penetration is classified into two subgroups: SM1 (<500 μm penetration into submucosa or T1b1) and SM2 (≥500 μm or T1b2) (Fig. 12.11) [2, 5]. The abovementioned vertical infiltration distance is measured

- Common types
  - Tubular adenocarcinoma
    - Well-differentiated (tub1)
    - Moderately-differentiated (tub2)
  - Papillary adenocarcinoma (pap)

    } Differentiated type

  - Poorly differentiated adenocarcinoma
    - Solid type (por1)
    - Non-solid type (por2)
  - Signet ring cell carcinoma (sig)
  - Mucinous carcinoma (muc)

    } Undifferentiated type

- Special types

Fig. 12.10 The Japanese classification of gastric carcinoma (JCGC): histological types

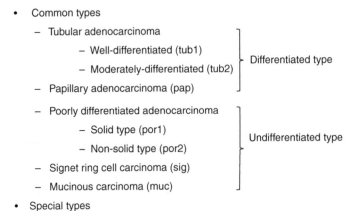

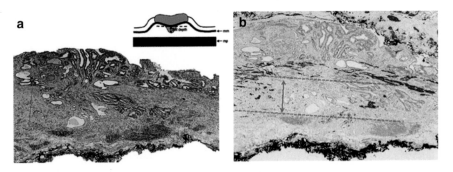

Fig. 12.11 The depth of submucosal invasion (red arrows between two red dashed lines) is measured from the lowest point of the muscularis mucosae to the deepest point of invasion (**a**), as shown in the insert on the right upper corner. Anti-desmin immunohistochemical staining is useful to identify the muscularis mucosae that are stained brown (**b**)

using a microscope equipped with an ocular scale bar. If the muscularis mucosae is obscure and indiscernible due to tumor ulceration or an ulcerated scar within the lesion, an imaginary continuous line may need to be mentally drawn between the residual muscularis mucosae in the adjacent mucosa at the two sides of an ulcerated lesion for the measurement of the vertical invasion depth. Immunohistochemical staining with the anti-desmin antibody is also useful in identifying the residual muscularis mucosae (Figs. 12.11 and 12.12). In cases with massively submucosal invasive tumors, the depth of submucosal invasion is measured (estimated) from the surface of the tumor to the deepest invasion point (Fig. 12.13).

When the vertical margin is involved, there is no need for measuring the invasive depth, but the possibility of deeper invasion should be described in the pathological report. In cases in which muscularis mucosae is irregular or partially destroyed by cancer infiltration as part of desmoplasia, it is hard to choose a reliable method to

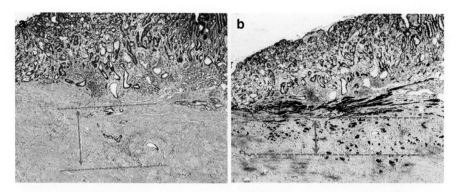

Fig. 12.12 In cases in which the muscularis mucosae is destroyed due to an ulcer or scar within the lesion (**a**), anti-desmin immunohistochemical staining (**b**) is helpful for drawing an imaginary continuous line between the residual muscularis mucosae in the adjacent mucosa to determine the vertical depth of invasion (red arrows between the two red dashed lines)

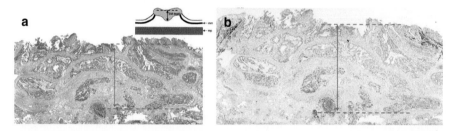

Fig. 12.13 When the muscularis mucosae is completely destroyed by carcinoma (**a**), the depth of submucosal invasion is measured from the surface of the lesion to the deepest point of invasion, as shown in the insert on the right upper corner. Anti-desmin immunohistochemical staining high-lights the residual muscularis mucosae (**b**). *mm* muscularis mucosae, *mp* muscularis propria, *arrows* depth of invasion

measure the depth of submucosal invasion. In fact, discrepancies in invasion depth measurement may be related to different measurement methods. For instance, Kim et al. [10] recently reported that differences in depth of tumor invasion depended upon whether the measurement was started from the bottom of the muscularis mucosae (which was termed as the classic method in their paper) or from an imaginary line at the muscularis mucosae (as the alternative method). In their study, the mean depth of invasion was greater in the nodal positive group than in the nodal negative group when the depth of invasion was evaluated by the alternative method ($P = 0.012$). However, there was no significant difference between the groups when the classic measurement method was used ($P = 0.128$). In addition, they categorized the muscularis mucosae in submucosal invasive EGC as normal with well-preserved muscularis mucosae (Fig. 12.14a), as hypertrophic with thickened or expanded muscularis mucosae secondary to the infiltration of tumor cells (Fig. 12.14b), or as

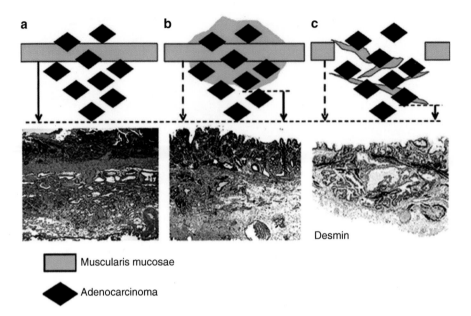

Muscularis mucosae

Adenocarcinoma

Fig. 12.14 Three morphological patterns of the muscularis mucosae in early gastric carcinoma with submucosal invasion: (**a**) normal, (**b**) hypertrophic, and (**c**) discontinuous. Measuring from the bottom of muscularis mucosae in patients with normal muscularis mucosa (**a**) or from an imaginary line of the muscularis mucosae in patients with irregular, hypertrophic muscularis mucosae (**b**) or with discontinuous muscularis mucosae (dashed arrows) (**c**), the measurement methods highlighted with dashed arrows in **b** and **c**, not the method with solid arrows, are recommended

discontinuous with irregular muscularis mucosae due to disruption of its continuity by infiltrating tumor cells (Fig. 12.14c) or even disappeared in the cancerous invasive area (Fig. 12.13). Receiver operating characteristic (ROC) curve analysis demonstrated a difference between the methods of measurement as well. The area under the ROC curve using the alternative method was greater than the classic method (0.652 vs. 0.620) among all morphologic patterns of muscularis mucosae. The differences were magnified when evaluating discontinuous and hypertrophic type (0.672 vs. 0.601), compared to normal muscularis mucosa (0.543 vs. 0.581), separately. Finally, they recommended measuring the submucosal depth of invasion from an imaginary line of the muscularis mucosae in patients with irregular muscularis mucosae (discontinuous, hypertrophic) and from the bottom of muscularis mucosae in patients with normal muscularis mucosae.

Ulceration in the stomach is defined as a loss of mucosal tissue to the muscularis mucosae and, sometimes, deep to the submucosa and even muscularis propria. Oftentimes, it is necessary to determine whether or not tumor ulceration or an ulcerated scar is present within the lesion for accurate evaluation on whether or not an ESD resection has been curative. In this setting, the diagnosis of intralesional ulceration becomes critically important. Ulcer should not be confused and misdiagnosed with erosion that does not involve the muscularis mucosae.

It must be pointed out that discrepancies in tumor size and other risk factors related to lymph node metastasis are considerable between pre- and post-ESD procedures for EGC. A recent multicenter Korean study of 737 EGC cases reported an overall discrepancy rate of 20.1% (148/737) [10], most frequently related to the tumor size (8.7%, 64/736), depth of deep submucosal invasion (SM2, 6.9%, 51/737), and ulceration (4.6%, 34/737). The most problematic issue was related to ulceration, in which depth of tumor invasion was significantly deeper in the cases with ulceration than those without. Because depth of invasion was significantly correlated with tumor size, ulceration, differentiation, lymphovascular invasion, and endoscopic tumor gross types, it is critically important for the responsible pathologist to carefully measure and accurately determine the depth of tumor invasion in ESD-resected EGC specimens [10]. Because of 20–30% shrinkage of gastric mucosal tissue after formalin fixation, the most accurate determination of tumor size is best carried out by the ESD endoscopist in the endoscopy unit immediately after the specimen is appropriately pinned down on a plate. The endoscopic differentiation between "ulceration" and "erosion" is oftentimes difficult, and the histologic diagnosis of ulceration or erosion remains the gold standard.

Assessment of lymphovascular invasion should be carried out using immunohistochemical staining with anti-vascular endothelial antibodies, such as CD31 to identify vessels (v), and anti-lymphatic endothelial antibody (D2–40) for lymphatic channels (ly) (Fig. 12.15). Elastic fiber staining (Elastica van Gieson) is useful for illustration of the elastic fiber in a vessel and identifying intravascular cancerous emboli (Fig. 12.16).

Other pathologic changes should also be recorded, such as precancerous lesions (e.g., intraepithelial neoplasia), *H. pylori* infection, chronic atrophic gastritis, intestinal metaplasia, pancreatic metaplasia, etc. Gastritis cystica profunda involving submucosa should be reported, distinguished with invasive well-differentiated adenocarcinoma, and also thoroughly inspected for the presence or absence of epithelial dysplasia [11]. Any pathologic lesions in the distal esophagus such as columnar-lined esophagus, intestinal metaplasia, dysplasia, and carcinoma unrelated to early gastric cardiac carcinoma must be reported. In our practice, Barrett's esophagus and distal esophageal Barrett's adenocarcinoma should be clearly scrutinized in the ESD

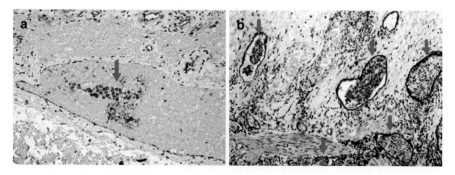

Fig. 12.15 Intravascular tumor emboli (red arrows) identified on the routine hematoxylin and eosin stain can be highlighted by anti-CD31 (**a**) or D2–40 (**b**) immunostains

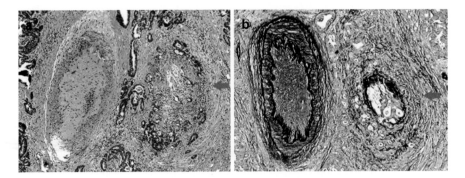

Fig. 12.16 Intravenous cancerous embolus (red arrow) suspected on a routine hematoxylin and eosin stained section (**a**) can be diagnosed by the Elastica van Gieson stain (**b**)

specimen for the extent of the disease along with the endoscopic/clinical findings. In general, columnar-lined esophagus with intestinal metaplasia within 1 cm above the EGJ line should not be interpreted as Barrett's esophagus, if given non-specific clinical presentation and unremarkable endoscopic findings. For adenocarcinoma in the distal esophagus, a careful investigation into the origin of this tumor should be meticulously conducted, including identification of the tumor epicenter, the distance and relationship to the EGJ line, associated components of uncommon histology subtypes, and intestinal metaplasia, dysplasia in the adjacent esophageal columnar-lined esophagus. By definition, Barrett's adenocarcinoma derives from Barrett's intestinal metaplasia and shows primarily tubular and papillary adenocarcinoma phenotypes but most unlikely presents as adenosquamous carcinoma, signet ring cell carcinoma, mucinous carcinoma, neuroendocrine carcinoma, and carcinoma with lymphoid stroma, among other uncommon types of malignancy, which belongs to gastric cardiac carcinoma [12, 13].

Summary

Optimal pathologic evaluation of the ESD specimen for early gastric cardiac carcinoma is crucial for determination of whether or not additional surgery with lymph node dissection is indicated and how the patient will be triaged and managed. A comprehensive accurate pathology report on the ESD specimen provides valuable information for clinical decision-making and determines (1) the histopathological type, (2) tumor size, (3) whether ulceration is present, (4) depth of invasion, (5) lymphovascular and perineural invasion, (6) horizontal and vertical margin involvement, (7) associated other gastric diseases, and (8) distal esophageal lesions. It requires close communication and collaboration between the endoscopist and the pathologist with the standardized pathologic tissue processing protocol to ensure the best management of patients with early gastric cardiac carcinoma.

References

1. Choi KS, Jung HY, Choi KD, et al. EMR versus gastrectomy for intramucosal gastric cancer: comparison of long-term outcomes. Gastrointest Endosc. 2011;73(5):942–8.
2. Ono H, Yao K, Fujishiro M, et al. Guidelines for endoscopic submucosal dissection and endoscopic mucosal resection for early gastric cancer. Dig Endosc. 2016;28(1):3–15.
3. Park YM, Cho E, Kang HY, et al. The effectiveness and safety of endoscopic submucosal dissection compared with endoscopic mucosal resection for early gastric cancer: a systematic review and meta-analysis. Surg Endosc. 2011;25(8):2666–77.
4. Chinese Society of Digestive Endoscopy. Chinese consensus on the screening, endoscopic diagnosis and treatment of early gastric cancer. Chin J Dig Endosc. 2014;31(7):361–77.
5. Japanese Gastric Cancer Association. Japanese classification of gastric carcinoma: 3rd English edition. Gastric Cancer. 2011;14(2):101–12.
6. Lauwers GY, Carneiro F, Graham DY, et al. Gastric carcinoma. In: Bosman FT, Carneiro F, Hruban RH, Theise ND, editors. WHO classification of tumours of the digestive system. Lyon: IARC Press; 2010. p. 48–58.
7. Inoue H, Kashida H, Kudo S, et al. The Paris endoscopic classification of superficial neoplastic lesions: esophagus, stomach, and colon: November 30 to December 1, 2002. Gastrointest Endosc. 2003;58(6 Suppl):S3–S43.
8. Huang Q, Fang C, Shi J, et al. Differences in clinicopathology of early gastric carcinoma between proximal and distal location in 438 Chinese patients. Sci Rep. 2015;5:134–9.
9. Huang Q, Shi J, Sun Q, et al. Clinicopathologic characterization of small (≤ 2 cm) proximal and distal gastric carcinomas in a Chinese population. Pathology. 2015;47(6):526–32.
10. Kim JM, Sohn JH, Cho MY, et al. Pre- and post-ESD discrepancies in clinicopathologic criteria in early gastric cancer: the NECA-Korea ESD for Early Gastric Cancer Prospective Study (N-Keep). Gastric Cancer. 2016;19(4):1104–13.
11. Xu G, Peng C, Huang Q, et al. Endoscopic resection of gastritis cystica profunda: preliminary experience with 34 patients from a single center in China. Gastrointest Endosc. 2015;81(6):1493–8.
12. Huang Q, Fan XS, Agoston AT, et al. Comparison of gastroesophageal junction carcinomas in Chinese versus American patients. Histopathology. 2011;59(2):188–97.
13. Huang Q, Sun Q, Fan XS, et al. Recent advances in proximal gastric carcinoma. J Dig Dis. 2016;17(7):421–32.

Chapter 13
Surgical Therapy

Jun Qian, Yu Gong, Qin Huang, A. Travis Manasco, Liming Tang, and Jason S. Gold

Introduction

Gastric cardiac cancer (GCC) possesses unique pathobiology, epidemiology, histopathology, and molecular biology as well as having characteristic features for malignant degeneration, invasion, and metastasis. Advanced GCC is able to metastasize to lymph nodes in the lower para-esophagus, mediastinum, abdominal cavity, diaphragm, paragastric mesenteries, and adjacent abdominal tissues and organs.

J. Qian (✉)
Department of General Surgery, Center of Gastrointestinal Surgery, Changzhou No 2 People's Hospital, Affiliated Hospital of Nanjing Medical University,
Changzhou, Jiangsu, People's Republic of China

Y. Gong
Department of Gastrointestinal Surgery, Affiliated Changzhou No 2 Peoples Hospital Nanjing Medical University, Changzhou, Jiangsu, People's Republic of China

Q. Huang
Pathology and Laboratory Medicine, Veterans Affairs Boston Healthcare System,
West Roxbury, MA, USA

Harvard Medical School and Brigham and Women's Hospital,
Boston, MA, USA

A. T. Manasco
Department of Anesthesiology, Washington University in St. Louis School of Medicine,
Barnes Jewish Hospital, St. Louis, MO, USA

L. Tang
Department of Gastroenterology, Changzhou Second Hospital, Nanjing Medical University,
Changzhou, People's Republic of China

J. S. Gold
Department of Surgery, Harvard Medical School/Brigham and Women's Hospital,
Boston, MA, USA

Veterans Affairs Boston Healthcare System, West Roxbury, MA, USA
e-mail: jgold@bwh.harvard.edu

© Springer International Publishing AG, part of Springer Nature 2018   243
Q. Huang (ed.), *Gastric Cardiac Cancer*, https://doi.org/10.1007/978-3-319-79114-2_13

Local recurrence and distant organ metastasis frequently lead to fatal outcomes after resection. The correct surgical procedure may improve post-resection prognosis and survival of the patients.

Methods for radical surgical resection of advanced GCC have been controversial. As research progresses, a standardized surgical approach for advanced GCC has been gradually accepted. At present, The US National Comprehensive Cancer Network (NCCN) [1] and The International Gastric Cancer Association (IGCA) [2] recommend endoscopic resection for certain early GCC tumors. In contrast, for advanced GCC, radical surgical resection is advocated. Because of the higher morbidity without increased benefit associated with thoracic operations for advanced GCC, abdominal surgery with D2 nodal dissection has been gradually accepted as the mainstay for radical resection of advanced GCC [3, 4].

Endoscopic Resection of Early Gastric Cardiac Carcinoma

Endoscopic resection is utilized only in cases of early gastric carcinoma without lymph node metastasis. Endoscopic resection has fewer complications with a faster post-procedure recovery. This technique has been widely used in East Asian countries such as Japan, Korea, and China. Considerable success has been made in this approach, although experience remains limited.

Indication for Endoscopic Resection

In 2015, the Japan Gastroenterological Endoscopy Society (JGES) in collaboration with the Japanese Gastric Cancer Association (JGCA) published practice guidelines on endoscopic resection of early gastric carcinoma [5] which include the absolute and extended criteria:

1. Absolute indications include clinical intramucosal carcinoma (cT1a) with a size smaller than 2 cm, intestinal (differentiated) histology, and a non-ulcerative gross endoscopic appearance.
2. Extended criteria for endoscopic resection are (1) intramucosal carcinoma (cT1a) with a size greater than 2 cm, a non-ulcerative gross appearance, and intestinal (differentiated) histology; (2) intramucosal carcinoma (cT1a) with a size smaller than 3 cm, but with ulcer and intestinal (differentiated) histology; and (3) intramucosal carcinoma (cT1a) with a size smaller than 2 cm, ulcerative gross appearance, and diffuse (undifferentiated) histology, without lymphovascular invasion [5].

In general, if the tumor does not fit the absolute and extended criteria, open surgical resection is indicated because of the increased risk of nodal metastasis. It must be pointed out that GCC is uncommon in Japan, where Siewert II and III carcinomas account for about 2.5% of cases in gastrectomy with nodal dissection [2]. Apparently, the Japanese guidelines are based on the research results primarily for early distal non-cardiac carcinoma. In contrast, GCC is common in China and accounts for over 25% of all gastrectomies for early gastric carcinoma [6]. Thus, the most appropriate practice guidelines among different patient populations for endoscopic resection of early GCC remain to be established.

For cases of early GCC not fitting the criteria for endoscopic resection, open surgical or laparoscopic resection is used for the following situations:

1. Endoscopic resection specimens show the involvement of carcinoma at the vertical (deep) margin.
2. Intramucosal carcinoma in size of >3 cm discovered in an endoscopic resection specimen with intestinal (differentiated) histology and ulcer.
3. Early carcinoma in size of <3 cm but invading into the superficial submucosal layer (SM1 <0.5 mm in depth), if the tumor is resected in a piecemeal fashion or en bloc but with the involvement of carcinoma at the resection margins.
4. Submucosal lymphovascular invasion.
5. Poorly cohesive carcinoma, including signet-ring cell carcinoma, invading the muscularis mucosae and submucosa.
6. Patient preference.

The current practice guidelines on endoscopic therapy are summarized in Fig. 13.1.

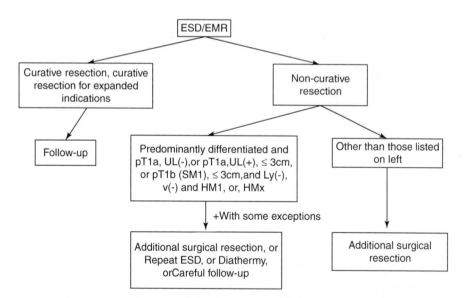

Fig. 13.1 The flowchart on the decision of endoscopic resection with either endoscopic submucosal dissection (ESD) or endoscopic mucosal resection (EMR), modified from Reference [5]. Note: *UL* ulcer, *SM1* superficial submucosal invasion up to 0.5 mm, *Ly* lymphatic invasion, *v* vascular invasion, *HM* horizontal margin

Laparoscopic Resection

Laparoscopic resection for early gastric carcinoma has been successfully carried out primarily for distal non-cardiac carcinoma with considerable success [7]. Advantages of laparoscopic resection for distal non-cardiac carcinoma include minimal injury to the patient, rapid recovery, and comparable curative efficacy. The efficacy and safety for laparoscopic resection of GCC remain to be scrutinized because of complicated anatomy, diverse nodal metastasis channels, and difficult reconstruction after resection. At present, it is prudent to use the laparoscopic technique to resect GCC for the following primary indications: (1) early GCC that failed endoscopic resection; (2) advanced GCC in patients with high risk for open surgical resection; and (3) select GCC cases that can be resected by skilled surgeons of high-volume medical centers. In GCC cases with tumor invading into the distal esophagus, laparoscopic surgery may not be an ideal option for resection.

Once laparoscopic surgery is chosen for GCC resection, total gastrectomy is the technique of choice [7]. During the resection procedure, the surgeon must strictly follow gastric cancer resection practice guidelines, meticulously dissecting lymph nodes at various nodal stations. For early GCC, the omentum may be spared in order to minimize surgical injury and reduce resection difficulty.

Most recently, Chinese surgeons compared the conventional open total gastrectomy with laparoscopic-assisted total gastrectomy for advanced GCC (i.e., Siewert II and III tumors) [8]. They reported that laparoscopic-assisted total gastrectomy significantly reduced operative time, blood loss, length of hospital stay, and increased the number of lymph nodes retrieved, compared to the open total gastrectomy. More importantly, both the 3-year survival and disease-free survival rates were significantly better in the laparoscopic-assisted (81.3% and 77.5%) than open (66.4% and 63.8%) total gastrectomy groups in patients with Siewert II tumors ($p < 0.05$) [8]. Apparently, advanced technology such as laparoscopic- and robot-assisted total gastrectomy will greatly improve post-resection outcomes in patients with advanced GCC.

Robot-Assisted Resection

The robotic surgical system has opened up a new era of minimally invasive surgery. For example, the da Vinci Surgical System has been widely used in urological, hepatobiliary, cardiovascular, and gynecological surgeries. In 2002, Hashizume [9] reported the first robot-assisted gastrectomy (RAG), followed by similar reports from China, Korea, Japan, and Italy, among others. A 2002 surgical study from China compared clinicopathological characteristics and short-term surgical outcomes between RAG and laparoscopic gastrectomy (LAG) for gastric cancer. Their results showed that RAG was associated with a longer operative time ($P < 0.001$), lower blood loss ($P = 0.001$), and a larger number of harvested lymph nodes

($P = 0.047$). Clinical parameters such as negative proximal and distal resection margins, hospital stay, day of first flatus, and day of taking a liquid diet were similar between RAG and LAG groups [10]. A meta-analysis shows similar results [11]. In 2011, Alberto et al. assessed the feasibility and safety of laparoscopic robot-assisted radical surgery for GCC using the four-arm da Vinci Surgical System. Seventeen laparoscopic robot-assisted operations were completed without conversion (14 extended gastrectomies, 2 transhiatal distal esophagectomies, and 1 transthoracic distal esophagectomy). The mean operative time was 327.2 (±93.4) min and blood loss was 279 (±199) mL. The mean number of nodes retrieved was 28 (±9). All resection margins were negative. There was no mortality and overall morbidity was acceptably low (41.1%). During a mean follow-up time of 20 months, four recurrences were recorded (two to multi-abdominal organs, one to the lung, and one to lymph nodes) with two associated deaths [12]. The results of these studies suggest that robot-assisted laparoscopic radical surgical resection of GCC is safe. Further randomized studies are needed to evaluate long-term prognosis with this technique.

Radical Surgical Resection

The current guidelines for radical surgical resection of advanced gastric carcinoma primarily follow Japanese gastric cancer treatment guidelines on the basis of tumor staging. Briefly, for stage IA (T1a) tumors, endoscopic resection is recommended; for tumors staged at IA (T1b), II, and III (including T1b–T4b), radical resection is the primary therapy; for tumors staged at IV, surgical resection is not recommended, and the patients are treated primarily by chemotherapy, radiation therapy, or both, along with symptomatic management. For young patients (<40 years old) with advanced stage IV tumors, radical resection with D2 nodal dissection has been found to be able to significantly improve post-resection survival, compared to those with palliative therapy [13].

Surgical Approach

The optimal surgical approach and methods for advanced GCC have been debated between thoracic and abdominal surgeons. At present, the abdominal approach via the esophageal opening is preferred, based on the data from two major randomized controlled clinical trials conducted in Netherlands in 2002 [14] and Japan in 2006 [15]. In the randomized Dutch prospective study, the investigators compared the pros and cons between right thoracic approach (RTA) and transhiatal esophagectomy (TE) for radical resection of Siewert types I and II carcinomas. They reported the significantly superior outcomes for the abdominal TE approach, compared to the RTA approach, for radical resection (Table 13.1). In 2007, the same team published

Table 13.1 The randomized prospective Dutch study on surgical approach

Parameter	Right thoracic approach	Transhiatal esophagectomy	P value
Post-resection complications (%)	57	27	<0.001
Intensive care unit stay (day)	6	2	<0.001
Total hospital stay (day)	19	15	<0.001

their follow-up study results with similar conclusions. For Siewert I adenocarcinoma, which is distal esophageal adenocarcinoma, the RTA group showed a higher overall 5-year survival rate (51% vs. 37% in the TA group) and a higher 5-year survival in patients with positive lymph nodes but tumor-free (64% vs. 23%); however, the differences were not statistically significant. The results clearly suggest that the right thoracic approach is able to easily dissect lymph nodes in the upper and lower mediastinum and should be recommended for patients with Siewert I adenocarcinoma [16]. In contrast, for advanced GCC, i.e., Siewert type II and some type III carcinomas, the TA approach is more appealing than the RTA approach because of better D2 nodal dissection after total gastrectomy with the anastomosis reconstruction procedure [3]. It should be noted that the Dutch trial included only 18% Siewert II tumors and thus was really an esophageal adenocarcinoma trial. Furthermore, the surgical procedure was esophagectomy (not gastrectomy) in both arms. Lastly, it should be noted that perhaps minimally invasive techniques allow for the thoracic lymphadenectomy without the morbidity of thoracotomy. For the Japanese trial, this included Siewert II and III tumors only. The procedure was total gastrectomy in both arms. Whether to perform esophagectomy versus total gastrectomy for Siewert II tumors is unanswered by these trials.

A most recent surgical study from the QingDao University in China compared post-resection outcomes and prognosis between transthoracic ($N = 140$) and transesophageal ($N = 194$) approaches for radical surgical resection with D2 nodal dissection of Siewert types II and III carcinomas [17]. Compared to the transthoracic approach, the transhiatal approach demonstrated significantly better post-resection short-term outcomes, such as shorter operative time, shorter length of resected esophagus, higher number of lymph nodes retrieved, shorter duration of antibiotic use, lower post-resection pain score, shorter hospital stay, and lower overall cost. No significant difference in 5-year overall survival was found between the patients with tumors staged at pI and pII; however, the patients with tumors staged at pIII demonstrated significantly better 5-year survival after transhiatal (37.2%) resection, compared to those with transthoracic (25.7%) resection ($p < 0.05$) [17]. The findings parallel to those reported previously also in Chinese patients [18, 19].

To compare the survival benefit between the left thoracic approach (LTA) and transhiatal approach (TH), Japanese investigators organized an open-labeled, randomized clinical trial in 1995 with a total of 167 patients enrolled. They reported a higher post-resection complication frequency (49%) with a lower survival (37%) in the LTA group, compared to the TH (34% and 51%, respectively) group. The trial was terminated prematurely. Ten years later, the same group of investigators reported a follow-up study with similar results, in which the 10-year overall survival rate was 24% in the LTA group, lower than that (37%) in the TH group; but the difference did not reach a statistically significant level [20]. The authors concluded that for Siewert II and III tumors (GCC) with esophageal invasion shorter than 3 cm in distance above the esophagogastric junction, the TH approach is preferred with a thorough nodal dissection in the para-esophageal region [20].

A meta-analysis compared the efficacy and safety of radical surgical resection of advanced GCC (Siewert types II and III) between transthoracic ($N = 639$) and transhiatal ($N = 516$) approaches in a total of eight qualified studies [21]. The pooled study data showed that although no significant differences were found between the two groups in the operative time, blood loss, anastomotic leak, cardiovascular complications, and the number of lymph nodes retrieved, the transhiatal approach group, compared to the transthoracic group, showed significantly shorter hospital stay ($P < 0.00001$), lower 30-day hospital mortality ($P = 0.03$), and decreased pulmonary complications ($P < 0.00001$). The investigators strongly recommend the transhiatal approach for advanced GCC [21].

In summary, surgical therapy for advanced GCC (Siewert II and III) is challenging and associated with a high frequency of post-resection complications. The choice of an optimal surgical method is dictated by the extent of tumor invasion, especially esophageal invasion. For tumor invasion into the distal esophagus more than 3 cm above the esophagogastric junction, nodal metastasis in the lower mediastinum needs to be thoroughly dissected, and the thoracic approach is recommended for achieving an R0 resection with distal esophagectomy of 6–7 cm in length, and anastomosis in the neck, which is the standard of practice; otherwise, the transhiatal approach is most preferable with D2 nodal dissection primarily in the abdomen.

Nodal Dissection

Because of the unique anatomic position of GCC, nodal metastasis occurs primarily in the abdomen and occasionally to the lower thorax (Fig. 13.2) [22]. Kakeji et al. in 2012 surveyed nodal metastasis in 129 GCC resection cases and reported the following frequency: 1% in the neck and 2% in the upper and lower mediastinum, in which the frequencies of nodal metastasis in nodal stations 110, 111, and 112 were 2%, 1%, and 1%, respectively [23]. In the abdomen, the frequency of nodal metastasis was over 20% for nodal stations 1, 2, and 3 and over 7% for stations 8, 9, 10, and 11. They further reported that in GCC cases with an esophageal invasion length of over 1 cm, the frequency of nodal metastasis was increased to 33%, 8%, 8%, 20%, and 20% for nodal stations 108, 104, 107, 110, and 112, respectively. This group of tumors is primarily related to Siewert I distal esophageal adenocarcinoma, in which the thoracic approach is able to thoroughly dissect lymph nodes in the mediastinum, as required by the Japan Esophageal Society. In a recent questionnaire-based national retrospective study in Japan, investigators studied nodal

Fig. 13.2 Thoracic and
abdominal lymph node
station numbers, created by
the Japan Esophageal
Society, reproduced with
permission [22]

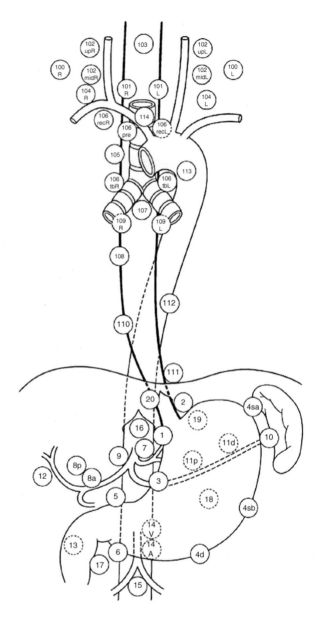

metastasis in 2807 advanced GCC (cancer in the esophagogastric junction) tumors
with the size smaller than 4 cm between 2001 and 2010 in patients without neoadjuvant therapy. They reported the predominant pattern of nodal metastasis in T3/T4
advanced GCC [$N = 523$] primarily in the abdominal lymph nodes (Table 13.2).

As illustrated in Table 13.2, the vast majority of nodal metastasis occurs in
abdominal nodal stations 1, 2, 3, and 7, regardless of the esophageal or gastric predominance of advanced GCC. In contrast, nodal metastasis to other nodal stations

Table 13.2 Frequency (%) of lymph node metastasis among the most common nodal stations in advanced T3/T4 gastric cardiac carcinoma (Siewert II and III) of 523 Japanese patients

Nodal station	110	1	2	3	7	8	9	11p
Esophageal-predominant tumor	12	42	23	34	25	4	9	5
Gastric-predominant tumor	2	42	22	36	17	5	5	7

Note: The data were based on the results in reference [24]

is minimal, ranging from 0 to 2%; the investigators emphasized that the right and left cardia and lesser curvature along the left gastric artery were the most vulnerable regions for nodal metastasis in advanced GCC. Because of the limited number of nodal dissection procedures carried out in the mid and/or upper mediastinum, no conclusive recommendation can be made for nodal dissection in those regions [24]. Celiac nodal metastasis in the distal paragastric region has been reported to be associated with worse prognosis in patients with advanced GCC [19]. The value of nodal dissection in that region remains to be further investigated, since the data recommending D2 nodal dissection are limited and controversial. The two randomized controlled trials showing the lack of benefit for D2 dissection (in Western patients) need to be noted.

As to nodal dissection at nodal stations 10 and 11 along with splenectomy, there are no definitive recommendations. A 2009 Japanese study suggested that nodal metastasis was correlated with the tumor invasion depth. Nodal metastasis frequency in station 10 was 8.8% for pT3 tumors, but increased to 12.8% for serosal invasion, and 40% for invasion into the adjacent organs. For nodal station 11, the nodal metastasis rate was 13.5% for pT2 tumors, 8.6% for subserosal invasion, 8.1% for serosal invasion, and 20% for invasion into the adjacent organs [25]. In a smaller Japanese study of 42 patients with total gastrectomy and D2 lymph node dissection for advanced GCC (Siewert type II) tumors, investigators reported a low incidence of 4.8% for splenic hilar lymph node metastasis with no increased benefit and thus recommended omitting splenic hilar lymph node dissection in advanced GCC patients [26].

Splenectomy

At present, splenectomy with nodal dissection in stations 10 and 11d in advanced GCC remains controversial. The Japanese practice guideline on gastric cancer resection requires nodal dissection in station 10 for upper and mid-gastric cancers, including GCC [7]. That guideline recommends performing splenectomy in addition to radical resection of advanced GCC involving the greater curvature. One Dutch study with 210 cases of Siewert I and II carcinoma resections reported that splenectomy was associated with significantly increased blood transfusions, prolonged operative time, post-resection stay in the intensive care unit, and decreased short-term survival [27].

In general, the indications for radical GCC resection with splenectomy are as follows: (1) tumor invasion into the spleen and splenic vessel, (2) enlarged and fused station 10 lymph nodes on imaging studies, and (3) operative injury to the spleen and splenic vessels leading to uncontrollable massive bleeding [28]. The laparoscopic approach may minimize these risks [29].

Para-aortic Lymph Node Dissection (PAND)

Radical surgical resection with D2 lymphadenectomy for primary nonmetastatic gastric carcinoma has become standard practice because of better survival benefit [30]. The addition of para-aortic nodal dissection (PAND) in nodal stations 8p, 12p, 13, 16a2, and 16b1 to D2 lymphadenectomy has been tested in a Japanese randomized controlled trial in 523 patients with advanced resectable gastric carcinoma [31]. Because of no significant differences in recurrence-free survival between the D2 alone and the D2 plus PAND groups, Japanese surgeons give up the additional PAND dissection. However, that study suffers from several limitations, including the exclusion of Borrmann IV tumors, case selection bias, discrepancy in nodal metastasis rates in station 16 between pre- and post-resection examinations, inadequate nodal dissection with few positive lymph nodes, as well as the inappropriate statistical stage-specific analysis for patient post-resection survival [31]. Based on a retrospective study from China [32], the nodal metastasis rate in station 16 is as high as 47.1% in patients with Borrmann IV tumors, 29.4% in cases with pT4 tumors, and 45.2% in cases with pN2–3 tumors, in sharp contrast to 16.1% in cases with pT1–3 tumors, and 6.2% in cases with pN0–1 tumors. They also reported that in cases with pN3 nodal metastasis, D2 plus PAND lymphadenectomy significantly increased the 5-year survival rate from 17.4 to 28.2% ($p < 0.05$) [33].

In a recent Italian study evaluating the pattern of carcinoma recurrence in 568 advanced gastric carcinoma patients, the investigators compared the impact between D2 and D3 (PAND) lymphadenectomies on locoregional recurrence and reported a significantly lower risk of recurrence for diffuse/mixed histologic types of advanced gastric carcinoma ($p < 0.01$) [34]. Because the diffuse-type advanced gastric carcinoma has a high propensity to metastasize to abdominal organs, posterior and para-aortic lymph nodes, the investigators concluded that D3 (including PAND) lymphadenectomy could be considered as a valid surgical option to reduce locoregional recurrence of the diffuse-type gastric carcinoma [34].

At the 11th World Conference on Gastric Cancer, Dr. Sasako specifically discussed the surgical issues related to PAND indications [35, 36]. Based on the data from JCOG0001 and JC0G0404 clinical trials in Japan, he proposed the following indications for PAND: (1) the enlarged and fused lymph nodes in the para-aortic and para-celiac artery regions after neoadjuvant therapy, (2) nodal metastasis confined to lymph nodes in stations 16a2 and 16b1 or pN2 tumors with fused nodes without

Table 13.3 Approaches of radical resection and lymphadenectomy for advanced gastric cardiac carcinoma

Siewert type	Surgical approach		Lymphadenectomy	
II	Length of esophageal invasion		Length of esophageal invasion	
	<3 cm	>3 cm	<3 cm	>3 cm
	Transhiatal total or upper partial gastrectomy with distal esophagectomy	Left thoracotomy with upper gastrectomy	Lower mediastinum and abdominal D2, D3	Mid-lower mediastinum plus abdominal D2
III	Total gastrectomy with conservation of pancreas but with splenectomy plus distal esophagectomy		D2 plus PAND and sampling nodes in the renal hilar region	

metastasis to para-aortic nodes, and (3) advanced GCC. However, despite many single-center-based studies, PAND lymphadenectomy in advanced GCC remains to be further investigated for efficacy, safety, and overall survival benefits.

At present, the consensus of radical surgical resection approaches for advanced, nonmetastatic, resectable GCC is listed in Table 13.3.

Extent of Distal Esophagectomy

The length of distal esophagectomy is an important issue for surgical therapy of GCC. A resected distal esophageal segment longer than 3.8 cm in length is an independent risk factor for prognosis [37]. Therefore, it is essential to secure a safe distance between the proximal resection margin of the distal esophagus and the esophagogastric junction. Barbour et al. studied the relationship between the length of the resected distal esophagus and the positive proximal margin of resection in 505 esophagectomy cases. They reported the average safe length to secure a negative proximal resection margin is 3.5 cm (range 0.2–16 cm), in contrast to the average length of 0.7 cm (range 0–8 cm) in cases with a positive proximal margin with involvement of carcinoma [37]. They also reported that the safe length to secure a free proximal resection margin in the distal esophagus is 3.5 cm, 4 cm, and 2.5 cm for Siewert types I, II, and III adenocarcinomas, respectively [37]. It is prudent for the surgeon to thoroughly understand the extent of esophageal involvement and possible nodal metastasis before making a decision on the resected length of the distal esophagus. The distance between the proximal resection margin and the tumor should be at least 5 cm in longitudinal length and the proximal margin may be examined intraoperatively by frozen section for evaluation of possible carcinoma involvement of the proximal esophageal margin. It may be warranted to know the fact that the relationship between positive margin and survival is tricky. Sometimes a positive margin is a surrogate for a more aggressive tumor with worse outcomes, and thus more radical resections with frozen section may not necessarily provide improved benefit [38–41].

Extent of Gastrectomy

To make an optimal decision on the extent of gastrectomy in advanced GCC, the surgeon needs to know the exact relationship between the tumor and the esophago-gastric junction as well as the depth of tumor infiltration. In general, Siewert III tumors are resected with the methods for gastric cancer resection. However, for Siewert II tumors, the recommendation for partial proximal or total gastrectomy is unclear. This is related to the difficulty understanding nodal metastasis in the greater curvature, para-pylorus, as well as para-aortic/para-celiac artery regions. Japanese scholars recommend using the distance between the tumor distal edge and esopha-gogastric junction to guide the decision-making process: (1) if the distance is shorter than 3 cm, the tumor location at the greater curvature, and the possibility of para-pyloric nodal metastasis smaller than 2.2%, partial proximal gastrectomy is pre-ferred; (2) in contrast, if the distance between the tumor distal edge and the esophagogastric junction is over 5 cm and the possibility of para-pyloric nodal metastasis over 20%, total gastrectomy is recommended. However, a meta-analysis with two randomized trials and nine retrospective studies showed similar 5-year survival between proximal and total gastrectomies for GCC, but proximal gastrec-tomy was associated with higher rates of local recurrence and anastomotic stenosis than total gastrectomy, in addition to worse reflux disease [42], which explains why many surgeons have abandoned partial proximal gastrectomy for GCC.

Reconstruction of Upper Digestive Tract

After successful radical resection of nonmetastatic advanced GCC, reconstruction of the upper digestive tract becomes crucial. Because of complexity of the anatomy, the goal for the optimal surgical reconstruction procedure is to ensure the best func-tionality with the highest safety margin and the lowest iatrogenic reflux disease incidence.

Reconstruction After Total Gastrectomy

There are three major reconstruction anastomosis methods after total gastrectomy. Roux-en-Y anastomosis is the most frequently used reconstructive technique. The procedure is started with transection of the jejunum at 15–20 cm distal to the liga-ment of Treitz. Then, the distal jejunum is anastomosed in the end-side fashion with the distal esophagus. Subsequently, the second end-side anastomosis is carried out at 40–60 cm distal to the previous esophagojejunal anastomosis site. As illustrated in Fig. 13.3, the efferent limb of this procedure serves as the primary recipient of food after the surgery, while the afferent limb functions as the recipient for biliary

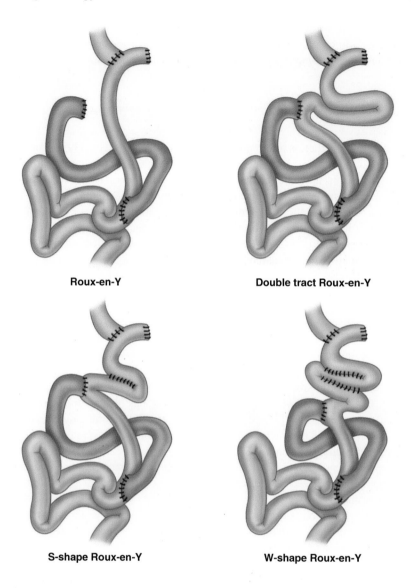

Roux-en-Y

Double tract Roux-en-Y

S-shape Roux-en-Y

W-shape Roux-en-Y

Fig. 13.3 Schematic drawing of four types of Roux-en-Y anastomosis between the distal esophagus and jejunum after total gastrectomy. The stomach has been removed. The transverse colon is not shown here for a better illustration of the reconstruction

secretions to aid digestion to ensure appropriate preservation of digestive function after reconstruction. The major limitations of Roux-en-Y anastomosis are preservation of the gastric reservoir and digestive dysfunction after total gastrectomy, leading to dietary restriction, malnutrition, early satiety, postprandial fullness, vomiting, heartburn, and diarrhea [43].

Other two reconstruction methods include jejunal pouch interposition and double-tract jejunal interposition, which are much less frequently used in this setting because of the complexity of surgery and high complications.

Reconstruction After Partial Proximal Gastrectomy

The key for reconstruction after partial proximal gastrectomy is to choose an appropriate method to minimize iatrogenic gastroesophageal reflux. After proximal gastrectomy, the vagus nerve has been resected along with tumor, the lower esophageal smooth muscle sphincter, and the His angle between the fundus and the distal esophagus. Therefore, the most important complication after resection is gastric dysfunction and dysmotility in the residual distal stomach, leading to symptomatic gastroesophageal reflux disease. Because of the unique anatomic location, the operative reconstruction is considerably difficult. At present, the most common reconstruction methods are the esophagogastric anastomosis and jejunal interposition. Each method has its own advantages and disadvantages. A surgeon may make a decision based on personal experience and postoperative functional outcomes. Classical esophagogastric anastomosis is safe, easy-to-do, and widely used worldwide (Fig. 13.4). However, because of the surgical removal of the lower esophageal smooth muscle sphincter, part of the diaphragm, diaphragm-esophageal ligament, and the angle of His, post-resection-related iatrogenic gastroesophageal reflux is inevitable, due to the loss of normal structure in the gastroesophageal junction. In addition, reconstruction with a smaller anastomosis has also been reported to be able to cause severe reflux [44–46]. Furthermore, the failure of the pylorus to relax due to transection of the vagus nerve is another problem associated with partial proximal gastrectomy. Therefore, at present, there is no convincing evidence for either method in preservation of function or prevention of stump gastric carcinoma. As such, no universally accepted recommendation for the optimal size of the residual distal stomach exists.

Jejunal interposition is used to connect the esophagus and jejunum to maintain jejunal continuity and duodenal food passage after gastrectomy. As shown in Fig. 13.5, this anastomosis is effective in minimizing the risk of major post-gastrectomy complications such as dumping syndrome, bile reflux, and malabsorption. However, patients frequently complain of upper abdomen discomfort.

In a recent retrospective study in functional outcomes between the conventional Roux-en-Y ($N = 79$) and the jejunal interposition ($N = 71$) anastomosis procedures in China [47], the investigators compared the nutritional status and incidence of complications at 3 and 12 months after a reconstruction procedure. They reported significant increases in serum levels of hemoglobin and total proteins, less body weight reduction, and fewer incidences of complications, such as reflux esophagitis, dumping syndrome, in the jejunal interposition group, compared to the conventional Roux-en-Y group [47].

Fig. 13.4 Schematic
drawing of esophagogastric
anastomosis

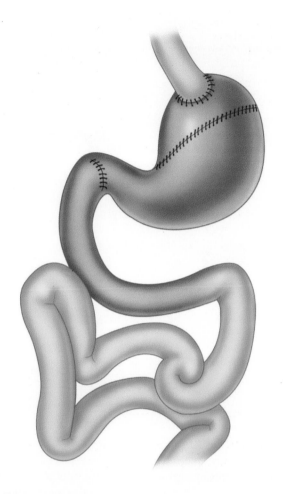

Laparoscopic-Assisted Reconstruction

With the advances in new technology, laparoscopic-assisted reconstruction after
gastrectomy has rapidly become a safe, economic, and effective alternative method
to open surgical reconstruction [48–50]. This procedure is especially attractive
because of the minimal post-reconstruction-related bile reflux disease, according to
a recent observational study carried out in Japan [50]. Hosoda et al. used a novel
laparoscopic "open-door" technique to carry out reconstruction after proximal gastrectomy in 20 patients. In this novel technique, the surgeon pulled up the remnant
stomach to the esophageal hiatus and fixed the superior end of the mucosal "window" to the esophagus at 4 cm above the resection site. Then, the mucosal "window" was opened, and continuous suturing was performed between the posterior
wall of the esophagus and the superior opening of the remnant gastric mucosa.

Fig. 13.5 Schematic
drawing of jejunal
interposition anastomosis

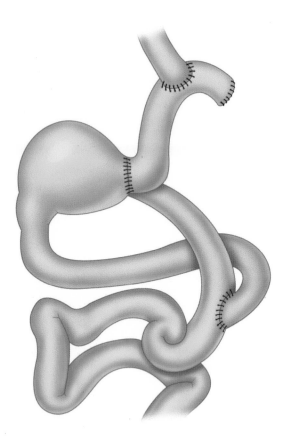

Subsequently, interrupted sutures were placed between the anterior esophagus and inferior remnant gastric mucosa. Then, continuous suturing was carried out between muscular layers of the esophagus and stomach. The inferior ends on both sides of the seromuscular flaps were fixed at position 1 cm below the mucosal "window" to complete the reconstruction procedure with both side ends of anastomosis sutured upward. Thus, the anastomosis site was completely covered by the flaps. Although the procedure needs a longer operation time (up to 330 min because of difficulty), post-reconstruction outcomes are encouraging with no anastomotic leaks and minimal reflux esophagitis (<1.1%) [50]. Because of the small sample size, the results remain to be validated in larger samples.

Risk Factors for Worse Prognosis After Radical Resection

Due to a high frequency of nodal metastasis, GCC has a high propensity to recur after radical resection. On average, carcinoma recurrence occurs within 24 months. Over 45% of patients relapse within 2 years. Metastasis occurs by hematogenous spread in 43% of cases and peritoneal spreading in 41% [51]. The median survival time in patients with early (within 2 years after resection) recurrence (16.6 months) was significantly shorter than that in patients with late (over 2 years) recurrence (55.2 months) ($p < 0.001$). Interestingly, patients with proximal gastrectomy, poorly differentiated histology, advanced pT stage, and lymph node metastasis were prone to early recurrence, while those with total gastrectomy were more likely to suffer late recurrence [51]. The overall prognosis of patients with advanced GCC after radical resection for curative intent was poor with a 5-year survival rate varied between 27.5 and 52% [19, 51]. A retrospective study of 142 Chinese patients with advanced GCC identified several independent risk factors for worse prognosis, including age over 70 years, over 16 lymph nodes with metastasis, distant metastasis, and advanced pathologic stage [19]. According to a retrospective study of 99 patients with recurrent GCC after radical resection, the patients with locoregional nodal metastasis demonstrated significantly longer progression-free survival than those with hematogenous spread and peritoneal diseases. The liver is the organ most commonly involved by hematogenous metastasis [51, 52]. As expected, patients with distant nodal recurrence had significantly worse overall survival (13.5 months) than those with locoregional (48.5 months), hematogenous (29.9 months), and peritoneal (31.4 months) diseases ($p < 0.01$) [51]. The data from several studies seem to show a lower recurrence frequency in patients treated with total gastrectomy and D2 or even D3 lymphadenectomy [51, 52].

Multidisciplinary Team Approach

Advanced GCC is much more complicated in pathology, staging, surgical approach, lymphadenectomy, recurrence, and prognosis than distal gastric or esophageal carcinoma. Thus, it requires a multidisciplinary approach for patient management and surgical therapy with specialists from surgical oncology, medical oncology, radiation oncology, radiology, pathology, and gastroenterology. At the preoperative stage, a multidisciplinary team needs to determine an accurate carcinoma diagnosis, the extent of the disease including esophageal involvement, lymph node status, functional status, choice of an appropriate surgical approach, and the decision on use of neoadjuvant chemoradiation therapy. After resection, a complete pathological examination of the resected specimen is vital for determination of future patient management options. The goal of the multidisciplinary team is to help patients reserve quality of life and improve post-resection outcomes and prognosis.

Summary

The incidence of GCC is rising, especially in East Asian countries [53]. This carcinoma, corresponding to Siewert types II and some III carcinomas, is poorly understood. At present, there exist no universally accepted optimal radical resection guidelines among different patient populations. An accumulating body of evidence suggests, however, the transhiatal abdominal approach is preferred for advanced, nonmetastatic resectable GCC with esophageal invasion in length of shorter than 3 cm above the esophagogastric junction. In that situation, splenectomy with lymphadenectomy to station 10 may not be necessary. Although traditional open surgical resection remains the mainstay, advanced endoscopic resection, such as endoscopic submucosal dissection, and laparoscopic-assisted procedure have become promising options as a safe, economic, minimally invasive alternative. As more surgeons are learning new techniques and operative experience grows, there will be more high-quality data acquired from multicenter, prospective, randomized, controlled clinical trials to help establish an internationally recognized surgical practice guideline on this potential fatal cancer.

References

1. Ajani JA, D'Amico TA, Almhanna K, et al. Esophageal and esophagogastric junction cancers, version 1.2015. J Natl Compr Cancer Netw. 2015;13(2):194–227.
2. Sano T, Coit DG, KIim HH, et al. Proposal of a new stage grouping of gastric cancer for TNM classification: International Gastric Cancer Association staging project. Gastric Cancer. 2017;20(2):217–25. https://doi.org/10.1007/s10120-016-0601-9.
3. Orditura M, Galizia G, Fabozzi A, et al. Preoperative treatment of locally advanced esophageal carcinoma (Review). Int J Oncol. 2013;43(6):1745–53. https://doi.org/10.3892/ijo.2013.2118.
4. Huang L, Xu AM. Adenocarcinoma of esophagogastric junction: controversial classification, surgical management, and clinicopathology. Chin J Cancer Res. 2014;26(3):226–30.
5. Ono H, Yao K, Fujishiro M, et al. Guidelines for endoscopic submucosal dissection and endoscopic mucosal resection for early gastric cancer. Dig Endosc. 2016;28(1):3–15.
6. Huang Q, Fang C, Shi J, et al. Differences in clinicopathology of early gastric carcinoma between proximal and distal location in 438 Chinese patients. Sci Rep. 2015;5:13439. https://doi.org/10.1038/srep13439.
7. Japanese gastric cancer treatment guidelines 2014 (ver. 4). Gastric Cancer. 2017;20(1):1–19.
8. Huang CM, Lv CB, Lin JX, et al. Laparoscopic-assisted versus open total gastrectomy for Siewert type II and III esophagogastric junction carcinoma: a propensity score-matched case-control study. Surg Endosc. 2017;31(9):3495–503. https://doi.org/10.1007/s00464-016-5375-y.
9. Hashizume M, Shimada M, Tomikawa M, et al. Early experiences of endoscopic procedures in general surgery assisted by a computer-enhanced surgical system. Surg Endosc. 2002;16(8):1187–91.
10. Shen W, Xi H, Wei B, et al. Robotic versus laparoscopic gastrectomy for gastric cancer: comparison of short-term surgical outcomes. Surg Endosc. 2016;30(2):574–80.
11. Shen WS, Xi HQ, Chen L, et al. A meta-analysis of robotic versus laparoscopic gastrectomy for gastric cancer. Surg Endosc. 2014;28(10):2795–802.
12. Patriti A, Ceccaralli G, Ceribelli C, et al. Robot-assisted laparoscopic management of cardia carcinoma according to Siewert recommendations. Int J Med Robot. 2011;7(2):170–7.
13. Zhou F, Shi J, Fang C, et al. Gastric carcinomas in young (younger than 40 years) Chinese patients: clinicopathology, family history, and postresection survival. Medicine (Baltimore). 2016;95(9):e2873.
14. Hulscher JB, van Sandwick JW, de Boer AG, et al. Extended transthoracic resection compared with limited transhiatal resection for adenocarcinoma of the esophagus. N Engl J Med. 2002;347(21):1662–9.

15. Sasako M, Sano T, Yamamoto S, et al. Left thoracoabdominal approach versus abdominal-transhiatal approach for gastric cancer of the cardia or subcardia: a randomised controlled trial. Lancet Oncol. 2006;7(8):644–51.

16. Omloo JM, Lagarde SM, Hulscher JB, et al. Extended transthoracic resection compared with limited transhiatal resection for adenocarcinoma of the mid/distal esophagus: five-year survival of a randomized clinical trial. Ann Surg. 2007;246(6):992–1000; discussion 1000–1001.

17. Zhou J, Wang H, Niu Z, et al. Comparisons of clinical outcomes and prognoses in patients with gastroesophageal junction adenocarcinoma, by transthoracic and transabdominal hiatal approaches: a teaching hospital retrospective cohort study. Medicine (Baltimore). 2015;94(50):e2277.

18. Huang Q, Fan X, Agoston AT, et al. Comparison of gastro-oesophageal junction carcinomas in Chinese versus American patients. Histopathology. 2011;59(2):188–97.

19. Zhang YF, Shi J, Yu HP, et al. Factors predicting survival in patients with proximal gastric carcinoma involving the esophagus. World J Gastroenterol. 2012;18(27):3602–9.

20. Kurakowa Y, Sasako M, Sano T, et al. Ten-year follow-up results of a randomized clinical trial comparing left thoracoabdominal and abdominal transhiatal approaches to total gastrectomy for adenocarcinoma of the oesophagogastric junction or gastric cardia. Br J Surg. 2015;102(4):341–8.

21. Wei MT, Zhang YC, Deng XB, et al. Transthoracic vs transhiatal surgery for cancer of the esophagogastric junction: a meta-analysis. World J Gastroenterol. 2014;20(29):10183–92.

22. Okholm C, Svendsen LB, Achiam MP. Status and prognosis of lymph node metastasis in patients with cardia cancer—a systematic review. Surg Oncol. 2014;23(3):140–6.

23. Kakeji Y, Yamamoto M, Ito S, et al. Lymph node metastasis from cancer of the esophagogastric junction, and determination of the appropriate nodal dissection. Surg Today. 2012;42(4):351–8.

24. Yamashita H, Seto Y, Sano T, et al. Results of a nation-wide retrospective study of lymphadenectomy for esophagogastric junction carcinoma. Gastric Cancer. 2017;20(Suppl 1):69–83. https://doi.org/10.1007/s10120-016-0663-8.

25. 速藤和也, 褚地吉弘, 前原喜彦. 胃癌:噴朋部胃癌治療. 消化器外科. 2009;32(5):738–44.

26. Goto H, Tokunaga M, Sugisawa N, et al. Value of splenectomy in patients with Siewert type II adenocarcinoma of the esophagogastric junction. Gastric Cancer. 2013;16(4):590–5.

27. Pultrum BB, van Bastelaar J, Schreurs LM, et al. Impact of splenectomy on surgical outcome in patients with cancer of the distal esophagus and gastro-esophageal junction. Dis Esophagus. 2008;21(4):334–9.

28. Sano T, Yamamoto S, Sasako M. Randomized controlled trial to evaluate splenectomy in total gastrectomy for proximal gastric carcinoma: Japan Clinical Oncology Group study JCOG 0110-MF. Jpn J Clin Oncol. 2002;32(9):363–4.

29. Huang CM, Chen QY, Lin JX, et al. Huang's three-step maneuver for laparoscopic spleen-preserving No. 10 lymph node dissection for advanced proximal gastric cancer. Chin J Cancer Res. 2014;26(2):208–10.

30. Mocellin S, McCulloch P, Kazi H, et al. Extent of lymph node dissection for adenocarcinoma of the stomach. Cochrane Database Syst Rev. 2015;(8):CD001964.

31. Sasako M, Sano T, Yamamoto S, et al. D2 lymphadenectomy alone or with para-aortic nodal dissection for gastric cancer. N Engl J Med. 2008;359(5):453–62.

32. Wang L, Liang H, Wang X, et al. Risk factors for metastasis to para-aortic lymph nodes in gastric cancer: a single institution study in China. J Surg Res. 2013;179(1):54–9.

33. Liang XY, Liang H, Ding XW, et al. N3 gastric cancer D2 combined with para-aortic lymph node dissection on the prognosis of patients with survival. Chin J Surg. 2013;51(12):1071–6.

34. de Manzoni G, Verlato G, Bencivenga M, et al. Impact of super-extended lymphadenectomy on relapse in advanced gastric cancer. Eur J Surg Oncol. 2015;41(4):534–40.

35. Yoshikawa T, Sasako M, Yamamoto S, et al. Phase II study of neoadjuvant chemotherapy and extended surgery for locally advanced gastric cancer. Br J Surg. 2009;96(9):1015–22.

36. Tsubaraya A, Mizusawa J, Tanakay Y, et al. Neoadjuvant chemotherapy with S-1 and cisplatin followed by D2 gastrectomy with para-aortic lymph node dissection for gastric cancer with extensive lymph node metastasis. Br J Surg. 2014;101(6):653–60.

37. Barbour AP, Rizk NP, Gonen M, et al. Adenocarcinoma of the gastroesophageal junction: influence of esophageal resection margin and operative approach on outcome. Ann Surg. 2007;246(1):1–8.
38. Bickenbach KA, Gonen M, Strong V, et al. Association of positive transection margins with gastric cancer survival and local recurrence. Ann Surg Oncol. 2013;20(8):2663–8.
39. Squires MH, Kooby DA, Pawlik TM, et al. Utility of the proximal margin frozen section for resection of gastric adenocarcinoma: a 7-Institution Study of the US Gastric Cancer Collaborative. Ann Surg Oncol. 2014;21(13):4202–10.
40. Postlewait LM, Squires MH, Kooby DA, et al. The importance of the proximal resection margin distance for proximal gastric adenocarcinoma: a multi-institutional study of the US Gastric Cancer Collaborative. J Surg Oncol. 2015;112(2):203–7.
41. Squires MH, Kooby DA, Poultsides GA, et al. Is it time to abandon the 5-cm margin rule during resection of distal gastric adenocarcinoma? A multi-institution study of the U.S. Gastric Cancer Collaborative. Ann Surg Oncol. 2015;22(4):1243–51.
42. Pu YW, Gong W, Wu YY, et al. Proximal gastrectomy versus total gastrectomy for proximal gastric carcinoma. A meta-analysis on postoperative complications, 5-year survival, and recurrence rate. Saudi Med J. 2013;34(12):1223–8.
43. Fein M, Fuchs KH, Thalheimer A, et al. Long-term benefits of Roux-en-Y pouch reconstruction after total gastrectomy: a randomized trial. Ann Surg. 2008;247(5):759–65.
44. Tsiouris A, Hammoud Z, Velanovich V. Barrett's esophagus after resection of the gastroesophageal junction: effects of concomitant fundoplication. World J Surg. 2011;35(8):1867–72.
45. Ishigami S, Uenosono Y, Arigami T, et al. Novel fundoplication for esophagogastrostomy after proximal gastrectomy. Hepato-Gastroenterology. 2013;60(127):1814–6.
46. Nakamura M, Nakamori M, Ojima T, et al. Reconstruction after proximal gastrectomy for early gastric cancer in the upper third of the stomach: an analysis of our 13-year experience. Surgery. 2014;156(1):57–63.
47. Ding X, Yan F, Liang H, et al. Functional jejunal interposition, a reconstruction procedure, promotes functional outcomes after total gastrectomy. BMC Surg. 2015;15:43.
48. Ahn SH, Lee JH, Park DJ, et al. Comparative study of clinical outcomes between laparoscopy-assisted proximal gastrectomy (LAPG) and laparoscopy-assisted total gastrectomy (LATG) for proximal gastric cancer. Gastric Cancer. 2013;16(3):282–9.
49. Chen K, Pan Y, Cai JQ, et al. Totally laparoscopic versus laparoscopic-assisted total gastrectomy for upper and middle gastric cancer: a single-unit experience of 253 cases with meta-analysis. World J Surg Oncol. 2016;14:96.
50. Hosoda K, Yamashita K, Moriya H, et al. Laparoscopically assisted proximal gastrectomy with esophagogastrostomy using a novel "Open-Door" technique: LAPG with novel reconstruction. J Gastrointest Surg. 2017;21(7):1174–80. https://doi.org/10.1007/s11605-016-3341-6.
51. Bilici A, Selcukbiricik F. Prognostic significance of the recurrence pattern and risk factors for recurrence in patients with proximal gastric cancer who underwent curative gastrectomy. Tumour Biol. 2015;36(8):6191–9.
52. Li F, Zhang R, Liang H, et al. The pattern and risk factors of recurrence of proximal gastric cancer after curative resection. J Surg Oncol. 2013;107(2):130–5.
53. Huang Q, Sun Q, Fan XS, et al. Recent advances in proximal gastric carcinoma. J Dig Dis. 2016;17(7):421–32.

Chapter 14
Chemical Therapy

Kequn Xu, Yang Yang, Qin Huang, Hua Jiang, and Valia Boosalis

Introduction

Survival of patients with gastroesophageal junctional or gastric cardiac carcinomas (GCC) is poor because their tumors are frequently locally advanced or with distant metastasis at diagnosis. Even after radical resection with curative intent, a high proportion of the patients with GCC develop recurrence. Unlike conventional distal esophageal adenocarcinoma or gastric noncardiac carcinoma, a standardized, one-size-fits-all protocol on adjuvant, or neoadjuvant chemotherapy or chemoradiotherapy, is not available at present for GCC. Therefore, we will review the published data on chemotherapy or chemoradiotherapy for locally advanced or metastatic GCC and provide the readers with the most recent research results on this poorly investigated carcinoma.

K. Xu (✉) · H. Jiang
Department of Oncology, the Affiliated Changzhou No.2 People's Hospital of Nanjing
Medical University, Changzhou, People's Republic of China

Y. Yang
Nanjing Drum Tower Hospital, Nanjing University, Nanjing, People's Republic of China

Q. Huang
Pathology and Laboratory Medicine, Veterans Affairs Boston Healthcare System,
West Roxbury, MA, USA

Harvard Medical School and Brigham and Women's Hospital,
Boston, MA, USA

V. Boosalis
Department of Hematology, VA Boston Healthcare System, Jamaica Plain, MA, USA

© Springer International Publishing AG, part of Springer Nature 2018   263
Q. Huang (ed.), *Gastric Cardiac Cancer*, https://doi.org/10.1007/978-3-319-79114-2_14

Adjuvant Chemotherapy

The most frequent site of recurrence after radical resections in patients with GCC is the liver, not regional lymph nodes [1, 2]. Therefore, it is important to prevent the development of distant micrometastasis by administering systemic chemotherapy (Table 14.1).

In Japan, the randomized clinical phase III trial on adjuvant chemotherapy with the S-1 oral fluoropyrimidine derivative in patients with stage II–III GCC found that the 5-year overall survival (OS) rate was 71.7% in the S-1 arm, compared with 61.1% in the surgery-alone arm (HR, 0.68; 95% CI, 0.52–0.87; $P = 0.003$) [3]. The same result was obtained in the final analysis after a 5-year follow-up period (HR, 0.669; 95% CI, 0.540–0.828) [4]. In South Korea, the CLASSIC study reported a higher 3-year disease-free survival (DFS) rate in patients with stage II or III gastric cancer who received adjuvant chemotherapy treatment with capecitabine plus oxaliplatin, compared to patients who underwent only D2 gastrectomy (3-year DFS rate, 74% vs. 59%; HR, 0.56; 95% CI, 0.44–0.72; $P < 0.0001$) [5]. Finally, a meta-analysis by the Global Advanced/Adjuvant Stomach Tumor Research International Collaboration (GASTRIC) group with the combined data from 3838 patients in 17 trials showed a benefit of 5-fluorouracil (FU)-based adjuvant chemotherapy vs. surgery alone on overall survival (OS) (55.3% vs. 49.6%; HR, 0.82; 95% CI, 0.76–0.90; $P < 0.001$) and DFS (HR, 0.82; 95% CI, 0.75–0.90; $P < 0.001$) with results at 10-year follow-ups (48% vs. 40%, respectively) [6]. For this reason, 5-FU-based adjuvant chemotherapy is now considered as a therapeutic option and has been included in the French National Thesaurus of Digestive Oncology for patients with resected GCC.

Table 14.1 Phase III trials of adjuvant chemotherapy or chemoradiotherapy for patients with gastric cardiac carcinoma and gastric noncardiac carcinoma

Trial	Year	N	Treatment	Survival	HR (95% CI)	P
INT-0116	2001	275	Surgery alone	41% (3-year OS)	1.35 (1.09–1.66)	0.005
[11]		281	Surgery + postoperative CRT (5-FU/leucovorin + 45 Gy)	50% (3-year OS)		
MAGGIC	2006	253	Surgery alone	23% (5-year OS)		0.009
[8]		250	3 cycles ECF preoperative + surgery + 3 cycles ECF postoperative	36% (5-year OS)	0.75 (0.60–0.93)	
ACTS-GC	2007	530	Surgery alone (D2)	61% (5-year OS)		0.003
[4]		529	Surgery (D2) + postoperative CT (S-1)	72% (5-year OS)	0.68 (0.52–0.87)	
CLASSIC	2012	515	Surgery alone (D2)	59% (3-year OS)		<0.0001
[5]		520	Surgery (D2) + postoperative CT (XELOX)	74% (3-year OS)	0.56 (0.44–0.72)	

Note: *HR* hazard ratio, *OS* overall survival, *CI* confidence interval, *CT* chemotherapy, *CRT* chemoradiotherapy, *ECF* epirubicin/cisplatin/5-FU, *XELOX* capecitabine/cisplatin, *DOS* docetaxel/oxaliplatin/S-1, *ECX* epirubicin/cisplatin/capecitabine, *CC* cisplatin/capecitabine, *SOX* S-1/oxaliplatin, *OS* overall survival, *DFS* disease-free survival

Neoadjuvant Chemotherapy

Postoperative adjuvant chemotherapy seems to be effective for patients with locally advanced GCC. However, systemic chemotherapy to the patients before surgery of resectable GCC is mainly based on the possibility of improved R0 resections and primary tumor de-bulking. Systemic neoadjuvant therapy may improve the R0 resection rate, reduce occult micrometastatic diseases, and assess the preoperative chemosensitivity. Possible disadvantages of neoadjuvant systemic therapies include the risk of disease progression until surgery, the increased morbidity and chemotherapy-related toxicity, and the difficulty in assessing the treatment responses. Deterioration in physical fitness and complications after gastroesophageal surgery sometimes make it impossible for patients to receive an adequate dose of postoperative adjuvant chemotherapy. Therefore, there is a trend toward preoperative, rather than postoperative, neoadjuvant therapy (Table 14.2).

In Japan, although the data were retrospectively collected from a single center, the study results showed that preoperative chemotherapy using the DCS regimen (docetaxel, cisplatin, and S-1) provided benefits for patients with GCC. The 5-year relapse-free survival (RFS) rate was 55%, and the median follow-up period was 36 months. Cox regression analysis regarding RFS identified two significant independent risk factors for poor prognosis: (1) performance of perioperative transfusion (HR, 4.71; 95% CI, 1.69–11.88) and (2) no preoperative chemotherapy (HR, 3.75; 95% CI, 1.22–14.26) [7]. In Europe, the MAGIC trial showed that perioperative chemotherapy using ECF (epirubicin, cisplatin, and 5-FU) in patients with localized gastric or lower esophageal adenocarcinoma was associated with significantly improved overall survival. The pathological analysis of the resected specimens showed significant tumor downsizing in the chemotherapy group, compared to the surgery-alone group (mean tumor size, 3 cm vs. 5 cm; $P < 0.001$). A significant improvement of T stage ($P = 0.009$) and N stage ($P = 0.01$) was also reported in the chemotherapy group. The 79% R0 resection rate was significantly higher in the chemotherapy group than in the surgery-alone group (70%; $P = 0.03$). Progression-free survival was significantly longer in the chemotherapy group than in the surgery-alone group (HR, 0.66; 95% CI, 0.53–0.81, $P = 0.0001$). The perioperative chemotherapy group had a higher likelihood of overall survival than did the surgery-alone group (HR, 0.75; 95% CI, 0.60–0.93; $P = 0.009$; the 5-year survival rate, 36% vs. 23%, respectively) [8]. However, the flaw of this trial is that the study population comprised of only 40% of patients who underwent D2 lymph node dissection, which is currently the standard operation in the East Asia. On the other hand, the FNCLCC/FFCD trial showed that in patients after perioperative chemotherapy using fluorouracil plus cisplatin, the R0 resection rate was 87% in the chemotherapy group, significantly higher than that (74%) in the surgery-alone group ($P = 0.004$). The 5-year disease-free survival rate was 34% (95% CI, 26–44%) vs. 19% (95% CI, 13–28%), and the 5-year OS rate was 38% (95% CI, 29–47%) vs. 24% (95% CI, 17–33%) (HR, 0.69; 95% CI, 50–95%, $P = 0.02$) [9]. These two trials (MAGIC and FNCLCC) are the first studies to demonstrate better survival rates with a perioperative systemic

Table 14.2 Phase III trials of adjuvant chemotherapy or chemoradiotherapy for patients with gastric cardiac carcinomas and esophageal cancer

Trial	Year	Histology		N	Treatment	Overall survival	HR (95% CI)	P
		Adenocarcinoma	SCC					
CALGB-9781 [17]	2008	42 (75%)	14 (25%)	26	Surgery	16% (5 year)	Not reported	0.002
				30	Preoperative CRT (CF+ 50.4 Gy)	39% (5 year)		
FNCLCC/FFCD [9]	2011	224 (100%)	0	111	Surgery	24% (5 year)		0.02
				113	Preoperative CT (CF)	38% (5 year)	0.69 (0.50–0.95)	
CROSS [19]	2012	275 (75%)	84 (23%)	366	Surgery	44% (3 year)		0.003
					Preoperative CRT (carboplatin/paclitaxel +41.4 Gy)	58% (3 year)	0.66 (0.50–0.87)	

Note: *CT* chemotherapy, *CRT* chemoradiotherapy, *CF* cisplatin/5-FU

approach for the treatment of localized GCC (Table 14.1). These results have been confirmed in the meta-analysis [10]. Thus, neoadjuvant chemotherapy is now considered as standard treatment for GCC in Europe and some centers in North America.

Adjuvant Chemoradiotherapy

In the United States, the INT-0116 trial showed that postoperative chemoradiotherapy using 5-FU plus leucovorin followed by concurrent 45 Gy radiotherapy in patients with localized GCC was associated with significantly improved overall survival. The administration of adjuvant chemoradiotherapy resulted in an improvement of the 5-year OS rate, compared with the surgery alone (40% vs. 26%; HR, 1.31; 95% CI, 1.09–1.39; $P = 0.005$) and of the median disease-free survival (27 months vs. 19 months; HR, 1.52; 95% CI, 1.25–1.53, $P < 0.0001$), with a median follow-up of more than 10 years. The risk of death was reduced by 31%, and relapses were decreased by 52% [11, 12]. However, of all included patients, only 10% had undergone D2 lymphadenectomy in this trial. Moreover, only 64% of patients completed all planned therapies. However, the ARTIST trial in South Korea demonstrated that the addition of radiation therapy to capecitabine plus cisplatin chemotherapy did not significantly prolong disease-free survival (DFS; $P = 0.0862$) [13]. Therefore, this treatment modality has not been accepted in East Asia where D2 lymphadenectomy is widely performed. In Western countries, the effect of postoperative radiotherapy performed in addition to perioperative chemotherapy in patients with localized GCC is currently being evaluated in the CRITICS prospective randomized study (NCT00407186). In South Korea, a phase III trial evaluating the benefit of the addition of radiotherapy to postoperative capecitabine plus cisplatin after curative D2 resection in patients with pathologically node-positive gastric adenocarcinoma or GCC (ARTIST II) is currently underway (NCT01761461).

Neoadjuvant Chemoradiotherapy

Considering the improvement brought by systemic neoadjuvant chemotherapy for the management of patients with GCC and lower esophageal adenocarcinoma, several randomized phase III studies assessed the benefit of neoadjuvant chemoradiotherapy, compared to surgery alone. The results of those clinical trials were self-contradictory. The trials by Urba et al. [14] and Burmeister et al. [15] did not show any benefit of chemoradiotherapy, compared with surgery alone, concerning the 3-year OS rate (30% vs. 16%; $P = 0.16$) and the median OS (21.7 months vs. 18.5 months; $P = 0.38$) in patients with GCC or lower esophageal adenocarcinoma. However, one phase III trial found that chemoradiotherapy before surgery improved survival. After a median follow-up of 10 months, the median OS (16 months vs. 11 months, $P = 0.01$) and the 3-year OS rates (32% vs. 6%, $P = 0.01$) were

Table 14.3 Neoadjuvant chemoradiotherapy results on resectable gastric cardiac carcinoma and lower esophagus adenocarcinomas

Trial	Patients (N)	Pathology	CRT	5-year overall survival (%)	P
Walsh 1996	CRT = 58	AC (100%)	CDDP/5-FU	CT-RT 32%	0.01
[16]	S = 55		40 Gy	S 6% (3 year OS)	
Urba 2001	CRT = 50	AC (75%)	CDDP/VLB/5-FU	CT-RT 30%	0.15
[14]	S = 50	SCC	45 Gy	S 16% (3 year OS)	
Burmeister 2005	CRT = 128	AC (62%)	CDDP/5-FU	CT-RT 22 months	0.38
[15]	S = 128	SCC	35 Gy	S 19 months	
Tepper 2008	CRT = 30	AC (75%)	CDDP/5-FU	CT-RT 39%	<0.0008
[17]	S = 26	SCC	50.4 Gy	S 16%	
CROSS 2010	CRT = 180	AC (75%)	Paclitaxel-carboplatin	CT-RT 47%	0.03
[19]	S = 188	SCC	41.4 Gy	S 34%	

Note: *CT-RT* chemoradiotherapy, *S* surgery, *AC* adenocarcinoma, *SCC* squamous cell carcinoma, *VLB* vinblastine

significantly higher in the combination treatment arm than in the surgery-alone arm; the pathologic complete response rate was 25% in the chemoradiotherapy plus surgery arm [16]. However, this monocentric study was closed prematurely after an interim analysis with an unusually low survival rate in the surgery-alone arm. Therefore, it is unclear how its results could be generalized (Table 14.3).

In the United States, the CALGB 9781 trial was conducted between 1997 and 2000 to compare preoperative chemoradiotherapy with cisplatin, 5-FU, and 50.4 Gy of radiation plus surgery (trimodality therapy) with surgery alone for patients with GCC or distal esophageal carcinoma. The median survival time was significantly longer in the trimodality therapy group than in the surgery-alone group (4.48 vs. 1.79 years, $P = 0.002$). The 5-year survival rate was 39% vs. 16%. The results were in favor of trimodality therapy [17]. An Australian randomized phase II study reported a significant reduction of the R1 resection rate in a similar patient population treated with neoadjuvant chemoradiotherapy vs. neoadjuvant chemotherapy alone (0% vs. 11%, $P = 0.04$); pathological complete response rates were 31% and 8%, respectively ($P = 0.01$) [18]. In Europe, the CROSS trial was conducted between 2004 and 2008 to evaluate the efficacy of preoperative chemoradiotherapy for patients with localized esophageal adenocarcinoma or GCC. An R0 resection margin was achieved in 92% of patients in the chemoradiotherapy-surgery group vs. 69% in the surgery group ($P < 0.001$). A pathological complete response was reported in 29% of patients who underwent radical resection after chemoradiotherapy. Median overall survival was 49.4 months in the chemoradiotherapy plus surgery group vs. 24.0 months in the surgery-alone group. Overall survival was significantly better in the chemoradiotherapy plus surgery group (HR, 0.657; 95% CI, 0.50–0.87; $P = 0.003$) [19]. Some meta-analyses have also shown that preoperative chemoradiotherapy contributes to better survival in patients with localized GCC

[20–22]. However, postoperative mortality was significantly higher in the preoperative chemoradiotherapy group than in the surgery-alone group [20, 22]. In the POET trial, which was conducted mainly in Germany, preoperative chemoradiotherapy comprising 5-FU, cisplatin, leucovorin, and radiation was compared with preoperative chemotherapy with 5-FU, cisplatin, and leucovorin-only for patients with Siewert types I, II, and III gastroesophageal junction adenocarcinomas. Patients in the preoperative chemoradiotherapy group had a significantly higher probability of a pathologic complete response than patients in the preoperative chemotherapy group (15.6% vs. 2.0%, respectively). Preoperative radiation therapy improved the 3-year survival rate from 27.7 to 47.4% (HR, 0.67; 95% CI, 0.41–1.07; $P = 0.07$). However, the postoperative mortality rate in the preoperative chemoradiotherapy group was much higher than that in the preoperative chemotherapy-only group (10.2% vs. 3.8%, respectively) [23]. Thus, the necessity of radiotherapy remains unclear. Some clinical studies are currently evaluating the effect of preoperative radiotherapy performed in addition to perioperative chemotherapy (TOPGEAR, NCT01924819) or the superiority of preoperative chemoradiotherapy over postoperative chemotherapy (NCT01962246).

Taken together, comparing perioperative chemotherapy vs. preoperative chemoradiation therapy for localized, advanced but resectable, GCC, the latter has the potential to be the mainstay.

Chemotherapy for Rare Cancers

Adenosquamous Carcinoma

Adenosquamous carcinoma (ASC) is rare malignancy with both adenocarcinoma (AC) and squamous cell carcinoma (SCC) components within the same tumor [24, 25]. Primary ASCs develop most commonly in the lung, pancreas, and cervix [26–28]. Due to its rarity in the gastric cardia, most of the literatures are primarily in the form of case reports. Surgical resection is the main treatment method, and the overall survival rate is no worse than that reported for SCC. The postoperative adjuvant treatment results in a decline of the 5-year survival rate, compared with surgery alone (22.2% vs. 62.9%; HR, 4.036; 95% CI, 1.167–13.957, $P = 0.028$) [29]. Therefore, adjuvant therapy appears to be inferior and may not be used in this carcinoma in the gastric cardia.

Primary High-Grade Neuroendocrine Carcinoma

Primary high-grade neuroendocrine carcinoma, i.e., small cell carcinoma, is rare in the esophagus, accounting for only 1–1.5% of all esophageal cancers [30, 31], as also scarce in the gastric cardia [32–34]. There is a wide range of opinions on treatment of high-grade neuroendocrine carcinoma in the gastric cardia, but most regimens clinically consist of chemotherapy, radiotherapy, surgery, and various combinations of these strategies. Despite the lack of a well-established standard guideline of care, many investigators have recommended that chemotherapy regimens for this rare carcinoma are those for small cell lung cancer because of clinicopathological similarities in tumors between these two different organs [35]. Chemoradiotherapy is effective in some cases with gastric cardiac high-grade neuroendocrine carcinoma [36, 37]. Some patients even achieved a complete response [37]. A case of combination therapy with neoadjuvant chemotherapy, surgery, and adjuvant chemotherapy has been reported to be successful with this combination strategy, particularly neoadjuvant chemotherapy, which provides the patient with an opportunity to receive radical surgery resection with curative intent [38]. Because of the rarity, there have been universally accepted protocols of small cell lung cancer for treatment of this carcinoma in the gastric cardia.

Carcinosarcoma

Carcinosarcoma of the esophagus and the stomach is very rare and characterized by the simultaneous presence of carcinomatous and sarcomatous elements in the same cancer [39]. In the gastric cardia, this cancer is exceedingly rare. As such, most of the literatures are primarily in the form of case reports. Surgical resection, if feasible, is the treatment of choice for carcinosarcoma [40]. Adjuvant therapy seems to have a role in the eradication of residual microscopic disease and local control. One case report of carcinosarcoma in the gastric cardia described successful treatment with radical resection alone [41]. At present, radiotherapy may be a potential treatment of this cancer in the gastric cardia.

Carcinoma with Lymphoid Stroma

Gastric carcinoma with lymphoid stroma (GCLS) is a distinct histologic subtype of gastric cancer and characterized by poorly differentiated adenocarcinoma mixed with prominent lymphoid infiltration [42]. More than 80% of GCLS cases are associated with Epstein-Barr virus (EBV) infection [43] and showed a better prognosis than EBV-negative conventional adenocarcinomas [44]. It is known that EBV-positive tumor cells may be more sensitive to chemotherapy that induces tumor cell apoptosis [45, 46]. However, the well-accepted clinical study results on chemotherapy for this carcinoma in the gastric cardia are not available at this time.

Lymphoma

Primary gastric lymphoma is a rare malignant tumor. Occurrence in the gastric cardia is particularly sparse. Histologically, 70–80% of cases are extranodal marginal zone lymphoma of mucosa-associated lymphoid tissue (MALT) lymphoma or diffuse large B-cell lymphoma (DLBCL) [47].

Gastric MALT Lymphoma

Gastric MALT lymphoma is almost always curable. A recent large prospective study from Japan revealed a 10-year overall survival of 95% and disease-free survival of 86%, respectively [48].

H. pylori Eradication

According to a recent meta-analysis, 77.5% of patients with stages I and II gastric MALT lymphomas achieved complete regression after eradication of H. pylori [49]. H. pylori eradication therapy is recommended as the first-line treatment in all H. pylori-positive and H. pylori-negative MALT lymphomas at all stages [50–52]. Successful eradication of H. pylori cures the majority of patients from gastric MALT lymphoma. The 10-year follow-up data of a large prospective trial showed that 80% of patients with stage II gastric MALT lymphoma achieved complete remission after H. pylori eradication and remained disease-free [53–55]. Patients, who do not respond to H. pylori eradication and are classified as no change or progression for post-eradication evaluation, should be treated by radiation or chemotherapy [56].

Radiotherapy

Radiation offers a curative option to patients with localized gastric lymphoma at stages I and II that do not respond to H. pylori eradication therapy [57, 58].

Chemotherapy and Immunotherapy

In some European countries, chemotherapy is considered an alternative to radiation therapy in MALT lymphoma at stages I and II. In other countries, chemotherapy is restricted to the tumors at disseminated stages III and IV [49]. At present, there is no generally accepted standard chemotherapy for gastric MALT lymphoma. In a recent prospective randomized trial, the combination of rituximab and bendamustine was shown to be more effective in terms of progression-free survival and less toxic than R-CHOP in patients with indolent lymphoma. Median progression-free survival was significantly longer in the bendamustine plus rituximab group than in the R-CHOP group (69.5 months vs. 31.2 months; HR, 0.58; 95% CI, 0.44–0.74; $p < 0.0001$) [59].

Surgery

At present, surgery no longer plays a role in the therapy of gastric MALT lymphoma, except for very rare complications such as perforation or bleeding that cannot be controlled endoscopically [60].

Treatment of *H. pylori*-Negative Gastric MALT Lymphoma

As mentioned above, very few patients with gastric MALT lymphoma with a negative *H. pylori* status (including serology) can also be initially treated by *H. pylori* eradication therapy with some chance of success [52–54]. In case of nonresponse, depending on the stage of the disease, radiotherapy and immunochemotherapy represent therapeutic options with a promising outcome comparable to that of patients with *H. pylori*-positive gastric MALT lymphoma [50, 61–64]. The current treatment strategy is summarized in Fig. 14.1.

Gastric Diffuse Large B-Cell Lymphoma (DLBCL)

There have been several preliminary studies describing effective treatment of DLBCL after *H. pylori* eradication therapy [65, 66]. In those reports, 27–60% of *H. pylori*-positive patients with stage I/II DLBCL achieved a curative response after *H.*

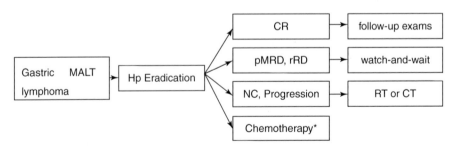

Fig. 14.1 The treatment strategy of gastric MALT lymphoma. *Hp H. pylori*, *CR* complete remission, *pMRD* probable minimal residual disease, *rRD* responding residual disease, *NC* no change, *RT* radiotherapy, *CT* chemotherapy, * EIII/IV/N3 M1 [71, 72]

pylori eradication. Therefore, *H. pylori* eradication should be tried in *H. pylori*-positive patients with DLBCL. Patients with DLBCL, who do not respond to *H. pylori* eradication, should immediately undergo immunochemotherapy with or without radiotherapy. Cases in stage I/II should be treated by three cycles of cyclophosphamide, doxorubicin, vincristine, and prednisone (CHOP) plus anti-CD20 antibody rituximab (R-CHOP) therapy, followed by radiotherapy. In DLBCL cases at advanced stages, six cycles of R-CHOP are regarded as standard treatment of high-grade gastric lymphoma [67].

Anti-HER2 and Anti-VEGFR-2 Therapies

More recently, molecular-targeted therapies have received increasing attention. HER2 is a member of the human epidermal growth factor receptor family and is amplified or overexpressed in 7–34% of patients with gastric noncardiac adenocarcinoma or GCC [68–70]. The proportion of patients with HER2 amplification or overexpression is reported higher in GCC than in gastric noncardiac adenocarcinoma [68, 71]. The HER2-positivity rate was 22.1% across analyzed tumor samples. The rates were similar between European and Asian patients (23.6% vs. 23.9%) but higher in the intestinal-type vs. the diffuse-type carcinomas (31.8% vs. 6.1%) and in GCC than in gastric noncardiac carcinomas (32.2% vs. 21.4%) [72]. In the NCT01041404 randomized, multicenter ToGA trial, in patients with the tumor overexpressing HER2, the addition of trastuzumab, a monoclonal antibody, to HER2, to the capecitabine plus cisplatin chemotherapy regimen, was associated with significantly better overall survival than chemotherapy alone (HR, 0.74; 95% CI, 0.60–0.91; P = 0.0046; median overall survival, 13.8 months vs. 11.1 months, respectively) [73]. In the NCT01364493 trial, in patients with HER2-positive tumors, addition of trastuzumab in combination with oxaliplatin/capecitabine in first-line treatment in advanced gastric cancer achieved a median progress-free survival (PFS) of 9.2 months (95% CI, 6.5–11.6) and a median OS of 19.5 months (95% CI, 15.5–26.0) [74]. Therefore, anti-HER2 therapy is a new, effective, and well-tolerated treatment for HER2-positive GCC [75]. On the other hand, the efficacy of adding trastuzumab to perioperative chemotherapy comprising 5-FU, leucovorin, docetaxel, and oxaliplatin in patients with locally advanced gastric noncardiac adenocarcinoma or GCC is being investigated in a phase II study (HerFLOT, NCT01472029).

The efficacy of many molecular-targeted agents for metastatic or unresectable, locally advanced gastric noncardiac adenocarcinoma or GCC has been investigated. Among them, one promising agent is anti-vascular endothelial growth factor receptor-2 (anti-VEGFR-2) antibody. VEGF- and VEGFR-2-mediated signaling and angiogenesis pathways seem to have an important role in the pathogenesis of gastric cancer. Ramucirumab is a fully humanized IgG1 monoclonal antibody VEGFR-2 antagonist that prevents ligand-binding and receptor-mediated pathway activation in endothelial cells. Ramucirumab showed single-agent activity and a favorable toxicity profile in a phase III study (REGARD) conducted in pretreated patients with metastatic or unresectable locally advanced gastric noncardiac adenocarcinoma or GCC. The ramucirumab group had a higher likelihood of overall survival than did the best supportive care group (median, 5.2 months vs. 3.8 months, respectively; HR, 0.776; 95% CI, 0.603–0.998; $P = 0.0473$) [76]. Another randomized phase III study (RAINBOW) compared the efficacy of ramucirumab in combination with paclitaxel vs. placebo plus paclitaxel in second-line treatment of metastatic or unresectable locally advanced gastric noncardiac adenocarcinoma or GCC. The ramucirumab plus paclitaxel group had a higher likelihood of overall survival than did the placebo plus paclitaxel group (median, 9.6 months vs. 7.4 months, respectively; HR, 0.807; 95% CI, 0.678–0.962; $P = 0.017$) [77]. Apatinib is a small-molecule tyrosine kinase inhibitor (TKI) that highly selectively binds to and strongly inhibits vascular endothelial growth factor receptor-2 (VEGFR-2), with a decrease in VEGF-mediated endothelial cell migration, proliferation, and tumor microvascular density [78]. Apatinib treatment significantly improved OS and PFS with an acceptable safety profile in patients with advanced gastric cancer refractory to two or more lines of prior chemotherapy. Median OS was significantly improved in the apatinib group, compared with the placebo group (6.5 months; 95% CI, 4.8–7.6 months vs. 4.7 months; 95% CI, 3.6–5.4; $P = 0.0149$; HR, 0.709; 95% CI, 0.537–0.937; $P = 0.0156$). Similarly, apatinib significantly prolonged median PFS, compared with placebo (2.6 months; 95% CI, 2.0–2.9 months vs. 1.8 months; 95% CI, 1.4–1.9; $P < 0.001$; HR, 0.444; 95% CI, 0.331–0.595; $P < 0.001$) [79]. Compared with the HER2 treatment pathway, the VEGF pathway may be an equally valid treatment target. Such molecular targeting may be applied to neoadjuvant and adjuvant therapies in patients with GCC in the near future.

Immune Checkpoint Inhibitors

T cells are the core performers of antitumor immunity. Their activation requires not only the stimulation of the first signal provided by antigen-presenting cells (APCs), but also the stimulation of the second signal provided by the co-stimulatory molecules. However, co-stimulatory molecules can also provide a repressive signal that inhibits immunization, as immune checkpoints. Immune checkpoints are a group of important elements of the immune system in long-term gradual evolution of the regulatory mechanism. Important members of immune checkpoints can be expressed in many human tumor tissues and tumor-infiltrating immune cells and involved in tumor immune escape. They can negatively regulate T-cell-mediated tumor responses. On the other hand, they can also regulate the biological behavior of tumor cells, participating in occurrence and development of tumors.

Antibody therapies that block the three important immune checkpoints, CTLA4 (cytotoxic T lymphocyte-associated antigen 4), PD1 (programmed death receptor 1), and PD-L1 (programmed death receptor ligand 1), have been approved by the US Food and Drug Administration to be used to treat several types of tumors, such as melanoma, non-small cell lung carcinoma, malignant mesothelioma, and urothelial carcinoma [80]. Gastric cancer ranks highly among solid tumors for having many DNA alterations, and approximately 18% of gastric microsatellite instability-high tumors show favorable responses to immune checkpoint inhibitors [81]. Numerous studies of immune checkpoint therapies for gastric cancer are ongoing. The KEYNOTE-059 study is a global, multi-cohort, phase II trial for the efficacy and safety of anti-PD1 monoclonal antibody, pembrolizumab (pembro), in patients with advanced gastric cancer. Study cohort 1 [82] enrolled 259 patients with measurable recurrent or metastatic gastric or gastroesophageal adenocarcinoma (GCC) who had progressed on ≥2 prior chemotherapy regimens. All patients received pembro 200 mg, three times per week (Q3W) for up to 2 years, or up to disease progression, or investigator's or patients' decision to withdrawal, and or unacceptable toxicity. Of 259 patients, 51.7% and 48.3% received pembro as third-line and fourth-line therapy, respectively. Over 57% of patients had PD-L1-positive tumors. At the data collection cutoff day (October 19, 2016), median duration of follow-up was 5.4 months (range, 0.5–18.7). Overall relapse-free (ORR) (CR + PR) survival was 11.2% (95% CI, 7.6–15.7%). Median duration of response (DOR) was 8.1 months (range, 1.4–15.1). ORR was 14.9% (95% CI, 9.4–22.1%) in third-line patients and 7.2% (95% CI, 3.3–13.2) in fourth-line patients. In patients with PD-L1-positive tumors, ORR was 15.5% (95% CI, 10.1%–22.4%); in patients with PD-L1-negative tumors, ORR was 5.5% (95% CI, 2.0–11.6%). In third-line patients with PD-L1-positive tumors, ORR was 21.3% (95% CI, 12.7%–32.3%). Pembro showed encouraging efficacy and manageable safety in patients with advanced gastric or gastroesophageal cancer (GCC) after ≥2 prior lines of therapy.

Study cohort 2 enrolled patients with HER2-negative recurrent or metastatic gastric or gastroesophageal adenocarcinoma (GCC), measurable disease, and no prior therapy [83]. All patients received pembro 200 mg on day 1 of each 21-day cycle plus cisplatin 80 mg/m^2 for six cycles, plus 5-FU 800 mg/m^2 (or capecitabine 1000 mg/m^2 in Japan) Q3W, for up to 2 years or until disease progression, or investigator's or patients' decision to withdrawal, and/or unacceptable toxicity. Of 25 enrolled patients, 64% had PD-L1-positive tumors. At the data collection cutoff date (October 19, 2016), ORR (CR + PR) was 60% (95% CI, 38.7–78.9%) in all patients. Overall, 32% of patients had stable disease (SD) (95% CI, 14.9–53.5%), 4% had progressive disease (PD) (95% CI, 0.1–20.4%), and 4% were not evaluable (95% CI, 0.1–20.4%). ORR was 68.8% (95% CI, 41.3–89.0%) in patients with PD-L1-positive tumors and 37.5% (95% CI, 8.5–75.5%) in patients with PD-L1-negative tumors. Median DOR was 4.6 months (range, 2.6 to 14.4+) in all patients, 4.6 months (3.2 to 14.4+) in patients with PD-L1-positive tumors, and 5.4 months (2.8 to 8.3+) in patients with PD-L1-negative tumors.

In the phase III ONO-12 study, third- or later-line nivolumab, another anti-PD1 monoclonal antibody, monotherapy prolonged OS vs. placebo in Asian patients with advanced gastric or gastroesophageal junctional (GCC) cancer (median OS, 5.3 vs. 4.1 months; HR, 0.63; $P < 0.0001$) [84]. The following phase I/II CheckMate 032 study showed favorable clinical activity of nivolumab with or without ipilimumab in Western patients with advanced chemotherapy-refractory gastric, esophageal, or

Table 14.4 Overall relapse-free (ORR) and DOR survival of phase III ONO-12 study of third- or later-line anti-PD1 nivolumab on gastric, gastroesophageal junctional carcinoma against placebo controls

Group	Nivolumab 3 mg/kg	Nivolumab 1 mg/kg plus ipilimumab 3 mg/kg	Nivolumab 3 mg/kg plus ipilimumab 1 mg/kg
PD-L1-positive tumors (ORR, %)	12	24	8
PD-L1+ tumors (ORR, %)	19	40	23
PD-L1-negative tumors (ORR, %)	12	22	0
All tumors (DOR, month)	7.1	7.9	0

gastroesophageal junction cancer (GCC) [85]. A total of 160 heavily pretreated patients (79% had ≥ 2 prior treatments) were enrolled for the study and divided into 3 groups: (1) nivolumab 3 mg/kg Q2W (the N3 group), (2) nivolumab 1 mg/kg plus ipilimumab 3 mg/kg Q3W (the N1+I3 group), and (3) nivolumab 3 mg/kg plus ipilimumab 1 mg/kg Q3W (the N3+I1 group). Among 24% patients with PD-L1-positive tumors, ORR was 12% in the N3 group, 24% in the N1+I3 group, and 8% in the N3+I1 group. In patients with PD-L1+, ORR was 19% (3/16) in the N3 group, 40% (4/10) in the N1+I3 group, and 23% (3/13) in the N3+I1 group. In patients with PD-L1-negative tumors, ORR was 12% (3/26) in the N3 group, 22% (7/32) in the N1:I3 group, and 0% (0/30) in the N3+I1 group, respectively. Median DOR was 7.1 months in the N3 group, 7.9 months in the N1+I3 group, and no response in the N3+I1 group. The study showed that nivolumab with or without ipilimumab led to durable responses and long-term OS in heavily pretreated patients with advanced gastric, esophageal, or gastroesophageal junction cancer (GCC) (Table 14.4). In short, immune checkpoint inhibitors have showed potential application value in gastric cancer treatment.

Summary

Currently, two main therapeutic options are used for the treatment of resectable GCC: (1) adjuvant chemoradiotherapy [12] and (2) perioperative chemotherapy with 5-FU and platinum salt-based regimens [9, 10]. Because the most frequent site of GCC recurrence is the liver [2], adjuvant chemotherapy is preferred to chemoradiotherapy in patients with locally advanced GCC. Additionally, because of the clinical deterioration associated with postoperative complications after radical resection, neoadjuvant chemotherapy is preferable to postoperative adjuvant chemotherapy and expected to become the mainstay of treatment for GCC. However, for patients with a good prognosis, a preoperative approach may be overtreated; on the other hand, for a postoperative approach in which patients may have a high risk of recurrence and poor nutritional status after surgery, their tumors may be under-treated. A randomized, multicenter study is urgently needed for establishment of optimal therapy guidelines for GCC.

More recently, targeted therapies have been investigated for gastric noncardiac adenocarcinoma and GCC. In the adjuvant setting, a phase II study evaluated the addition of trastuzumab to chemotherapy of gastric noncardiac adenocarcinoma, or GCC with HER2 overexpression is underway. The anti-VEGFR-2 antibody ramucirumab is another promising agent. Further insight into the pathobiology of GCC is expected to enable the progression of treatment for this devastating disease. Immune checkpoint inhibitors (PD-L1) have showed potential values in gastric cancer treatment. We recommend making the therapeutic management decision for each individual patient in a multidisciplinary team approach before the primary tumor surgery is started. Future applications of cytotoxic therapies, e.g., oxaliplatin, capecitabine, or docetaxel, or targeted therapies may help in improving outcomes of patients with GCC after curative resection.

References

1. Yamashita H, Katai H, Morita S, et al. Optimal extent of lymph node dissection for Siewert type II esophagogastric junction carcinoma. Ann Surg. 2011;254(2):274–80.
2. Wayman J, Bennett MK, Raimes SA, et al. The pattern of recurrence of adenocarcinoma of the oesophago-gastric junction. Br J Cancer. 2002;86(8):1223–9.
3. Sakuramoto S, Sasako M, Yamaguchi T, et al. Adjuvant chemotherapy for gastric cancer with S-1, an oral fluoropyrimidine. N Engl J Med. 2007;357(18):1810–20.
4. Sasako M, Sakuramoto S, Katai H, et al. Five-year outcomes of a randomized phase III trial comparing adjuvant chemotherapy with S-1 versus surgery alone in stage II or III gastric cancer. J Clin Oncol. 2011;29(33):4387–93.
5. Bang Y-J, Kim Y-W, Yang H-K, et al. Adjuvant capecitabine and oxaliplatin for gastric cancer after D2 gastrectomy (CLASSIC): a phase 3 open-label, randomised controlled trial. Lancet. 2012;379(9813):315–521.
6. Paoletti X, Oba K, Burzykowski T, et al. Benefit of adjuvant chemotherapy for resectable gastric cancer: a meta-analysis. JAMA. 2010;303(17):1729–37.
7. Hosoda K, Yamashita K, Katada N, et al. Benefit of neoadjuvant chemotherapy for Siewert type II esophagogastric junction adenocarcinoma. Anticancer Res. 2015;35(1):419–25.
8. Cunningham D, Allum WH, Stenning SP, et al. Perioperative chemotherapy versus surgery alone for resectable gastroesophageal cancer. N Engl J Med. 2006;355(1):11–20.
9. Ychou M, Boige V, Pignon JP, et al. Perioperative chemotherapy compared with surgery alone for resectable gastroesophageal adenocarcinoma: an FNCLCC and FFCD multicenter phase III trial. J Clin Oncol. 2011;29(143):1715–21.
10. Li W, Qin J, Sun YH, et al. Neoadjuvant chemotherapy for advanced gastric cancer: a meta-analysis. World J Gastroenterol. 2010;16(44):5621–8.
11. Macdonald JS, Smalley SR, Benedetti J, et al. Chemoradiotherapy after surgery compared with surgery alone for adenocarcinoma of the stomach or gastroesophageal junction. N Engl J Med. 2001;345(10):725–30.
12. Lee J, Limdo H, Kim S, et al. Phase III trial comparing capecitabine plus cisplatin versus capecitabine plus cisplatin with concurrent capecitabine radiotherapy in completely resected gastric cancer with D2 lymph node dissection: the ARTIST trial. J Clin Oncol. 2012;30(3):268–73.

13. Smalley SR, Benedetti JK, Haller DG, et al. Updated analysis of SWOG-directed intergroup study 0116: a phase III trial of adjuvant radiochemotherapy versus observation after curative gastric cancer resection. J Clin Oncol. 2012;30(19):2327–33.

14. Urba SG, Orringer MB, Turrisi A, et al. Randomized trial of preoperative chemoradiation versus surgery alone in patients with locoregional esophageal carcinoma. J Clin Oncol. 2001;19(2):305–13.

15. Burmeister BH, Smithers BM, Gebski V, et al. Surgery alone versus chemoradiotherapy followed by surgery for resectable cancer of the oesophagus: a randomised controlled phase III trial. Lancet Oncol. 2005;6(9):659–68.

16. Walsh TN, Noonan N, Hollywood D, et al. A comparison of multimodal therapy and surgery for esophageal adenocarcinoma. N Engl J Med. 1996;335(7):462–7.

17. Tepper J, Krasna MJ, Niedzwiecki D, et al. Phase III trial of trimodality therapy with cisplatin, fluorouracil, radiotherapy, and surgery compared with surgery alone for esophageal cancer: CALGB 9781. J Clin Oncol. 2008;26(7):1086–92.

18. Burmeister BH, Thomas JM, Burmeister EA, et al. Is concurrent radiation therapy required in patients receiving preoperative chemotherapy for adenocarcinoma of the oesophagus? A randomised phase II trial. Eur J Cancer. 2011;47(3):354–60.

19. van Hagen P, Hulshof MC, van Lanschot JJ, et al. Preoperative chemoradiotherapy for esophageal or junctional cancer. N Engl J Med. 2012;366(22):2074–84.

20. Fiorica F, Di Bona D, Schepis F, et al. Preoperative chemoradiotherapy for oesophageal cancer: a systematic review and meta-analysis. Gut. 2004;53(7):925–30.

21. Gebski V, Burmeister B, Smithers BM, et al. Survival benefits from neoadjuvant chemoradiotherapy or chemotherapy in oesophageal carcinoma: a meta-analysis. Lancet Oncol. 2007;8(3):226–34.

22. Sjoquist KM, Burmeister BH, Smithers BM, et al. Survival after neoadjuvant chemotherapy or chemoradiotherapy for resectable oesophageal carcinoma: an updated meta-analysis. Lancet Oncol. 2011;12:681–92.

23. Stahl M, Walz MK, Stuschke M, et al. Phase III comparison of preoperative chemotherapy compared with chemoradiotherapy in patients with locally advanced adenocarcinoma of the esophagogastric junction. J Clin Oncol. 2009;27(6):851–6.

24. Bombi JA, Riverola A, Bordas JM, et al. Adenosquamous carcinoma of the esophagus: a case report. Pathol Res Pract. 1991;187(4):519–21.

25. Yachida S, Nakanishi Y, Shimoda T, et al. Adenosquamous carcinoma of the esophagus. Clinicopathologic study of 18cases. Oncology. 2004;66(3):218–25.

26. Maeda H, Matsumura A, Kawabata T, et al. Japan National Hospital Organization Study Group for Lung Cancer. Adenosquamous carcinoma of the lung: surgical results as compared with squamous cell and adenocarcinoma cases. Eur J Cardiothorac Surg. 2012;41(2):357–61.

27. Boyd CA, Benarroch-Gampel J, Sheffield KM, et al. 415 Patients with adenosquamous carcinoma of the pancreas: a population-based analysis of prognosis and survival. J Surg Res. 2012;174(1):12–9.

28. Baek MH, Park JY, Kim D, et al. Comparison of adenocarcinoma and adenosquamous carcinoma in patients with early-stage cervical cancer after radical surgery. Gynecol Oncol. 2014;135(3):462–7.

29. Sun YH, Lin SW, Chen CH, Liang WY, Hsieh CC, et al. Adenosquamous carcinoma of the esophagus and esophagogastric junction: clinical manifestations and treatment outcomes. J Gastrointest Surg. 2015;19(7):1216–22.

30. Huang Q, Wu HY, Nie L, et al. Primary high-grade neuroendocrine carcinoma of the esophagus: a clinicopathologic and immunohistochemical study of 42 resection cases. Am J Surg Pathol. 2013;37(4):467–83.

31. Law SY, Fok M, Lam KY, et al. Small cell carcinoma of the esophagus. Cancer. 1994;73(12):89–94.

32. Huang Q, Zhang LH. The histopathologic spectrum of carcinomas involving the gastroesophageal junction in the Chinese. Int J Surg Pathol. 2007;15:38–52.

33. Huang Q, Fan XS, Agoston AT, et al. Comparison of gastroesophageal junction carcinomas in Chinese versus American patients. Histopathology. 2011;59(2):188–97.
34. Richards D, Davis D, Yan P, et al. Unusual case of small cell gastric carcinoma: case report and literature review. Dig Dis Sci. 2011;56(4):951–7.
35. Brenner B, Tang LH, Shia J, et al. Small cell carcinoma of the gastrointestinal tract: clinico-pathological features and treatment approach. Semin Oncol. 2007;34(1):43–50.
36. Liu H, Xie YB, Xu Q, et al. Clinical analysis of 17 cases of gastric small cell carcinoma. Zhonghua Zhong Liu Za Zhi. 2013;35(4):292–4.
37. Matsunaga M, Miwa K, Noguchi T, et al. Small cell carcinoma of gastro-oesophageal junction with remarkable response to chemo-radiotherapy. BMJ Case Rep. 2012;2012. https://doi.org/10.1136/bcr-2012-006361.
38. Xin K, Wei J, Wang H, et al. Neoadjuvant chemotherapy followed by D2 gastrectomy and esophagojejunal Roux-en-Y anastomosis in gastric small cell carcinoma: a case report. Oncol Lett. 2014;8(6):2549–52.
39. Ziauddin MF, Rodriguez HE, Quiros ED, et al. Carcinosarcoma of the esophagus: pattern of recurrence. Dig Surg. 2001;18(3):216–8.
40. Yamazaki K. A gastric carcinosarcoma with neuroendocrine cell differentiation and undif-ferentiated spindle-shaped sarcoma component possibly progressing from the conventional tubular adenocarcinoma; an immunohistochemical and ultrastructural study. Virchows Arch. 2003;442(1):77–81.
41. Solerio D, Ruffini E, Camandona M, et al. Carcinosarcoma of the esophagogastric junction. Tumori. 2008;94(3):416–8.
42. Watanabe H, Enjoji M, Imai T. Gastric carcinoma with lymphoid stroma. Its morphologic characteristics and prognostic correlations. Cancer. 1976;38(1):232–43.
43. Murphy G, Pfeiffer R, Camargo MC, et al. Meta-analysis shows that prevalence of Epstein-Barr virus-positive gastric cancer differs based on sex and anatomic location. Gastroenterology. 2009;137(3):824–33.
44. Lim H, Park YS, Lee JH, et al. Features of gastric carcinoma with lymphoid stroma associated with Epstein-Barr virus. Clin Gastroenterol Hepatol. 2015;13(10):1738–44.
45. Matsunou H, Konishi F, Hori H, et al. Characteristics of Epstein-Barr virus-associated gastric carcinoma with lymphoid stroma in Japan. Cancer. 1996;77(10):1998–2004.
46. Murray PG, Billingham LJ, Hassan HT, et al. Effect of Epstein-Barr virus infection on response to chemotherapy and survival in Hodgkin's disease. Blood. 1999;94(2):442–7.
47. Nakamura S, Matsumoto T, Iida M, et al. Primary gastrointestinal lymphoma in Japan: a clinicopathologic analysis of 455 patients with special reference to its time trends. Cancer. 2003;97(10):2462–73.
48. Nakamura S, Sugiyama T, Matsumoto T, et al. Long-term clinical outcome of gastric MALT lymphoma after eradication of Helicobacter pylori: a multicentre cohort follow-up study of 420 patients in Japan. Gut. 2012;61(4):507–13.
49. Zullo A, Hassan C, Cristofari F, et al. Effects of Helicobacter pylori eradication on early stage gastric mucosa-associated lymphoid tissue lymphoma. Clin Gastroenterol Hepatol. 2010;8(2):105–10.
50. Ruskoné-Fourmestraux A, Fischbach W, Aleman BMP, et al. EGILS consensus report. Gastric extranodal marginal zone B cell lymphoma of MALT. Gut. 2011;60(6):747–58.
51. Raderer M, Streubel B, Wöhrer S, et al. Successful antibiotic treatment of Helicobacter pylori negative gastric mucosa associated lymphoid tissue lymphomas. Gut. 2006;55(5):616–8.
52. Al-Taie O, Al-Taie E, Fischbach W. Patients with Helicobacter pylori negative gastric mar-ginal zone B-cell lymphoma (MZBCL) of MALT have a good prognosis. Z Gastroenterol. 2014;52(12):1–5.
53. Fischbach W, Goebeler-Kolve ME, Dragosics B, et al. Long term outcome of patients with gastric marginal zone B cell lymphoma of mucosa associated lymphoid tissue (MALT) follow-ing exclusive Helicobacter pylori eradication: experience from a large prospective series. Gut. 2004;53(1):34–7.

54. Wündisch T, Thiede C, Morgner A, et al. Long-term follow-up of gastric MALT lymphoma after Helicobacter pylori eradication. J Clin Oncol. 2005;23(31):8018–24.

55. Wündisch T, Dieckhoff P, Greene B, et al. Second cancers and residual disease in patients treated for gastric mucosa-associated lymphoid tissue lymphoma by Helicobacter pylori eradication and followed for 10 years. Gastroenterology. 2012;143(4):936–42.

56. Copie-Bergman C, Gaulard P, Lavergne-Slove A, et al. Proposal for a new histological grading system for post-treatment evaluation of gastric MALT lymphoma. Gut. 2003;52(11):1656.

57. Koch P, Probst A, Berdel WE, et al. Treatment results in localized primary gastric lymphoma: data of patients registered within the German multicenter study (GIT NHL 02/96). J Clin Oncol. 2005;23(28):7050–9.

58. Tsang RW, Gospodarowicz MK, Pintilie M. Localized mucosa-associated lymphoid tissue lymphoma treated with radiation therapy has excellent clinical outcome. J Clin Oncol. 2003;21(22):4157–64.

59. Rummel MJ, Niederle N, Maschmeyer G, et al. Bendamustine plus rituximab versus CHOP plus rituximab as first-line treatment for patients with indolent and mantle-cell lymphomas: an open-label, multicentre, randomised, phase3 non-inferiority trial. Lancet. 2013;381(9873):1203–10.

60. Fischbach W. MALT lymphoma: forget surgery? J Dig Dis. 2013;31(1):38–42.

61. Akamatsu T, Mochizuki T, Okiyama Y, et al. Comparison of localized gastric mucosa associated lymphoid (MALT) lymphoma with and without Helicobacter pylori infection. Helicobacter. 2006;11(2):86–95.

62. Chung SJ, Kim JS, Kim H, et al. Long-term clinical outcome of Helicobacter pylori-negative gastric mucosa-associated lymphoid tissue lymphoma is comparable to that of H. pylori-positive lymphoma. J Clin Gastroenterol. 2009;43(4):312–7.

63. Park HS, Kim YJ, Yang WI, et al. Treatment outcome of localized Helicobacter pylori-negative low-grade gastric MALT lymphoma. World J Gastroenterol. 2010;16(17):2158–62.

64. Fischbach W, Malfertheiner P, Hoffmann JC, et al. S3-guideline "helicobacter pylori and gastroduodenal ulcer disease" of the German society for digestive and metabolic diseases (DGVS) in cooperation with the German society for hygiene and microbiology, society for pediatric gastroenterology and nutrition e.V., German society for rheumatology, AWMF-registration-no. 021/001. Z Gastroenterol. 2009;47(12):1230–63.

65. Morgner A, Miehlke S, Fischbach W, et al. Complete remission of primary high-grade B-cell gastric lymphoma after cure of Helicobacter pylori infection. J Clin Oncol. 2001;19(7):2041–8.

66. Kuo SH, Yeh KH, Wu MS. Helicobacter pylori eradication therapy is effective in the treatment of early-stage H. pylori-positive diffuse large B-cell lymphomas. Blood. 2012;119(21):4838–44.

67. NCCN Clinical Practice Guidelines in Oncology: Non-Hodgkin's lymphomas, version 2.2012. http://www.nccn.org/professionals/physician_gls/pdf/nhl.pdf

68. Tanner M, Hollmen M, Junttila TT, et al. Amplification of HER-2 in gastric carcinoma: association with Topoisomerase IIalpha gene amplification, intestinal type, poor prognosis and sensitivity to trastuzumab. Ann Oncol. 2005;16(2):273–8.

69. Gravalos C, Jimeno A. HER2 in gastric cancer: a new prognostic factor and a novel therapeutic target. Ann Oncol. 2008;19(9):1523–9.

70. Hofmann M, Stoss O, Shi D, et al. Assessment of a HER2 scoring system for gastric cancer: results from a validation study. Histopathology. 2008;52(7):797–805.

71. Van Cutsem E, Bang YJ, Feng-Yi F, et al. HER2 screening data from ToGA: targeting HER2 in gastric and gastroesophageal junction cancer. Gastric Cancer. 2015;18(3):476–84.

72. Bang Y, Chung H, Xu J, et al. Pathological features of advanced gastric cancer (GC): relationship to human epidermal growth factor receptor 2 (HER2) positivity in the global screening programme of the ToGA trial. J Clin Oncol. 2009;20(27):4556.

73. Bang YJ, Van Cutsem E, Feyereislova A, et al. Trastuzumab in combination with chemotherapy versus chemotherapy alone for treatment of HER2-positive advanced gastric or gastro-oesophageal junction cancer (ToGA): a phase 3, open-label, randomised controlled trial. Lancet. 2010;376(9742):687–97.

74. Gong J, Liu T, Fan Q, et al. Optimal regimen of trastuzumab in combination with oxali-platin/capecitabine in first-line treatment of HER2-positive advanced gastric cancer (CGOG1001): a multicenter, phase II trial. BMC Cancer. 2016;16:68. https://doi.org/10.1186/s12885-016-2092-9.

75. Van Cutsem E, Kang Y, Chung H, et al. Efficacy results from the ToGA trial: a phase III study of trastuzumab added to standard chemotherapy (CT) in first-line human epider-mal growth factor receptor 2 (HER2)-positive advanced gastric cancer (GC). J Clin Oncol. 2009;20(27):LBA4509.

76. Fuchs CS, Tomasek J, Yong CJ, et al. Ramucirumab monotherapy for previously treated advanced gastric or gastro-oesophageal junction adenocarcinoma (REGARD): an international, randomised, multicentre, placebo-controlled, phase 3 trial. Lancet. 2014;383(9911):31–9.

77. Wilke H, Muro K, Van Cutsem E, et al. Ramucirumab plus paclitaxel in patients with previ-ously treated advanced gastric or gastrooesophageal junction adenocarcinoma (RAINBOW): a double-blind, randomised phase 3 trial. Lancet Oncol. 2014;15(11):1224–35.

78. Tian S, Quan H, Xie C, et al. YN968D1 is a novel and selective inhibitor of vascular endothe-lial growth factor receptor-2 tyrosine kinase with potent activity in vitro and in vivo. Cancer Sci. 2011;102(7):1374–80.

79. Li J, Qin S, Xu J, et al. Randomized, double-blind, placebo-controlled phase III trial of apa-tinib in patients with chemotherapy-refractory advanced or metastatic adenocarcinoma of the stomach or gastroesophageal junction. J Clin Oncol. 2016;34(13):1448–54.

80. Ajani JA, Lee J, Sano T, et al. Gastric adenocarcinoma. Nat Rev Dis Primers. 2017;3:17036.

81. Alexandrov LB, Nik-Zainal S, Wedge DC, et al. Signatures of mutational processes in human cancer. Nature. 2013;500(7463):415–21.

82. Charles SF, Toshihiko D, Raymond WJJ, et al. KEYNOTE-059 cohort 1: efficacy and safety of pembrolizumab (pembro) monotherapy in patients with previously treated advanced gastric cancer. J Clin Oncol. 2017;35(suppl; abstract):4003.

83. Yung-Jue B, Kei M, Charles SF, et al. KEYNOTE-059 cohort 2: safety and efficacy of pem-brolizumab (pembro) plus 5-fluorouracil (5-FU) and cisplatin for first-line (1L) treatment of advanced gastric cancer. J Clin Oncol. 2017;35(suppl; abstract):4012.

84. Kang YK, Satoh T, Ryu MH, et al. Nivolumab (ONO-4538/BMS-936558) as salvage treat-ment after second or later-line chemotherapy for advanced gastric or gastro-esophageal junc-tion cancer (AGC): a double-blinded, randomized, phase III trial. J Clin Oncol. 2017;35(suppl 4S):2–2.

85. Yelena Y, Patrick AO, Emiliano C, et al. Nivolumab ± ipilimumab in patients with advanced/metastatic chemotherapy refractory (CTx-R) gastric (G), esophageal (E), or gastroesophageal junction (GEJ) cancer: CheckMate 032 study. J Clin Oncol. 2017;35(suppl; abstract):4014.

Chapter 15
Radiotherapy and Chemoradiotherapy

Xingchu Ni and Kun (Kim) Huang

Introduction

Gastric cardiac cancer (GCC) encompasses Siewert type II and some type III gastroesophageal junction (GEJ) cancers [1]. Although endoscopic or surgical resection still plays the decisive role in the treatment of nodal-negative early tumors at stage T1, standard radical surgical resection for locally advanced T3 and T4 tumors or cases with node-positive diseases is frequently unsuccessful to cure the disease because of local-regional recurrence and distant metastasis. At present, the 5-year post-resection survival rate after surgical resection of locally advanced diseases is only about 25% [2–5]. However, randomized studies such as the INT0116 trial [4] and the CROSS trial [3, 6] have given new impetus to the debate on the value of radiotherapy (RT) or chemoradiotherapy (CRT) in GCC. Most clinical trials have demonstrated that there is a value in the use of neoadjuvant and/or adjuvant RT or CRT in the treatment of GCC on the basis of limited small samples studied previously (Table 15.1) [7–9]. Recent genomic studies on gastric adenocarcinoma and esophageal adenocarcinoma showed GCC carried the same genetic signature as gastric and esophageal chromosomal instable-type adenocarcinomas, implying that they are the same disease entity [10]. In the United States, esophageal adenocarcinoma is traditionally treated with a neoadjuvant approach combining CRT, followed by surgery. In contrast, gastric cancer is treated with surgery followed by CRT but

X. Ni (✉)
Department of Radiotherapy, Affiliated Changzhou No 2 People's Hospital, Nanjing Medical University, Changzhou, Jiangsu, People's Republic of China
e-mail: nixinchu@163.com

K. (K.) Huang
Department of Radiation Oncology, Harvard Medical School, Boston University School of Medicine, VA Boston Healthcare System, Jamaica Plain, MA, USA
e-mail: kun.huang@va.gov

© Springer International Publishing AG, part of Springer Nature 2018
Q. Huang (ed.), *Gastric Cardiac Cancer*, https://doi.org/10.1007/978-3-319-79114-2_15

Table 15.1 Phase III trials of neoadjuvant and adjuvant RT or CRT for GCC (GEJ cancer)

Trial	Year	N GCC/total	Treatment	Survival	HR (95% CI)	P
China – Beijing [7]	1998	370/370	Surgery	19.75% (5-y OS) 13.3% (10-y OS)		0.009
			Neoadjuvant RT 40 Gy + surgery	30.1% (5-y OS) 20.26% (10-y OS)		
INT-0116 trial [4]	2001	39/556	Surgery	41% (3-y OS)	1.35 (1.09–1.66)	0.005
			Adjuvant CRT (5-FU/leucovorin + 45 Gy)	50% (3-y OS)		
POET trial [8]	2009	54/120	Neoadjuvant chemotherapy + surgery	27.7% (3-y OS) 23% (5-y OS)	0.67 (0.41–1.07)	0.07
			Neoadjuvant CRT (PFL + 30 Gy) + surgery	47.4% (3-y OS) 37% (5-y OS)		
ARTIST trial [9]	2012	Not reported/458	Adjuvant chemotherapy + surgery	74% (3-y DFS)	Not reported	
			Adjuvant chemotherapy (XP) + CRT (capecitabine + 45 Gy)	78% (3-y DFS)		
CROSS trial [3, 6]	2012	Not reported/366	Neoadjuvant CRT (weekly CP + 41.4 Gy)	49.4 months (median overall survival)	0.657 (0.495–0.871)	0.003
			Surgery	24.0 months (median overall survival)		
CRITICS	Underway	Not reported/788	Perioperative chemotherapy (ECX)			
			Preoperative chemotherapy (ECX) + adjuvant CRT (CX + 45 Gy)			
TOPGEAR	Underway	Not reported/752	Perioperative chemotherapy (ECF or ECX) + Neoadjuvant CRT (5-FU + 45 Gy) + perioperative chemotherapy (ECF or ECX)			
			Adjuvant CT (S-1)			
ARTIST II	Underway	Not reported/900	Adjuvant chemotherapy (SOX)			
			Adjuvant chemotherapy (SOX) plus CRT (S-1 + 45 Gy)			

Note: *y* year, *OS* overall survival, *HR* hazard ratio, *CI* confidence interval, *GEJ* gastroesophageal junction

increasingly managed with chemotherapy alone before and after surgery. In this chapter, we will analyze and present the most recent progress on the role of RT or CRT in the treatment of GCC from a radiation oncological perspective.

Neoadjuvant RT or CRT

Purposes

The primary purposes of neoadjuvant RT or CRT include tumor de-bulking, down-grading pathological tumor and nodal stages, increasing the possibility of R0 resection, and sterilizing micrometastasis. For locally advanced GCC staged at T4 Nx M0, preoperative RT or CRT may decrease the pathological stage and increase the chance of R0 radical resection. Some studies revealed that neoadjuvant RT or CRT improved the local control rate and overall survival of patients with advanced tumors and did not increase the risk of postoperative complications and death [3, 11].

Comparison on Complications and Mortality of Neoadjuvant RT or CRT Between Chemotherapy and Surgery-Alone Therapies

The published studies show similar incidence of morbidity and mortality in GCC patients treated with neoadjuvant RT or CRT, compared to those with other therapies. van Hagen and colleagues [3] reported that the postoperative complications were similar in the two treatment groups, i.e., CRT followed by surgery and surgery alone; in-hospital mortality was 4% in both. Most recently, Klevebro and colleagues [11] conducted a seven-center trial in Sweden and Norway to compare the incidence and severity of postoperative complications after esophagectomy for carcinoma of the esophagus and gastroesophageal junction, including GCC, after randomized accrual to neoadjuvant chemotherapy or neoadjuvant CRT. In that study, 181 patients were randomly assigned to neoadjuvant chemotherapy ($N = 91$) and neoadjuvant CRT ($N = 90$) groups. Among 155 patients who underwent surgical resections of their carcinomas, 78 had neoadjuvant chemotherapy and 77 had neoadjuvant CRT. The investigators reported no statistically significant differences between the groups in the incidence of surgical or nonsurgical complications ($P = 0.69$ and 0.13, respectively), including 30- and 90-day mortality. However, the median Clavien-Dindo complication severity grade was significantly higher in the CRT group.

Badgwell and colleagues [12] evaluated postoperative morbidity and mortality rates after preoperative CRT in 500 patients who underwent gastrectomy. Successful total gastrectomy was carried out in 33% of 200 patients with the surgery-alone therapy, 43 of 65 cases with neoadjuvant chemotherapy, and 58% of 235 treated with neoadjuvant CRT. Neoadjuvant CRT significantly increased the proportion of cases with total gastrectomy ($p < 0.01$) without significantly increased complications in 90-day morbidity and 90-day mortality. Overall, postoperative morbidity and mortality in the patients with neoadjuvant CRT were similar to those treated with surgery alone and neoadjuvant chemotherapy. To evaluate all-cause mortality with resectable gastroesophageal cancer (including GCC), a meta-analysis, including nine published phase III trials, four with preoperative RT, and five with postoperative CRT, reported that the patients treated with surgery combined with preoperative RT, compared to those in the surgery-alone group, had significantly reduced 3-year (odds ratio, OR, 0.57; 95% confidence interval, CI, 0.43–0.76; $p = 0.0001$) and 5-year (OR, 0.62; 95% CI, 0.46–0.84; $p = 0.002$) mortality rates. In addition, a significant reduction of the 5-year (OR, 0.45; 95% CI, 0.32–0.64; $p < 0.00001$) mortality rate was found in the patients treated with surgery followed by CRT, compared to those in the surgery-alone group [13].

Neoadjuvant RT or CRT

Randomized trials testing neoadjuvant RT or CRT have been performed in many clinical centers. When unresectable local disease is diagnosed preoperatively, neoadjuvant RT or CRT would preferably be adopted before an attempt for resection of all gross primary and lymph node diseases. Most of the trials have shown a positive survival benefit, compared with surgery-alone or preoperative chemotherapy control arms.

In 1980s, Zhang and colleagues [7] (see Table 15.1) randomly assigned 370 patients with GCC either to neoadjuvant RT therapy ($N = 171$) or to surgery alone ($N = 199$). In that study, RT was given to cover anterior-posterior/posterior-anterior fields with a dose of 40 Gy in 20 fractions of 2 Gy over 4 weeks by using 8-MV photons or cobalt. Two to four weeks after RT, surgical resection was performed. Compared with the surgery-alone group, the proportion of cases with successful cancer resection was significantly ($p = 0.009$) higher in patients in the preoperative RT therapy group (89.5% vs. 79.4%), with superior overall survival (5-year overall survival, OS, 30% vs. 20%; 10-year OS, 20% vs. 13%). The authors concluded that neoadjuvant RT therapy was able to downstage disease and improve radical resection rates without increasing treatment-related morbidity or mortality.

In the United States, the CALGB 9781 trial [14] was conducted to compare trimodality therapy, comprising cisplatin, 5-FU, and 50.4 Gy of RT plus surgery, to surgery alone for patients with esophageal or GEJ cancer (including GCC). Because of poor accrual, this study was closed with 56 patients enrolled. Of all the enrolled patients, 75% had adenocarcinomas. The median survival time was significantly longer in the trimodality therapy group than in the surgery-alone group (4.48 vs. 1.79 years, $P = 0.002$). Trimodality therapy for patients had longer 5-year survival (39%, 95% CI: 21–57%) than that of the surgery-alone group (16%, 95% CI: 5–33%).

In the POET phase III trial, Stahl and colleagues [8] recruited patients with T3–T4 lower esophageal adenocarcinoma or GCC ($N = 54$) (see Table 15.1) to compare neoadjuvant CRT, which consisted of 5-FU, cisplatin, leucovorin, and RT in a total dose of 30 Gy, given at 2.0 Gy per fraction, 5 fractions per week, with neoadjuvant chemotherapy comprising 5-FU, cisplatin, and leucovorin. They reported that neoadjuvant CRT improved the 3-year survival rate from 27.7 to 47.4% ($P = 0.07$, hazard ratio adjusted for randomization strata variables 0.67, 95% CI, 0.41–1.07). Because this study was closed early, due to a low accrual rate of only 126 patients enrolled, the difference in comparison between the two groups could not reach a statistical significant level. However, the improvement in both local tumor-free and overall survival rates seems to provide the evidence that neoadjuvant CRT appears to be more effective to cure patients with localized adenocarcinoma involving GEJ, including GCC.

The CROSS trial [3, 6] investigated the utilization of trimodality therapy for the treatment of cancers of the distal esophagus or GEJ, including GCC (see Table 15.1). Among 366 patients, 178 (39 GCC) were randomly assigned to CRT (weekly administration of carboplatin, an area under the curve of 2 mg per milliliter per minute, and paclitaxel, 50 mg per square meter of body-surface area, for 5 weeks and concurrent RT, 41.4 Gy in 23 fractions, 5 days per week) followed by surgery and 188 (49 GEJ tumor patients) to surgery alone. Overall survival was statistically significantly better in the CRT group, with a median overall survival of 49.4 months, compared with 24.0 months in the surgery-alone arm. For patients with adenocarcinomas, there was statistically significant difference in median overall survival: 43.2 months in the neoadjuvant CRT plus surgery group and 27.1 months in the surgery-alone group. Neoadjuvant CRT improved survival among patients with potentially curable esophageal or GEJ cancer including GCC.

Recently, Zhao and colleagues [15] investigated the efficacy of using a concurrent neoadjuvant CRT (a XELOX regimen) to treat GCC. Seventy-six patients with unresectable advanced GCC (pT3/4, pN+, pM0) were randomly assigned to either the CRT group or the surgery group. The adjuvant treatment consisted of orally given capecitabine (1000 mg/m^2, twice daily for 14 days, days 1–14) and intravenous oxaliplatin (130 mg/m^2 on day 1) for 2 cycles and 45 Gy radiation in 25 sessions for 5 weeks. As a result, the R0 resection rate was significantly higher in the CRT group (100%) than in the surgery group (80%, 32/40) ($P < 0.05$).

Some other clinical studies are currently evaluating the effects of preoperative CRT, compared with perioperative chemotherapy (TOPGEAR, NCT01924819) [16] or the superiority of preoperative CRT over adjuvant chemotherapy (NCT01962246) (see Table 15.1). Neoadjuvant CRT followed by surgery has the potential to be the mainstay of treatment for locally advanced GCC.

Perioperative Chemotherapy

The MAGIC trial used a regimen of epirubicin, cisplatin, and fluorouracil given as neoadjuvant as well as adjuvant regimens for resectable gastric and GEJ cancer. The perioperative chemotherapy arm showed a survival benefit of 36% versus 23% at

5 years [17]. This trial has established one standard of care which omits RT. Ongoing studies such as Critics, Topgear, and Artist II trials are evaluating whether addition of adjuvant or neoadjuvant CRT will improve outcomes, compared to perioperative chemotherapy.

Meta-analyses: Neoadjuvant RT, CRT, and Chemotherapy

A meta-analysis by Ronellenfitsch and colleagues [18] assessed the effects of peri-operative chemotherapy for gastroesophageal adenocarcinoma (GCC) on survival and other clinically relevant outcomes in the overall population of participants in randomized controlled trials. Fourteen such trials were identified with 2422 eligible patients. Individual patient data were available for analysis in eight trials with 1049 patients (43%). Perioperative chemotherapy was associated with significantly lon-ger overall survival (HR, 0.81; 95% CI, 0.73–0.89). This survival advantage was consistent across the subgroup of GEJ tumors, including GCC, for combined CRT, as compared to chemotherapy, while there was no significant association with peri-operative morbidity and mortality.

Another meta-analysis by Fu and colleagues [19] evaluated the efficacy and safety of neoadjuvant CRT therapy for advanced esophagogastric adenocarcinoma, including GCC. This meta-analysis systematically investigated seven randomized controlled trials including 1085 patients with 869 adenocarcinomas. They reported significant longer overall survival (HR, 0.74; 95% CI, 0.63–0.88), higher likelihood of R0 resection, greater chance of pathological complete responses, lower likeli-hood of lymph node metastasis, and postoperative recurrence for patients treated with neoadjuvant CRT, but no difference in surgical mortality.

Adjuvant RT or CRT

Adjuvant RT or CRT is intended for GCC patients with T3 or T4 tumors, lymph node-positive disease, postoperative positive tumor margin, and palliative resection or exploration. Adjuvant RT or CRT has been minimally evaluated in randomized phase III trials for cancer of the stomach or GEJ, among which the sample of GCC patients is so small that the results may not be convincing for GCC patients.

A phase III trial INT0116 by MacDonald and colleagues [4] assessed the effect of CRT after surgery, compared with surgery alone, for adenocarcinoma ($N = 556$) of the stomach or GEJ, including 18 GCC cases in the surgery-alone group and 21 in the surgery plus CRT group (see Table 15.1). The adjuvant treatment consisted of 425 mg of fluorouracil per square meter of body-surface area per day; 20 mg of leucovorin per square meter per day, for 5 days; and followed by 45 Gy in 25 frac-tions plus concurrent 5-FU and leucovorin, 4 days/week 1, 3 days/week 5. After the completion of RT, two 5-day cycles of fluorouracil (425 mg per square meter per day) plus leucovorin (20 mg per square meter per day) were given at 1-month interval. With a median follow-up period of 5 years, the median overall survival in the surgery-only group was 27 months, as compared with 36 months in the CRT group. The hazard ratio for death in the surgery-alone group, as compared with the CRT group, was 1.35 (95% CI, 1.09–1.66; $P = 0.005$). The hazard ratio for relapse in the surgery-alone group, as compared with the CRT group, was 1.52 (95% CI, 1.23–1.86; $P < 0.001$). The median duration of relapse-free survival was 30 months in the CRT group, compared to only 19 months in the surgery-alone group. This difference in relapse-free survival was significant between the two groups ($P < 0.001$).

In 2009, MacDonald and colleagues [20] reported long-term results of the INT0116 trial with a median follow-up of more than 10 years (see Table 15.1). Survival remains significantly improved in stage IB-IV (M0) gastric cancer patients treated with CRT with hazard ratios (HR) for survival (HR = 1.32, $p = 0.004$) and disease-free survival (HR = 1.51, $p < 0.001$). CRT benefited all subsets with the exceptions of women and diffuse histology. In women, the HR for therapy was 1.0 (95% CI, 0.68–1.45). The HR for therapy in diffuse histology cases was 0.97 (95% CI, 0.62–1.40). There were no increased late toxic effects caused by RT and/or chemotherapy.

The ARTIST trial by Lee and colleagues [9] assessed the role of adjuvant CRT in patients with curatively resected gastric cancer with D2 lymph node dissection (see Table 15.1). Of 458 patients, 228 were randomly assigned to the chemotherapy (XP) arm (capecitabine 2000 mg/m^2 per day on days 1–14 and cisplatin 60 mg/m^2 on day 1, repeated every 3 weeks for six cycles) and 230 patients to the chemotherapy-chemoradiation-chemotherapy (XP/XRT/XP) arm (two cycles of chemotherapy XP followed by CRT 45Gy with capecitabine and two cycles of chemotherapy XP). There was no statistical difference in disease-free survival between the two groups ($P = 0.0862$). However, in the subgroup of patients with pathologic lymph node metastasis at the time of surgery ($n = 396$), the chemotherapy-chemoradiation-chemotherapy (XP/XRT/XP) arm had significantly longer disease-free survival, compared with those who received chemotherapy alone ($P = 0.0365$). There was also statistical difference in post-resection survival by multivariate analysis (estimated HR, 0.6865; 95% CI, 0.4735–0.9952; $P = 0.0471$). The current ongoing trial (ARTIST II) will continue investigating differences in recurrence and survival between the two therapy groups. In this trial, the number of patients with proximal and diffuse-type gastric cancer was 62. A definitive conclusion for GCC requires studies with larger samples.

A population-based (SEER database) analysis by Coburn and colleagues [21] assessed the impact of adjuvant RT or CRT in 4041 patients with nonmetastatic gastric adenocarcinoma treated between May 2000 and December 2003. Patients treated with adjuvant RT or CRT versus surgery alone had significantly improved median overall survival for stage III (31 vs. 24 months; $p = 0.005$) and stage IV M0 (20 vs. 15 months; $p < 0.001$), and the difference approached, but not reached, the statistical significance level for stage II disease ($p = 0.0535$). However, there was no significant improvement in overall survival for stage Ib and II patients who had received adjuvant RT.

Definitive CRT and Palliative RT or CRT

RTOG 8501 randomized esophageal adenocarcinoma and squamous cell carcinoma patients to radiation alone versus CRT with 5-FU and cisplatin. The CRT arm received 50 Gy, while the RT-alone arm received 64 Gy. The 5-year overall survival rate was 0% for RT alone and 27% for CRT patients. There was no difference in survival based on histology [22, 23]. The INT0123 trial was designed to test dose escalation for CRT from 50 to 65 Gy. However, the trial was stopped early after an interim analysis showed higher treatment-related death in the high-dose group (10% vs. 2%). Of the 11 deaths in the high-dose group, 7 occurred at dose of $\leq$50 Gy. There were no significant differences in terms of 2-year overall survival (31% vs. 40%) and locoregional failure (56% vs. 52%). CRT at 50 Gy remains the standard dose for esophageal cancer patients in the United States.

Palliative RT or CRT is primarily used for patients with unresectable undifferentiated or poorly differentiated adenocarcinoma, and local recurrence after surgery, and the cases that are not suitable for reoperation. RT alone for adenocarcinoma of the stomach or GEJ is rarely utilized because of difficulty achieving curative effects even at the dose as high as 70–80 Gy. At a high dose, RT can easily cause radiation damage to the surrounding tissues and organs, leading to gastroduodenal ulcer, bleeding, perforation, and necrosis. Moderate dose of RT is recommended for RT or CRT for palliative treatment.

Although some GCC patients without surgery but treated with RT or CRT may have long-term survival, this is not a viable alternative option because of the limited RT tolerance of the stomach and surrounding organs. However, if a tumor is unresectable, RT or CRT is employed as a palliative procedure. The GI Tumor Study Group (GITSG) [24] reported that CRT followed by maintenance chemotherapy resulted in statistically superior long-term survival when compared with chemotherapy alone (3- and 4-year overall survival of 18% vs. 6%–7%; $p < 0.05$).

In a small published series with only 40 patients with localized gastric cancer treated at the Massachusetts General Hospital in the United States [25], RT plus concomitant 3 days of 5-FU, followed by maintenance 5-FU, or combined drugs for 26 patients and the other 14 patients, the sequence of RT and chemotherapy was alternated. A 3-year survival rate of about 20% was achieved for the total group of patients and 43% in the group with resection but at high risk for later failure. The data, although small in number, suggest the existence of advantage of CRT in palliative therapy for GCC patients.

In summary, the local-regional spread and distant metastasis of advanced GCC is characterized primarily by angiolymphatic flow in both the thoracic and abdominal directions with a wide range of lymph node metastasis. Neoadjuvant RT or CRT followed by surgery has the potential to be the mainstay of treatment for locally advanced GCC. Even after curative resection of advanced GCC, a high proportion of cases with local-regional lymph node and distant metastases should be treated with adjuvant therapy. The survival advantage of adjuvant RT or CRT plus surgery, compared to surgery alone for patients with advanced GCC, has been demonstrated in a series of phase III trials. However, the number of advanced GCC or GEJ carcinoma cases studied in those trials is too small to be generalized, and the results should be validated in multicenter studies with large case numbers. Nevertheless, RT or CRT has been shown to be more tolerable in patients with advanced GCC who cannot tolerate high morbidity of surgery. CRT followed by maintenance chemotherapy with acceptable tolerance has the potential of achieving symptomatic benefit from this palliative treatment.

RT Planning and Target Delineation for GCC

Preparation Before RT

Before RT planning, it is necessary to review preoperative barium roentgenography, CT, MRI, PET-CT, and other available imaging data to confirm the preoperative tumor volume and nodal groups to be treated. Surgical and pathology data should be considered to determine the risk of recurrence. Patients should fast for 2–3 h before planning CT scans. CT scan at 3–5 mm thickness should be performed with the patient in the supine position with arms placed overhead. The scan area should cover from the bifurcation of the trachea to the level of vertebrae L4/L5. Enhanced CT imaging is advantageous for distinguishing between blood vessels and lesions, particularly for lymph nodes. The RT target area from enhanced CT images should be focused into planning CT images, on which the physical plan is performed to avoid the slight change of doses due to contrast medium. Administration of oral contrast medium or water could result in gastric distension, which is only recommended for diagnostic CT, not for planning CT.

RT Field Design and Dose

Intensity-modulated radiotherapy (IMRT) has become the standard treatment for GCC and GEJ cancer. It has been shown to decrease cardiac dose for esophageal and GEJ cancer [26]. In cases of postoperative radiotherapy for GCC, IMRT can help reduce doses to critical organs such as the heart, kidneys, and liver. When contouring nodal regions, contouring atlases can be useful [27, 28].

Gross Tumor Volume (GTV)

GTV should include the primary tumor (GTV tumor), gross residual disease, and all involved lymph nodes (GTV nodal), according to the study results by preoperative CT and PET imaging, barium roentgenography, and surgical findings [8].

Clinical Target Volume (CTV)

For neoadjuvant RT, owing to the risk of submucosal or subserosal angiolymphatic spread, CTV for neoadjuvant RT should include a 4 cm margin superiorly and inferiorly and 1 cm radially, using the IMRT technique. If the tumor extends beyond the gastric cardiac/GEJ wall, a major portion of the left hemi-diaphragm should be included.

For adjuvant RT, other than for T4 lesions, the remnant stomach should not be routinely included within CTV. About 2 cm beyond the proximal and distal margins of surgical resection, the anastomosis or gastric stumps, and regional lymphatics must be identified as CTV for adjuvant RT.

CTV for regional lymphatics should contain lower esophageal, para-cardial, lesser curvature, greater curvature, left gastroepiploic, celiac trunk, left gastric, supra-pancreatic, splenic artery, and splenic hilar lymphatic drainage area for patients with pT3-T4 GCC, owing to the increased risk of microscopic nodal involvement in these nodal groups. The hepatogastric ligament should be treated because of high risk of recurrence at that location. It contains the left and right gastric lymph nodes that are not easily removed by surgery. Para-aortic nodes should be included for the entire length of the CTV [4, 9, 29, 30].

Planning Target Volume (PTV)

PTV should contain the CTV together with a 5 mm 3D margin to account for setup errors.

Prescription Dose of PTV

The dose is prescribed to a reference point within the PTV. The dose of PTV for neoadjuvant RT is typically 50.4 Gy, while the dose of PTV for adjuvant RT should be 45 Gy, up to 50.4–54 Gy for microscopic or gross disease, with 1.8–2.0 Gy daily fractions and 5 fractions per week. High-energy (>5 MeV) photons from a linear accelerator should be used. The dose may need to be boosted to 50.4–54 Gy for primary tumor, positive margin, or residual tumor, if the doses to the surrounding critical organs or structures are within the tolerance range [3, 8].

RT Techniques

There are important organs around the GEJ. As such, the conventional 2D RT technology of parallel-opposed anteroposterior-posteroanterior (AP-PA) fields is difficult to improve the target dose. With the wide availability of 3D conformal treatment planning systems in recent years, the conventional 2D RT has been replaced by the intensity-modulated radiotherapy (IMRT) that is able to target more accurately with the high-risk volume, to produce superior dose distributions, and to reduce the dose of organs at risk (ORA) surrounding the target field. Because of steep dose gradients and narrow margins around the PTV, IMRT should be supplemented with image-guided radiation therapy (IGRT), such as cone-beam CT (CBCT), ultrasound, and electromagnetic signals, among which CBCT is the most commonly used modality in GCC treatment (Fig. 15.1).

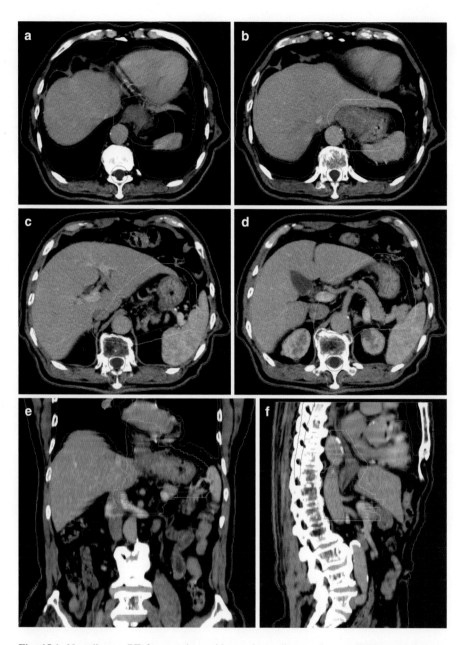

Fig. 15.1 Neoadjuvant RT for a patient with gastric cardiac carcinoma (GCC) treated at the Department of Radiotherapy of the Affiliated Changzhou Second Hospital of Nanjing Medical University. Panel 1: Clinical target volumes of the GCC patient. Transversal (**a–d**), coronal (**e**), and sagittal (**f**) planes are shown. Panel 2: Intensity-modulated radiotherapy (IMRT) plan (40 Gy in total dose). Transversal (**g**), sagittal dose distributions (**h**), coronal digitally reconstructed radiograph (DRR) (**i**), and dose-volume histograms (DVHs) (**j**) are shown

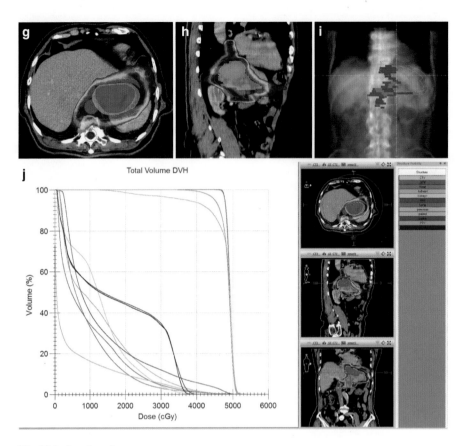

Fig. 15.1 (continued)

Dose-Limiting Organs/Structures

To reduce toxicity, the whole volume of all OAR should be drawn on the planning CT. Dose-limiting organs for radiation therapy in the lower chest and upper abdomen are numerous, including the lung, heart, stomach, small intestine, liver, kidneys, and spinal cord. Doses are limited in routine RT with 1.8–2.0 Gy daily fractions and 5 fractions per week (Table 15.2) [4, 31]. Less than 30% of the hepatic volume is exposed to more than 30 Gy of RT. The mean dose to the liver has to be limited to below 25 Gy. At least two thirds of one kidney should be spared from the field of RT. The mean dose to each kidney has to be limited to below 18 Gy. The volume of each kidney receiving more than 20 Gy should be less than 33%. About 30% of the cardiac volume is limited to the dose of more than 40 Gy of RT. Mean dose to the heart should be less than 25 Gy. The patient with a maximum 30% volume of the lung should receive a dose above 20 Gy. The maximum dose to the spinal cord should be 45 Gy.

Table 15.2 Scope of RT tolerance of OAR in routine RT

Liver	Maximum 30% volume >30 Gy, mean dose <25 Gy
Kidney	2/3 of one kidney is spared from the field of RT. The volume of kidneys receiving >20 Gy should be <33%
Heart	Maximum 30% volume >40 Gy, mean dose <25 Gy
Lung	Maximum 30% volume >20 Gy
Spinal cord	Maximum dose <45Gy

Summary

Local-regional spread and distant metastasis of advanced GCC is carried out primarily by angiolymphatic flow in both the thoracic and abdominal directions with a wide range of lymph node metastasis. Neoadjuvant RT or CRT followed by surgery has the potential to be the mainstay of treatment. Even after curative resection of advanced GCC, local-regional lymph node and distant metastases should be treated with adjuvant therapy. The survival advantage of adjuvant RT or CRT plus surgery, compared to surgery alone, for patients with advanced GCC has been demonstrated in a series of phase III clinical trials. However, the number of advanced GCC or GEJ carcinoma cases studied in those trials is too small to be generalized, and the results should be validated in multicenter studies with large case numbers. Nevertheless, RT or CRT has been shown to be more tolerable in patients with advanced GCC who may not endure high morbidity of surgery. CRT followed by maintenance chemotherapy with acceptable tolerance has the potential of achieving symptomatic relief as part of palliative care.

References

1. Siewert JR, Holscher AH, Becker K, et al. [Cardia cancer: attempt at a therapeutically relevant classification]. Chirurg. 1987;58(1):25–32.
2. Hulscher JB, van Sandick JW, de Boer AG, et al. Extended transthoracic resection compared with limited transhiatal resection for adenocarcinoma of the esophagus. N Engl J Med. 2002;347(21):1662–9.
3. van Hagen P, Hulshof MC, van Lanschot JJ, et al. Preoperative chemoradiotherapy for esophageal or junctional cancer. N Engl J Med. 2012;366(22):2074–84.
4. Macdonald JS, Smalley SR, Benedetti J, et al. Chemoradiotherapy after surgery compared with surgery alone for adenocarcinoma of the stomach or gastroesophageal junction. N Engl J Med. 2001;345(10):725–30.
5. Chou M, Boige V, Pignon JP, et al. Perioperative chemotherapy compared with surgery alone for resectable gastroesophageal adenocarcinoma: an FNCLCC and FFCD multicenter phase III trial. J Clin Oncol. 2011;29(13):1715–21.
6. Shapiro J, van Lanschot JJ, Hulshof MC, et al. Neoadjuvant chemoradiotherapy plus surgery versus surgery alone for oesophageal or junctional cancer (CROSS): long-term results of a randomised controlled trial. Lancet Oncol. 2015;16(9):1090–8.

7. Zhang ZX, Gu XZ, Yin WB, et al. Randomized clinical trial on the combination of preoperative irradiation and surgery in the treatment of adenocarcinoma of gastric cardia (AGC)—report on 370 patients. Int J Radiat Oncol Biol Phys. 1998;42(5):929–34.
8. Stahl M, Walz MK, Stuschke M, et al. Phase III comparison of preoperative chemotherapy compared with chemoradiotherapy in patients with locally advanced adenocarcinoma of the esophagogastric junction. J Clin Oncol. 2009;27(6):851–6.
9. Lee J, Lim DH, Kim S, et al. Phase III trial comparing capecitabine plus cisplatin versus capecitabine plus cisplatin with concurrent capecitabine radiotherapy in completely resected gastric cancer with D2 lymph node dissection: the ARTIST trial. J Clin Oncol. 2012;30(3):268–73.
10. Cancer Genome Atlas Research Network, Analysis Working Group, Asan University, BC Cancer Agency, et al. Integrated genomic characterization of oesophageal carcinoma. Nature. 2017;541(7636):169–75.
11. Klevebro F, Johnsen G, Johnson E, et al. Morbidity and mortality after surgery for cancer of the oesophagus and gastro-oesophageal junction: a randomized clinical trial of neoadjuvant chemotherapy vs. neoadjuvant chemoradiation. Eur J Surg Oncol. 2015;41(7):920–6.
12. Badgwell B, Ajani J, Blum M, et al. Postoperative morbidity and mortality rates are not increased for patients with gastric and gastroesophageal cancer who undergo preoperative chemoradiation therapy. Ann Surg Oncol. 2016;23(1):156–62.
13. Fiorica F, Cartei F, Enea M, et al. The impact of radiotherapy on survival in resectable gastric carcinoma: a meta-analysis of literature data. Cancer Treat Rev. 2007;33(8):729–40.
14. Tepper J, Krasna MJ, Niedzwiecki D, et al. Phase III trial of trimodality therapy with cisplatin, fluorouracil, radiotherapy, and surgery compared with surgery alone for esophageal cancer: CALGB 9781. J Clin Oncol. 2008;26(7):1086–92.
15. Zhao Q, Li Y, Wang J, et al. Concurrent neoadjuvant chemoradiotherapy for siewert II and III adenocarcinoma at gastroesophageal junction. Am J Med Sci. 2015;349(6):472–6.
16. Leong T, Smithers BM, Michael M, et al. TOPGEAR: a randomised phase III trial of perioperative ECF chemotherapy versus preoperative chemoradiation plus perioperative ECF chemotherapy for resectable gastric cancer (an international, intergroup trial of the AGITG/TROG/EORTC/NCIC CTG). BMC Cancer. 2015;15:532.
17. Cunningham D, Allum WH, Stenning SP, et al. Perioperative chemotherapy versus surgery alone for resectable gastroesophageal cancer. N Engl J Med. 2006;355(1):11–20.
18. Ronellenfitsch U, Schwarzbach M, Hofheinz R, et al. Perioperative chemo(radio)therapy versus primary surgery for resectable adenocarcinoma of the stomach, gastroesophageal junction, and lower esophagus. Cochrane Database Syst Rev. 2013;5:CD008107.
19. Fu T, Bu ZD, Li ZY, et al. Neoadjuvant chemoradiation therapy for resectable esophago-gastric adenocarcinoma: a meta-analysis of randomized clinical trials. BMC Cancer. 2015;15:322.
20. Macdonald JS, Benedetti J, Smalley S, et al. Chemoradiation of resected gastric cancer: a 10-year follow-up of the phase III trial INT0116 (SWOG 9008). J Clin Oncol. 2009;27(15_suppl):4515.
21. Coburn NG, Govindarajan A, Law CH, et al. Stage-specific effect of adjuvant therapy following gastric cancer resection: a population-based analysis of 4,041 patients. Ann Surg Oncol. 2008;15(2):500–7.
22. Herskovic A, Martz K, al-Sarraf M, et al. Combined chemotherapy and radiotherapy compared with radiotherapy alone in patients with cancer of the esophagus. N Engl J Med. 1992;326(24):1593–8.
23. Cooper JS, Guo MD, Herskovic A, et al. Chemoradiotherapy of locally advanced esophageal cancer: long-term follow-up of a prospective randomized trial (RTOG 85-01). Radiation Therapy Oncology Group. JAMA. 1999;281(17):1623–7.
24. Le Chevalier T, Smith FP, Harter WK, et al. Chemotherapy and combined modality therapy for locally advanced and metastatic gastric carcinoma. Semin Oncol. 1985;12(1):46–53.
25. Gunderson LL, Hoskins RB, Cohen AC, et al. Combined modality treatment of gastric cancer. Int J Radiat Oncol Biol Phys. 1983;9(7):965–75.

26. Kole TP, Aghayere O, Kwah J, et al. Comparison of heart and coronary artery doses associated with intensity-modulated radiotherapy versus three-dimensional conformal radiotherapy for distal esophageal cancer. Int J Radiat Oncol Biol Phys. 2012;83(5):1580–6.

27. Wu AJ, Bosch WR, Chang DT, et al. Expert consensus contouring guidelines for intensity modulated radiation therapy in esophageal and gastroesophageal junction cancer. Int J Radiat Oncol Biol Phys. 2015;92(4):911–20.

28. Wo JY, Yoon SS, Guimaraes AR, et al. Gastric lymph node contouring atlas: a tool to aid in clinical target volume definition in 3-dimensional treatment planning for gastric cancer. Pract Radiat Oncol. 2013;3(1):e11–9.

29. Meier I, Merkel S, Papadopoulos T, et al. Adenocarcinoma of the esophagogastric junction: the pattern of metastatic lymph node dissemination as a rationale for elective lymphatic target volume definition. Int J Radiat Oncol Biol Phys. 2008;70(5):1408–17.

30. Smalley SR, Gunderson L, Tepper J, et al. Gastric surgical adjuvant radiotherapy consensus report: rationale and treatment implementation. Int J Radiat Oncol Biol Phys. 2002;52(2):283–93.

31. Wieland P, Dobler B, Mai S, et al. IMRT for postoperative treatment of gastric cancer: covering large target volumes in the upper abdomen: a comparison of a step-and-shoot and an arc therapy approach. Int J Radiat Oncol Biol Phys. 2004;59(4):1236–44.

Chapter 16
Palliative Care

Qian Geng, Xiaolin Pu, Kun Yan, Qin Huang, and Ellen Hui Zhan

Introduction

Patients with gastric cardiac cancer (GCC) have distinct characteristics. First, the majority of patient with GCC, once diagnosed, are already at advanced stages of the disease in most parts of the world [1]. Secondly, in addition to the common symptoms of patients with advanced cancer, such as pain, gastrointestinal disturbances, dyspnea, weight loss, cachexia, and depression when informed of their terminal illnesses, patients with GCC are at high risk for gastric obstruction and gastric bleeding symptoms. These unique aspects of patients with GCC warrant a timely establishment of the palliative care program at early stages.

In order to provide the best care for the terminal ill cancer patients, healthcare professional should always consider offering a structured palliative therapeutic care regimen to improve the patient quality of life and help the patient and their family

Q. Geng (✉) · X. Pu
Department of Oncology, the Affiliated Changzhou No.2 People's Hospital of Nanjing Medical University, Changzhou, Jiangsu, People's Republic of China

K. Yan
VA North California Healthcare System, Mather, CA, USA
e-mail: kun.yan@va.gov

Q. Huang
Pathology and Laboratory Medicine, Veterans Affairs Boston Healthcare System, West Roxbury, MA, USA

Harvard Medical School and Brigham and Women's Hospital, Boston, MA, USA

E. H. Zhan
Harvard Medical School, VA Boston Healthcare System, Boston, MA, USA
e-mail: Hui.zhan@va.gov

© Springer International Publishing AG, part of Springer Nature 2018   299
Q. Huang (ed.), *Gastric Cardiac Cancer*, https://doi.org/10.1007/978-3-319-79114-2_16

to cope with the stressful situation [1, 2]. The purpose of palliative care is to relieve or reduce, rather than cure, mental and physical sufferings of patients with advanced cancer and/or chronic debilitating diseases, to assist patients and their families and loved ones to live with more autonomy, and even to prolong the patient limited life expectancy in certain cases.

The key of palliative care is to help patients affirm life during the normal dying process, neither to hasten nor to postpone death [3]. To that end, palliative care uses a multidisciplinary approach to integrate the medical, psychological, social, cultural, and spiritual aspects of patient care and offers a support system to help patients live as independently as possible until death. At the same time, the multidisciplinary team also supports and helps the family cope during the patient's illness, counsels bereavement, facilitates the family making decisions and choices, and positively influences the course of illness [4].

Palliative care can be provided in conjunction with other curative interventions including chemotherapy and radiation therapy as early as possible in order to better understand the disease, prevent clinical complication, and potentially prolong patient life [5].

Palliative care is an essential component of a comprehensive medical care package for cancer patients to relieve symptoms and sufferings, and reduce frequent visits to the hospital or clinic, and to achieve and maintain optimal physical, emotional, mental, and social behavioral status [6].

Symptom Management

Dysphagia or Obstruction

The main manifestation of patients with advanced GCC is dysphagia or obstruction due to stenosis. This can seriously affect the quality of life and the survival of patients. The loss of swallowing ability can seriously hinder patients' nutritional status, which in turn can result in death. Therefore, removing obstruction and restoring the function of swallowing are essential for patients who cannot tolerate systemic chemotherapy or radiation therapy or do not want to accept the above treatment for various reasons. To relieve the cancerous stenosis and create a clear passage of nutrients from the esophagus through the gastric cardia to the distal stomach and intestine, endoscopic placement of stents has become a widely accepted clinical practice (Fig. 16.1) [7]. A metallic stent can be used as a very useful and effective tool to relieve obstruction. This is particularly useful in elderly patients with advanced GCC and multiorgan dysfunction. In contrast to a placement of conventional stents, placement of self-expandable metallic stents (SEMS) does not require a large-bore bougienage [8], thereby minimizing the risk of perforation and facilitating the insertion procedure. Implantation of a 5-FU slow-releasing stent under endoscopy is another effective palliative treatment with little adverse reactions but good results [9].

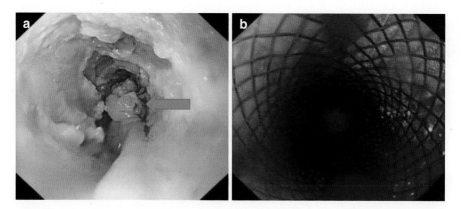

Fig. 16.1 An infiltrating gastric carcinoma (arrow) markedly narrows the lumen (**a**), which is kept patent with an endoscopic deployed self-expandable metallic stent (**b**)

Bleeding

Bleeding is one of the common complications in patients with advanced GCC as either a secondary effect of the tumor or part of adverse effects of the treatment. Bleeding seriously affects the quality of life in patients with inoperable cancer and may be even fatal. Multidisciplinary collaboration is needed for determining the cause of bleeding and providing effective intervention. Acute severe bleeding (in the forms of hematemesis or melena) should be immediately evaluated under upper endoscopy and at times with arteriography, if necessary. Recent studies have shown that endoscopic treatment, mainly endoscopic electrocoagulation hemostasis, is able to achieve a high efficiency of hemostasis for upper gastrointestinal bleeding in patients with advanced gastric cancer. The hemostatic rate was reported to be up to 92.9% (105/113) by endoscopic coagulation in 113 bleeding cases and patients with a median survival time of 3.2 months. After endoscopic therapy, 43 patients had recurrent bleeding (41.0%, 43/113), and the success rate of a second-time endoscopy treatment was 88.9% [10]. Despite the high success rate of endoscopic hemostasis demonstrated in that study, there is limited research on evaluating the safety of endoscopic hemostasis and the rate of postoperative rebleeding. A retrospective cohort study suggested that palliative radiation therapy could stop bleeding for a short period of time for gastric cancer patients who failed in blood transfusion and endoscopic hemostasis treatment [11]. Among all studied patients, 12 received palliative radiation therapy with the dose of 30 Gy/10 and 5 were treated with concurrent chemoradiation therapy with the dose of 40 Gy/20, 36 Gy/18, and 30 Gy/12, respectively. The results showed that 11 patients (64.7%) stopped bleeding with the median hemostasis time of 2 days. The median blood hemoglobin level was 6.0 g/L and rose to 9.0 g/L 30 days after radiation therapy. The study showed that radiation therapy had certain effects on gastric hemostasis, but the mechanism is still unclear, and the radiation dose remains to be further defined.

Pain

Pain adversely affects the quality of life in patients with advanced GCC. The goal of treatment is to improve the comfort, function, and quality of life of patients to the maximum. The three-step analgesic ladder guideline for cancer pain relief is followed worldwide. The degree of pain should be semiquantitatively measured and recorded, as shown in Fig. 16.2.

Once the level of pain is determined, appropriate therapy needs to be offered accordingly in the three-ladder system (Fig. 16.3). For patients with mild (scale 1–3) pain, the first-ladder drugs, known as nonsteroidal anti-inflammatory drugs, are recommended. In contrast, patients with moderate (scale 4–6) pain are prescribed the second-ladder drugs, known as weak opioid drugs, and those with severe (scale 7–10) pain are prescribed the third-ladder drugs, such as strong opioids. Because analgesic drugs cannot completely relieve the pain in cancer patients, non-

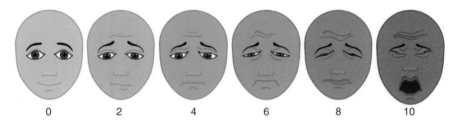

0	2	4	6	8	10

Fig. 16.2 The ten-scale pain assessment system (Adopted from the NCCN clinical practice guidelines in Oncology: Adult Cancer Pain Version 1.2017)

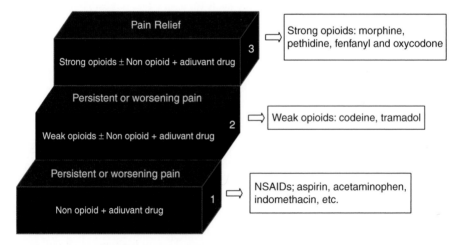

Fig. 16.3 Three-step analgesic ladder guideline for cancer pain (original) (Based on NCCN clinical practice guidelines in Oncology: Adult Cancer Pain Version 1.2017)

medication therapies may be useful, such as neurolytic celiac plexus [12], music therapy [13], psychological nursing intervention [14], meditation, moxibustion combined with auricular seeds [15], and massage and acupuncture [16], which may be able to reduce the pain to some extent.

Nausea and Vomiting

Nausea and vomiting are very common in gastric cancer patients due to various causes, such as chemotherapy, radiation therapy, gastric outlet obstruction, intestinal obstruction, constipation, and opioid drug abuse. These symptoms, especially related to chemoradiation therapy, seriously affect the quality of patient life and decrease their immune defense system and, therefore, should be treated, as required by the NCCN guidelines. The recommended antiemetic medications include a single-dose 5-HT3 receptor antagonist, dexamethasone, and an NK-1 receptor antagonist before initiation of high-emetic chemotherapy. Compared to granisetron, dexamethasone plus aprepitant and palonosetron in combination with dexamethasone and aprepitant have better antiemetic effects, when using high-emetic risk chemotherapy regimens [17, 18]. In addition, olanzapine has been shown to be able to effectively treat and prevent refractory chemotherapy-induced nausea and vomiting (Table 16.1) [19]. For patients with complaints of abdominal discomfort, nausea and occasional vomiting, a number of non-medication and medication therapies can be used (Table 16.2).

Table 16.1 Classification of antiemetic drugs (original)

Classification	Drug
NK-1 receptor antagonist	Aprepitant
	Fosaprepitant
5-HT3 receptor antagonist	Dolasetron
	Granisetron
	Ondansetron
	Palonosetron
Steroid	Dexamethasone
Atypical antipsychotic	Olanzapine
Benzodiazepine	Lorazepam
Cannabinoid	Dronabinol
	Nabilone
Other	Haloperidol
	Metoclopramide
	Scopolamine transdermal patch
Phenothiazine	Prochlorperazine
	Promethazine

Based on NCCN Clinical Practice Guidelines in Oncology: Antiemesis Version 2.2017

Table 16.2 Anticipatory anti-nausea/vomiting therapies

Anticipatory nausea/vomiting	
Prevention	Use optimal antiemetic therapy during every cycle of treatment
Behavioral therapy	Relaxation/systemic desensitization
	Hypnosis/guided imagery
	Music therapy
Acupuncture/ acupressure	
Consider anxiolytic therapy	Alprazolam 0.5–1.0 mg on the night before treatment
	Lorazepam 0.5–2.0 mg on the night before treatment or the next day 1–2 h before treatment begins

NCCN Clinical Practice Guidelines in Oncology: Antiemesis Version 2.2017

Nutritional Support

In recent years, nutritional support therapy has become a part of the comprehensive measures for cancer treatment. More than 40% of oncology patients develop signs of malnutrition during treatment [20], and nearly 20% of them die of malnutrition and/or its complications rather than from their primary diagnosis [21]. Nutritional support therapy can significantly improve the quality of life, expand the treatment effect, prevent complications, and prolong patients' survival.

Mechanism of Malnutrition in Cancer Patients

Abnormal Metabolism in Cancer Patients

Cancer patients usually have a high metabolic state or high consumption rate, leading to malnutrition, cachexia, and poor survival. In malignancy, glucose produces only a small amount of ATP molecules. As a result, glycogenic gluconeogenesis increases along with the increased fat and protein catabolism, causing protein depletion and impairing immunity. Increased nitrogen demand in cancer patients may exceed 50% of that of non-cancer patients [22]. A similar process also occurs for fat catabolism, resulting in accelerated endogenous lipolysis and fat utilization [23].

Results of Malnutrition in Patient with Advanced Cancer

Patients with advanced cancer are often in the state of malnutrition due to repetitive chemotherapy, radiation therapy, and/or surgery. In such situations, the absorption of chemotherapy drugs along with distribution, metabolism, and excretion also adversely affects and results in increased drug toxicity and decreased antitumor effects.

Malnutrition can lead to immune system dysfunction, which in turn accelerates the growth of malignant tumors, decreases the level of plasma albumin, and increases the levels of C-reactive protein. Patients would progress more rapidly toward cachexia, which is associated with a lower quality of life, more medical complications (infection, pressure sores, etc.), and a higher mortality rate [24].

Treatment of Malnutrition in Cancer Patients

Indications for Nutritional Support

Although tumor growth is stimulated by a variety of nutrients, limiting these tumor-preferred nutrients can be detrimental to the patient. If patients have moderate-to-severe malnutrition and are unable to meet their nutritional needs with oral intake alone, specialized nutrition support such as parenteral or enteral nutrition is indicated. In patients with advanced GCC, the anorexia-cachexia syndrome is mainly caused by obstruction of the upper digestive tract due to the mechanical effects of the tumor [25]. This syndrome is associated with shortened overall survival. In addition, symptoms such as nausea, vomiting, early satiety, and dysphagia following chemotherapy, radiation therapy, or surgery also contribute to cancer-related malnutrition [26, 27]. Thus, identifying and treating malnutrition early on in the course of GCC disease process is critical for improving patient outcomes. The indications of nutritional support are listed below in Table 16.3.

Screening for Nutritional Risk

The "nutritional risk" means the risk of leading to adverse clinical outcomes that are associated with malnutrition. The first step of nutritional therapy is the screening. The questionnaire of "Nutritional Risk Screening (NRS 2002)" is widely used and recommended by the American Society of Parenteral and Enteral Nutrition (ASPEN), European Society of Parenteral and Enteral Nutrition (ESPEN), and Chinese Society for Parenteral and Enteral Nutrition (CSPEN). According to NRS 2002, patients with a score of 3 or more have the risk of malnutrition and should be treated with nutritional support (Tables 16.4 and 16.5) [28, 29].

Table 16.3 Indication for nutrition support in cancer patients

	Indication
1	Tumor-induced gastrointestinal fistula, perforation, and mechanical/paralytic obstruction
2	Significant malignant ascites or intestinal dilatation
3	Chemoradiation therapy-related severe oral mucosal ulceration, leading to swallowing disorders, gastrointestinal mucositis, severe diarrhea, and gastrointestinal dysfunction
4	Postoperative gastrointestinal dysfunction
5	Radiation therapy-related tumor tissue adhesion, leading to gastrointestinal obstruction

Table 16.4 Initial screening of nutrition and scoring [28]

	Questions	Yes	No
1	Is BMI < 20.5?		
2	Has the patient lost weight within the last 3 months?		
3	Has the patient had a reduced dietary intake in the last week?		
4	Is the patient severely ill?		

Yes: If the answer is "Yes" to any question, the screening in Table 16.5 is performed
No: If the answer is "No" to all questions, the patient is rescreened at weekly intervals. If the patient is scheduled for a major operation, a preventive nutritional care plan is considered to avoid the associated risk status

Table 16.5 Final screening of nutrition and scoring of malnutrition [28]

Impaired nutritional status		Severity of disease (increased in requirements)	
Absent score 0	Normal nutritional status	Absent score 0	Normal nutritional requirement
Mild score 1	Weight loss >5% in 3 months or food intake below 50–75% of normal requirement in preceding week	Mild score 1	Hip fracture, chronic patients, in particular with acute complications: cirrhosis, COPD, chronic hemodialysis, diabetes, oncology
Moderate score 2	Weight loss >5% in 2 months or BMI 18.5–20.5 + impaired general condition or food intake 25–60% of normal requirement in preceding week	Moderate score 2	Major abdominal surgery, stroke, severe pneumonia, hematologic malignancy
Severe score 3	Weight loss >5% in 1 month or BMI < 18.5 + impaired general condition or food intake 0–25% of normal requirement in preceding week in preceding week	Severe score 3	Head injury, bone marrow transplantation, intensive care patients (APACHE > 10)

Score + score = total score
Age if >70 years: add 1 to total score above = age-adjusted total score
Score < 3: weekly rescreening of the patient. If the patient is scheduled for a major operation, a preventive nutritional care plan is considered to avoid the associated risk status
Score ≥ 3: the patient is nutritionally at risk and a nutritional care plan is initiated

Evaluation of Nutritional Status

After the screening of nutritional risk, the nutritional status of patients with the risk should be evaluated; this is termed "nutritional assessment." The questionnaire "Patient-Generated Subjective Global Assessment (PG-SGA)" is recommended by ESPEN, ASPEN, and CSPEN. The questionnaire includes weight, food intake, symptoms, activities and function, disease and its relation to nutritional requirements, metabolic demand, and physical exam. Patients' nutritional status is categorized into four groups, according to the scores (Table 16.6).

Table 16.6 Patient triage for nutritional intervention [29]

Score	Nutritional intervention
0–1	No intervention required at this time Reassessment on routine and regular basis during treatment
2–3	Patient and family education provided by a dietitian, nurse, or other clinicians. Pharmacologic intervention as indicated based on symptom survey and lab values as appropriate
4–8	Requires intervention by an interdisciplinary team, including dietitian, nurse, or physician as indicated based on patients' symptoms
≥9	Indicates a critical need for symptom management and/or nutrient intervention options

Methods of Nutritional Support

Nutritional support is recommended for patients with advanced gastric cancer in a variety of ways, including oral, enteral nutrition (EN), and parenteral nutrition (PN). Oral nutrition includes high-calorie and high-protein diet and oral supplementation. Due to a high percentage of GCC patients with obstructive dysphagia, an adequate oral nutritional intake can be difficult and sometimes unrealistic. As mentioned earlier in this chapter, in GCC patients with stenosis of the cardia, the placement of a metallic stent may allow oral nutrition, preserve the natural food intake pathway, and improve the quality of life.

EN (nourishment into the gut) is the next alternative intervention, which provides feeding via a tube placed by percutaneous endoscopic gastrostomy, percutaneous radiologic gastrostomy, or percutaneous endoscopic jejunostomy. EN preserves the structural and functional integrity of the gastrointestinal tract and represents a valid nutritional option for patients with dysphagia or obstruction when the oral intake does not satisfy the nutritional requirements [30]. The benefits of EN over PN have been well demonstrated, including fewer infection incidences, decreased levels of catabolic hormones, improved wound healing, shorter hospital stay, and maintenance of gut integrity. In other words, if the gut works, use it. To be successful, EN should be implemented as soon as possible. Prophylactic placement of gastrointestinal tubes can considerably reduce weight loss during radiation therapy and may reduce the need for hospitalization due to dehydration, weight loss, or other complications of mucositis caused by radiation. However, in patients with impaired gastrointestinal function, PN becomes a mandatory intervention. Although PN (nourishment by central and peripheral veins) ensures optimal nutrition, it increases the risk of infections, compared to EN [31]. Catheter-related bloodstream infection is the most common serious complication in patients receiving PN. Thus, in patients with terminal-stage diseases, the benefit of nutritional support may be limited and associated with an increased risk of complications (Table 16.7).

Nutritional counseling in cancer patients by a registered dietitian often helps to design a specific, individualized nutritional therapy plan in these patients. Ongoing

Table 16.7 Indication for enteral or parenteral nutrition [32]

Enteral nutrition EN	Functional GI tract but the patient is unable to meet nutritional needs orally	
	The malnourished patient cannot meet nutritional needs with enteral nutrition	
	The patient has failed the EN trial with appropriate tube placement	
Parenteral nutrition (PN)	Enteral nutrition is contraindicated due to underlying disease or treatment	Paralytic ileus
		Mesenteric ischemia
		Bowel obstruction
		GI fistula unless enteral access may be placed distal to the fistula or volume of output <200 mL/day

and early reassessment of both pharmacologic management and nutritional regimen can avoid more costly and risky nutritional support options. Nutritional intervention by a dietitian also includes patient and family education on individualized nutritional goals for energy, protein, and micronutrients, modification of foods and feeding schedules, fortification of foods with modular nutritional products, supplementation with meal-replacement products, or recommendations for appropriate nutritional support. In general, nutritional support treatment refers to the need to supplement the calories and nutrients, including parenteral, gastrointestinal nutritional supports, and dietary guidance to meet the nutritional requirements of cancer patients.

The European Society for Clinical Nutrition and Metabolism guidelines recommend the application of PN if inadequate food intake of less than 60% of the estimated energy intake is present for more than 10 days [31, 32]. For patients on chemotherapy who experience chemotherapy-related gastrointestinal side effects (i.e., anorexia, nausea, vomiting, constipation, and diarrhea), complementary home parenteral nutrition (HPN) is recommended for weight stabilization and therapy continuation [33]. Furthermore, short-term complementary HPN can be used safely and effectively for patients with weight loss and cancer cachexia, despite adequate oral intake, and also beneficiary for patients with EN intolerance with the symptoms such as nausea, abdominal pain, and diarrhea.

For patients with peritoneal carcinomatosis and severe impairment of gastrointestinal function, total HPN is mandatory [27]. Short bowel syndrome due to extensive surgical resection is another indication for HPN [34]. The success of PN depends on patient compliance, professional support, and a committed nutritionist. The collaboration among the patient, nutritionist, physician, and home care provider is crucial [35]. For patients with advanced GCC and for those who are not malnourished, the risks of PN may outweigh the benefits [36]. On the other hand, in patients with advanced cancer and moderate-to-severe malnutrition, HPN improves the quality of life, nutritional and functional status, irrespective of the tumor burden. The greatest benefit is seen in patients with 3 months of complementary HPN, even in patients receiving HPN for 1 or 2 months, who demonstrate significant improvements [37].

Psychological Intervention

One of the goals of palliative care is to provide support to patients and their families with continued psychological and social support. Cancer patients and their families are likely to experience various degrees of emotional stress and mental illnesses. The psychological intervention assists them during the end of the life period and beyond. It is aimed at reducing stress, making proper decisions regarding treatment options, maintaining open communication for symptom management, and dealing with grief and bereavement.

Classification of Psychological Therapy

Psychoanalysis

Psychoanalytic theory suggests that the root of many symptoms is the conflict of consciousness and subconscious and emotional and impulsive self-control mechanism disorders. Psychotherapists can help patients to understand the conflict process in the subconsciousness, to review the problems of the real world, and to accept and adapt to the real life of their own and natural environment.

Cognitive Behavior Therapy

Cognitive behavior theory believes that the root cause of clinical symptoms in patients with learning and thinking function problems is their peculiar understanding of things and the things outside the deviation. Irrational or erroneous cognition leads to abnormal emotions or behaviors. Through the cognitive behavior therapy, the therapist analyzes patient's thinking activities and helps the patient to design strategies to cope with reality and to adjust the cognitive structure and behavior. Cognitive behavioral therapy is very effective in the treatment of affective disorders, especially in patients with chronic diseases.

Humanistic Therapy

According to the theory, clinical symptoms are initiated by the fact that human growth is hindered in the process of self-actualization. The therapist creates unconditional support and encouragement to patients so that they are able to determine and discover their potential. Patients are encouraged to express sympathy, understanding, and love for others, thereby changing their views on their own. By improving self-awareness, the patient is able to fully affirm the self and to play a positive role in increasing the potential of changing the psychosomatic problems of maladjustment.

Meaning-Centered Psychotherapy

Meaning-centered psychotherapy is aimed to promote the patient's sense of life and sense of purposes of living. In recent years, more efforts have been taken to carry out meaning-centered psychotherapy for life-threatening patients. The goal is to reduce the patient's emotional and mental pain, increase their hope of living, their courage in face of adversity, and a sense of self-control and ultimately to mobilize their internal resources. Although the patients' life span is limited, they may wish to or need to redefine their future life goals. Psychological therapy helps them to strengthen their self-esteem and dignity, reduce loneliness, improve relationships with partners and family members, and enhance connections and collaboration with the multidisciplinary team.

Dignity as Center of Psychological Therapy

In palliative care, the expression of dignity and respect for patients and their care needs is an essential element. The patient's sense of dignity includes their sense of respect and worth in the context of increasing physical and psychological symptoms and is often affected by a number of internal and external factors. Dignity-centered treatment is specially designed for patients who are in the countdown of their life. According to the Chochinov's model of experience dignity, dignity treatment is aimed to reduce the suffering of patients; increase their emotional and spiritual well-being, quality of life, and sense of meaning; and encourage patients to recall the memories of life fragments.

Comprehensive Therapy

In the process of psychological treatment, therapists use two or more therapeutic strategies and treatment options, according to the individual circumstances of the patient, to achieve efficient and effective results.

Specific Measures of Psychotherapy for Patients with Advanced Gastric Cardiac Cancer

At the time when patients are informed of cancer diagnosis, their first reaction is suspicion and refusal, and some may even have emotional outbreaks, because they do not wish to believe the facts. When patients gradually accept the facts, they may become angry. They may not only blame on the people around them but also themselves. Subsequently, they may be fearful and frustrated and feel helpless. Once they accept the diagnosis, some of them begin to worry about the present and future and lose confidence with ample negative emotions. Every cancer patient reacts to stressful situation differently; therefore, a comprehensive understanding and assessment of their emotion state and needs is the first step of the psychological therapy. The assessment includes the following steps:

How to Inform Patients of Their Diseases

In many foreign countries, the law provides patients with the rights to know their conditions and disease diagnosis. As such, physicians cannot conceal the disease for any reasons to the patient. Because of the differences in cultural backgrounds, social values, ways of thinking, etc., healthcare providers should carefully deliver the "bad news" to patients and their families with a great deal of care, sympathy, and honesty.

Psychological therapy is the best example of the patient- and family-centered treatment intervention. It provides emotional support to both patients and their families. To minimize the trauma from hearing a devastating cancer diagnosis, it is reasonable to learn how a patient may react to the news from their family members. The presence of family members at the meeting may provide additional support to the patient. The environment where the people discuss the disease condition should be quiet and away from other patients. In certain cases, the information may need to be delivered in a stepwise approach.

One should also consider the language used in communicating such a complex medical condition and its disease process, treatment options, and prognosis. It has to be made comprehensible to patients and their families. Patients' cognitive functional and mental health states should be taken into consideration when a serious diagnosis is made available to them and their families.

A multidisciplinary approach to this important communication is required because patients and their families may typically have many questions regarding the medical, therapeutic, prognostic, social, emotional, and financial aspects of the process.

Supportive Psychotherapy

In the case of severe acute stress, the patient's emotional response should be acknowledged and respected. In major life events, especially death and separation, patients and their families may show strong emotional responses with anger, pain, and anxiety. They need to have the most direct, fundamental psychological support.

Quick Adjustment for Excessive Emotional Reactions

In some cases, the emotional response of a cancer patient may go beyond the ordinary people's emotional expression level and becomes exaggerated and dramatic. The efforts to comfort the patient by healthcare professionals and family members often have little effect. In some cases, a psychiatric situation or even syncope may occur, which may need a rapid intervention. A physician needs to respond quickly and indicate specific identity for the patient to follow the physician's orders and to do some simple activities, such as opening the mouth, opening eyes, showing the tongue, or holding the hands of a healthcare professional. This would diverse the patient's focus and reduce the tension. Then, the patient's vital signs should be quickly assessed to detect any serious abnormalities. The patient may be placed on a supine position, and the airway is kept open with oxygen and other supportive care, if indicated. In general, the patient would recover shortly.

Analysis of Deny Reaction

A denial response is one of defense mechanisms. Patients may suspect or disbelieve the cancer diagnosis, degree of seriousness, and dismal prognosis and even doubt the professional and medical authority of a physician. Through denial and suspicion, the patient would temporarily escape from the fear and threat and prevent from mental breakdown. However, this defense mechanism can only protect the patient for a short period of time, because it is illogical and unrealistic. Healthcare professionals need to work with patients and their families to disclose and explain the nature and severity of the disease and keep an open chain of communication throughout the disease and treatment process.

Treatment of Anxiety

Anxiety disorders are defined as cognitive-, emotional-, psychological-, and behavioral-related symptoms, such as excessive anxiety, difficulty focusing, irritability, shortness of breath, and so on. At clinical psychiatric examination, patients with advanced cancer have a probability of 6–14% to show generalized anxiety disorder, panic disorder, post-traumatic stress disorder, etc. The common causes for anxiety include suffering from life-threatening diseases, uncertainty of treatment and prognosis, inadaptability of hospital environment, broken singular law of life, etc.

Facing the patient with anxiety, healthcare professionals need to carefully observe and learn more about the patient's clinical manifestations and emotional reactions in order to find out the source of anxiety. This requires a close collaboration with the patient and the family. For patients with anxious symptoms, behavioral therapy can be utilized to coach patients and family members to manage anxiety and stress. Conditional biofeedback training can also be carried out.

Treatment of Depression

Depression is very common in patients with advanced cancer and occurs in the incidence from 14 to 37%. This is a part of natural responses to a devastating situation such as terminal illness, chronic debilitating diseases, and death. Depression is detrimental to patients with advanced cancer and to their families and requires timely diagnosis and treatment. Patients with severe depression may suffer from fatigue, poor appetite, flat mood, and insomnia. Some people may sigh or cry and even be suicidal. Patients with severe depression may benefit from the use of anti-depression medication.

Communication with Patients to Live Peacefully

Patients with advanced cancer can be or become very weak. They are either afraid of, or unwilling to, going out because of physical discomfort, such as vomiting, palpitation, shortness of breath, limb weakness, pain, etc. Some may visit a clinic or hospital repeatedly for the abovementioned symptoms or other medical complications. The palliative care team, especially social workers and home healthcare nurses, should maintain an ongoing communication with the patients and their families to provide effective medial and emotional support in a patient- and family-centered way. The goal of palliative care is to assist and support patients and their families to identify new issues, prevent and manage complications, make proper decisions, and maintain quality of life during and even after the end-of-life process.

Summary

The goal of palliative care in terminally ill patients with advanced gastric cardiac cancer is to relieve or reduce mental and physical sufferings induced by cancer and to help patients live more comfortably. This task includes three major aspects of palliative care: symptom management, nutritional support, and psychological intervention. Symptomatic relief is especially important for dysphagia, gastrointestinal tract obstruction, bleeding, pain, nausea, and vomiting. Nutritional support is strongly recommended in every patient and can be achieved via oral, enteral, and parenteral methods. Psychoanalysis, cognitive behavior therapy, humanistic therapy, meaning-centered psychotherapy, comprehensive therapy and so on are involved in psychological therapy. In general, palliative care should be provided in a multidisciplinary approach in conjunction with other interventions as early as possible.

References

1. Temel JS, Greer JA, Muzikansky A, et al. Early palliative care for patients with metastatic non-small-cell lung cancer. N Engl J Med. 2010;363:733–42.
2. Morita T, Miyashita M, Yamagashi A, et al. Effects of a program of interventions on regional palliative care for patients with cancer: a mixed-methods study. Lancet Oncol. 2013;14:638–46.
3. World Health Organization. Palliative care definition [R/OL]. http://www.who.int/cancer/palliative/definition/en/. Accessed 27 Sept 2017.

4. World Health Organization. WHO Definition of Palliative Care [EB/OL]. http://www.who.int/cancer/palliative/definition/en/. Accessed 1 Sept 2013.
5. World Health Organization. National cancer control program—Policies and managerial guidelines, 2nd Edn. Gevena [S]. 1995.
6. Maltoni M, Caraceni A, Brunelli C, et al. Prognostic factors in advanced cancer patients: evidence-based clinical recommendations: a study by the Steering Committee of the European Association for Palliative Care. J Clin Oncol. 2005;23(25):6240–8.
7. Shounak M, Navtej SB, Christopher C, et al. Lumen-apposing covered self-expanding metal stent for management of benign gastrointestinal strictures. Endosc Int Open. 2016;4(1):E96–E101.
8. Gaidos JK, Draganov PV. Treatment of malignant gastric outlet obstruction with endoscopically placed self-expandable metal stents. World J Gastroenterol. 2009;15(35):4365–71.
9. Xie JP, Zhan XJ, Dai YC, et al. Treatment of 20 cases of advanced esophageal and cardiac carcinoma with 5-Fu slow release particles. Gastroenterol Hepatol. 2010;19(9):798–9. (In Chinese).
10. Kim YI, Choi JJ, Cho SJ, et al. Outcome of endoscopic therapy for cancer bleeding in patients with unresectable gastric cancer. J Gastroenterol Hepatol. 2013;28(9):1489–95.
11. Kondoh C, Shitara K, Nomura M, et al. Efficacy of palliative radiotherapy for gastric bleeding in patients with unresectable advanced gastric cancer: a retrospective cohort study. BMC Palliat Care. 2015;4(1):14–37.
12. Fu S, Huang LX, Qu PS, et al. CT guided percutaneous celiac plexus block in the treatment of advanced gastric cancer. Chin Gen Pract. 2010;13(26):2928–30. (In Chinese).
13. Bradt J, Potvin N, Kesslick A, et al. The impact of music therapy versus music medicine on psychological outcomes and pain in cancer patients: a mixed methods study. Support Care Cancer. 2015;23(5):1261–71.
14. Meng CJ, Yu YH, Jiang YL. Effect of psychological nursing intervention on pain, quality of sleep and quality of life in patients with gastric cancer. Chin Modern Doctor. 2015;53(15):140–3. (In Chinese).
15. Cao Y, Chen YH. A clinical study on the effect of moxibustion combined with auricular seeds in pain relief of patients with advanced gastric cancer. Mod Med. 2015;31(17):2628–30. (In Chinese).
16. Zhang ST, Liu F. Clinical observation on acupuncture in combination with three-step analgesic method in the treatment of advanced gastric cancer. Emerg Tradit Chin Med. 2012;21(11):1848–28. (In Chinese)
17. Osawa H, Goto H, Myojo H. Comparison of antiemesis effects of granisetron, aprepitant and dexamethasone to palonosetron, aprepitant and dexamethasone in treatment of high-emetic risk chemotherapy-induced nausea and vomiting—a retrospective study for efficacy and safety in a single institute. Gan To Kagaku Ryoho. 2013;40(5):617–21.
18. Gao HF, Liang Y, Zhou NN, et al. Aprepitant plus palonosetron and dexamethasone for prevention of chemotherapy-induced nausea and vomiting in patients receiving multiple-day cisplatin chemotherapy. Intern Med J. 2013;43(1):73–6. (In Chinese)
19. Vig S, Seibert L, Green MR. Olanzapine is effective for refractory chemotherapy-induced nausea and vomiting irrespective of chemotherapy emetogenicity. J Cancer Res Clin Oncol. 2014;140(1):77–82.
20. Gyan E, Raynard B, Durand JP, et al. Malnutrition in patients with cancer. JPEN J Parenter Enteral Nutr. 2017. [Epub ahead of print].
21. Villar TR, Calleja FA, Vidal CA, et al. A short nutritional intervention in a cohort of hematological inpatients improves energy and protein intake and stabilizes nutritional status. Nutr Hosp. 2016;33(6):1347–53.
22. Yolanda LV, Serqio PD, Hugo ES, et al. Gastric cancer progression associated with local humoral immune responses. BMC Cancer. 2015;15:924.

23. Takano K, Kakuki T, Obata K, et al. The behavior and role of lipolysis-stimulated lipoprotein receptor, a component of tricellular tight junctions, in head and neck squamous cell carcinomas. Anticancer Res. 2016;36(11):5895–904.

24. Arthur ST, Van BA, Roy D, et al. Cachexia among US cancer patients. J Med Econ. 2016;19(9):874–80.

25. Donohoe CL, Ryan AM, Reynolds JV. Cancer cachexia: mechanisms and clinical implications. Gastroenterol Res Pract. 2011;2011:601434.

26. Tong H, Isenring E, Yates P. The prevalence of nutrition impact symptoms and their relationship to quality of life and clinical outcomes in medical oncology patients. Support Care Cancer. 2009;17:83–90.

27. Shahmoradi N, Kandiah M, Peng L. Impact of nutritional status on the quality of life of advanced cancer patients in hospice home care. Asian Pac J Cancer Prev. 2009;10:1003–9.

28. Kondrup J, Allison SP, Elia M, et al. ESPEN guidelines for nutrition screening 2002. Clin Nutr. 2003;22(4):415–21.

29. Bauer J, Capra S, Ferquson M. Use of the scored patient-generated subjective global assessment (PG-SGA) as a nutrition assessment tool in patients with cancer. Eur J Nutr. 2002;56(8):779–85.

30. Weimann A, Braga M, Harsanyi L, et al. ESPEN guidelines on enteral nutrition: surgery including organ transplantation. Clin Nutr. 2006;25:224–44.

31. Bozzetti F, Arends J, Lundholm K, et al. ESPEN guidelines on parenteral nutrition: non-surgical oncology. Clin Nutr. 2009;28:445–54.

32. Abraham J, Gulley JL, Allegra CJ. The Bethesda handbook of clinical oncology. 2014; p 355.

33. Arends J, Bertz H, Bischoff SC, et al. Committee S3-guideline of the German Society for Nutritional Medicine (DGEM). Aktuelle Ernahrungsmed. 2015;40:1–74.

34. Winkler MF, Smith CE. Clinical, social, and economic impacts of home parenteral nutrition dependence in short bowel syndrome. JPEN J Parenter Enteral Nutr. 2014;38(suppl):32S–7S.

35. Richter E, Denecke A, Klapdor S, et al. Parenteral nutrition support for patients with pancreatic cancer—improvement of the nutritional status and the therapeutic outcome. Anticancer Res. 2012;32:2111–8.

36. Koretz RL, Lipman TO, Klein S, American Gastroenterological Association. AGA technical review on parenteral nutrition. Gastroenterology. 2001;121:970–1001.

37. Vashi PG, Dahlk S, Popiel B, et al. A longitudinal study investigating quality of life and nutritional outcomes in advanced cancer patients receiving home parenteral nutrition. BMC Cancer. 2014;14:593.

Index

Printed by Printforce, the Netherlands